New Techniques in Gastrointestinal Imaging

edited by

Steve Halligan

St. Mark's Hospital
London, England

Helen M. Fenlon

Mater Misericordiae Hospital
Dublin, Ireland

MARCEL DEKKER, INC.   NEW YORK • BASEL

Transferred to Digital Printing 2005

Although great care has been taken to provide accurate and current information, neither the author(s) nor the publisher, nor anyone else associated with this publication, shall be liable for any loss, damage, or liability directly or indirectly caused or alleged to be caused by this book. The material contained herein is not intended to provide specific advice or recommendations for any specific situation.

Trademark notice: Product or corporate names may be trademarks or registered trademarks and are used only for identification and explanation without intent to infringe.

Library of Congress Cataloging-in-Publication Data
A catalog record for this book is available from the Library of Congress.

ISBN: 0-8247-5444-1

Headquarters
Marcel Dekker, 270 Madison Avenue, New York, NY 10016, U.S.A.
tel: 212-696-9000; fax: 212-685-4540

Distribution and Customer Service
Marcel Dekker, Cimarron Road, Monticello, New York 12701, U.S.A.
tel: 800-228-1160; fax: 845-796-1772

World Wide Web
http://www.dekker.com

The publisher offers discounts on this book when ordered in bulk quantities. For more information, write to Special Sales/Professional Marketing at the headquarters address above.

Preface

As our lives become busier it can be difficult to find the time to keep up with changes in medical practice. This is a particular challenge for radiologists because imaging technology waits for no one. No sooner have we become comfortable with one technique than it is replaced by another that is heralded as faster, better, and safer. But change and the challenges that accompany it are what make radiology the most attractive of all medical specialities.

This book is designed to summarise the most significant recent developments in gastrointestinal and abdominal radiology. It is not meant to be a review of the esoteric or obscure but rather a practical and common sense guide to new techniques that will be useful in everyday clinical practice. In planning the content of this book our aim was to cover a wide range of developments including those in abdominal ultrasound, CT, MRI, nuclear medicine, and interventional techniques. Practical information is provided, ranging from how to perform a particular technique through to image interpretation, with numerous handy tips thrown in and backed up by a little science where appropriate.

We have included contributions from authors of different backgrounds from both sides of the Atlantic so that this book has a truly international appeal. With so many competing demands on their time and expertise, we were very fortunate to have enlisted their help. Each has a proven track record in their specialty and is a recognised leader in the field: we are very grateful to them, especially for their speedy work.

We are acutely aware that what is today's "hot topic" rapidly becomes tomorrow's old news. For this reason we have attempted to keep this review as up-to-date as possible. At a time when radiologists face escalating workloads and demands, both clinical and administrative, we hope that this book will provide easy reading, and a concise but authoritative update for those interested in abdominal imaging.

Steve Halligan
Helen M. Fenlon

Contents

Contributors

Matthew Barish   Department of Radiology, Brigham & Women's Hospital, Harvard Medical School, Boston, Massachusetts, U.S.A.

Martin J. K. Blomley   Department of Imaging, Hammersmith Hospital, Imperial College Faculty of Medicine, London, England

David J. Breen   Department of Radiology, Southampton University Hospitals NHS Trust, Southampton, England

John Bruzzi   Department of Radiology, Mater Misericordiae Hospital, Dublin, Ireland

Gordon Buchanan   Department of Surgery and Intestinal Imaging Center, St. Mark's Hospital, London, England

Michela Celestre   Department of Radiological Sciences, University of Rome – "La Sapienza", Rome, Italy

David O. Cosgrove   Department of Imaging, Hammersmith Hospital, Imperial College Faculty of Medicine, London, England

Jörg F. Debatin   Department of Diagnostic and Interventional Radiology, University Hospital Essen, Essen, Germany

Helen Fenlon   Department of Radiology, Mater Misericordiae Hospital, Dublin, Ireland

Riccardo Ferrari   Department of Radiological Sciences, University of Rome – "La Sapienza", Rome, Italy

Nicholas C. Gourtsoyiannis   Department of Radiology, University Hospital of Iraklion, University of Crete Medical School, Iraklion, Crete, Greece

Steve Halligan   Intestinal Imaging Center, St. Mark's Hospital, London, England

Christopher J. Harvey   Department of Imaging, Hammersmith Hospital, Imperial College Faculty of Medicine, London, England

Franco Iafrate   Department of Radiological Sciences, University of Rome – "La Sapienza", Rome, Italy

Hoon Ji   Department of Radiology, Brigham & Women's Hospital, Harvard Medical School, Boston, Massachusetts, U.S.A.

Frederick M. Kelvin   Department of Radiology, Methodist Hospital of Indiana and Indiana University School of Medicine, Indianapolis, Indiana, U.S.A.

Christiane Kulinna   Department of Radiology, University of Vienna, Vienna, Austria

Andrea Laghi   Department of Radiological Sciences, University of Rome – "La Sapienza", Rome, Italy

Thomas C. Lauenstein   Department of Diagnostic and Interventional Radiology, University Hospital Essen, Essen, Germany

Adrian K. P. Lim   Department of Imaging, Hammersmith Hospital, Imperial College Faculty of Medicine, London, England

Andrea Maier   Department of Radiology, University of Vienna, Vienna, Austria

Koenraad J. Mortelé   Department of Radiology, Brigham & Women's Hospital, Harvard Medical School, Boston, Massachusetts, U.S.A.

Harpreet K. Pannu   The Russell H. Morgan Department of Radiology and Radiological Science, Johns Hopkins Medical Institutions, Baltimore, Maryland, U.S.A.

Pasquale Paolantonio   Department of Radiological Sciences, University of Rome – "La Sapienza", Rome, Italy

Nickolas Papanikolaou   Department of Radiology, University Hospital of Iraklion, University of Crete Medical School, Iraklion, Crete, Greece

Roberto Passariello   Department of Radiological Sciences, University of Rome – "La Sapienza", Rome, Italy

Hope Peters   Department of Radiology, Brigham & Women's Hospital, Harvard Medical School, Boston, Massachusetts, U.S.A.

Vassilios Raptopoulos   Department of Radiology, Beth Israel Deaconess Medical Center, Harvard Medical School, Boston, Massachusetts, U.S.A.

S. Ashley Roberts   Department of Radiology, University Hospital of Wales, Cardiff, Wales

Wolfgang Schima   Department of Radiology, University of Vienna, Vienna, Austria

Stephen J. Skehan   Department of Radiology, St Vincent's University Hospital, Dublin, Ireland

Brian Stedman   Department of Radiology, Southampton University Hospitals NHS Trust, Southampton, England

Andrew B. Williams   Department of Surgery and Intestinal Imaging Center, St. Mark's Hospital, London, England

1

CT Colonography (Virtual Colonoscopy)

John Bruzzi and Helen Fenlon
Mater Misericordiae Hospital, Dublin, Ireland

INTRODUCTION

CT colonography is a relatively new technique for imaging the entire colon using thin-section computed tomography (CT). First introduced in 1994 (1), it was immediately popularized as a form of "virtual colonoscopy" because of its capability to reconstruct the acquired images into three-dimensional (3D) views of the colonic lumen, allowing dynamic navigation through the colon in a manner simulating a "real" colonoscopy. Initial reports of diagnostic accuracies of CT colonography exceeding those of barium enema and approaching those of conventional colonoscopy generated intense excitement among radiologists and gastroenterologists alike (2–7). Further experience with the technique has led to widespread debate about the nature of colon cancer and revised thinking on the aims of colon surveillance. As CT colonography continues to undergo worldwide assessment and rapid refinement, it is increasingly being accepted as a routine tool for colon examination. This review of the performance of CT colonography to date will focus on the practical applications of the technique, pitfalls in image interpretation, and will attempt to discuss both consensus and controversial viewpoints on the role of CT colonography in colorectal cancer detection.

IMAGE ACQUISITION IN CT COLONOGRAPHY

CT colonography is based on acquiring thin-section CT slices of a clean, well-distended colon. For optimal studies, examinations are best performed using a multi-detector CT scanner. Patients should be scanned in both supine and prone positions to maximize visualization of the entire colonic lumen.

Patient Preparation

Adequate bowel cleansing is of utmost importance prior to CT colonography. Retained fecal material can simulate polyps and masses or hinder the detection of real pathology.

The most satisfactory experience with bowel cathartic agents has been with picosulfate-based preparations such as Fleet-Prep (De Witt International, David Mayers Ltd, Dublin, Ireland), which are traditionally used for barium enemas. Polyethylene glycol solutions, such as Kleen-Prep (Helsinki Birex Pharmaceuticals, Dublin, Ireland), which are commonly employed for conventional colonoscopy leave a large amount of residual fluid in the colon that can hide submerged pathology and hinder polyp detection.

A major component of patient discomfort associated with colon tests is attributable to the bowel cleansing process. Because patient acceptance of the technique is vital if CT colonography is to succeed as a tool for colon cancer screening, there has been widespread interest in developing ways of performing CT colonography with minimal or no bowel preparation. Encouraging results have been reported using oral contrast agents such as dilute barium sulfate or iodine-based solutions that become admixed with fecal material, thereby 'tagging' stool contents (8,9). At the moment, the optimal regime appears to involve diet modification and regular ingestion of oral contrast medium over a 48-hour period.

Muscle Relaxants

Although spasmolytic agents such as hyoscine n-butylbromide (Buscopan, Boehringer Ingelheim, Berkshire, UK) and glucagon (Eli Lilly, Indianapolis, Indiana) have been shown to be effective in overcoming spasm and improving colonic distension for barium enema, these agents have not been shown to benefit either colonic distention or polyp detection at CT colonography (10,11). They may have a selective role in patients who are known to suffer from diverticular disease, who are more susceptible to muscle spasm, but this is usually not known prospectively (12). While a reduction in colonic spasm should improve patient tolerance of rectal air insufflation, this has not been formally addressed. At the moment, available evidence does not support the routine use of spasmolytic agents for CT colonography and so one can avoid the added cost, need for direct venous injection or placement of a cannula, and potential associated side effects.

Scanning Parameters and Technique

For best results, patients should be scanned using a multidetector CT scanner, which can cover the entire abdomen and pelvis in a single breath-hold at a narrow collimation. CT colonography can be performed using a single-slice helical CT scanner, but this may involve use of thicker slices and/or multiple breath-holds or continuous breathing, which may result in artefact from respiratory movement and imperfect image overlap.

Patients are placed in a lateral decubitus position on the scanning table and a soft-tipped enema tube inserted into the rectum. Inflation of the tube balloon is recommended to prevent air leakage. Air is then insufflated into the colon using a hand pump up to maximum patient tolerance (generally 40–50 puffs). Carbon dioxide has been advocated by some investigators as being preferable to air, as it is reabsorbed by the mucosa relatively quickly and theoretically produces less patient discomfort (13). However, carbon dioxide must be administered from a gas cylinder increasing the complexity of the procedure and should be performed by a radiologist rather than by a radiographer.

The degree of distension of the colon can be assessed on the scout image and further air insufflated if necessary. The enema tube is left in place, and the patient is scanned in both supine and prone positions. Further air may be insufflated between supine and prone scans to overcome any loss of air from the rectum. Scanning the patient in two different positions leads to a redistribution of air and fluid within the colon, causing previously collapsed or submerged segments to open up, resulting in improved overall distension and better visualization of the entire colon. Studies have repeatedly emphasized the importance of this maneuver, highlighting the increased accuracy and confidence of polyp detection as a consequence of improved colonic distension (5,14).

Typical scanning parameters on a multislice CT scanner are 70–100 mA, 120 kVp, 2.5 mm × 4 collimation, and slice width reconstructions of 3 mm.

Radiation Dose Considerations

The radiation dose from CT colonography has been estimated to be equivalent to that incurred from a barium enema (15,16). Because of the inherent high-contrast resolution between luminal air and mucosal soft tissue at CT colonography, the mA can be reduced to as low as 50 mA or even further without significantly affecting image quality or diagnostic accuracy (15–17). With implementation of the recent European Communities (Medical Ionising Radiation Protection) Regulations 2002, attention has been focused on minimizing radiation dose exposure from CT colonography. This is particularly important in young patients who are at increased risk from colon cancer because of hereditary factors, who may require frequent colon examinations. It also becomes an issue if CT colonography is to be used in whole population screening programs. With further debate over the questionable benefit of detecting small polyps and greater research into the diagnostic performance of low-dose CT colonography, it is likely that CT colonography can be routinely performed at acceptably low radiation exposure values.

IMAGE INTERPRETATION

Image Display

Most studies now show that images from CT colonography studies can be reviewed primarily as axial 2D images, a format immediately familiar to most radiologists. Because of the large number of axial slices acquired and the nature of the interpretation process itself, studies should be read on a computer workstation rather than from hardcopy. By using a technique called lumen tracking, whereby the interpreting radiologist scrolls through the axial images, concentrating solely on the colonic lumen as it changes from slice to slice, the entire colon can be thoroughly mapped and examined from rectum to cecum (Fig. 1).

With current software capabilities, datasets from CT colonography studies can be additionally processed to provide a range of 2D and 3D display options. CT colonography has been popularized because of the ability to examine the colonic endolumen using 3D perspective–rendered techniques, allowing the radiologist to navigate through the colon in a simulated virtual colonoscopy (Fig. 2). The prospect of a quick, noninvasive method of examining the entire colon that produced images comparable to conventional colonoscopy had immediate appeal for referring gastroenterologists and the public alike. Early experience in the interpretation of CT colonography studies found that the use of 3D images complemented axial 2D images as the primary reading method, increasing reader confidence and leading to greater diagnostic accuracy in polyp detection (18,19).

There have been differing opinions, however, on the optimal employment of 3D images. A virtual fly-through examination of the entire colon is

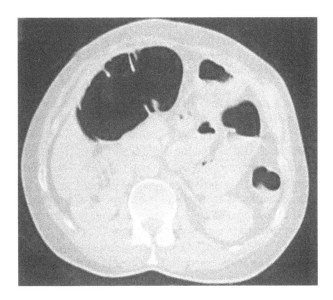

FIGURE 1   Supine scan in a patient with a well-distended colon. Haustral folds in the cecum are sharply defined gracile structures easily differentiated from polyps.

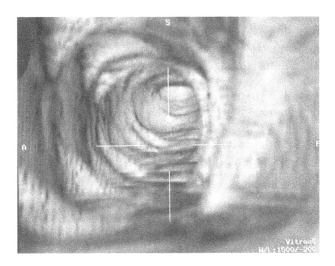

FIGURE 2   Three-dimensional endoluminal view of a normal well-distended descending colon demonstrating the normal appearance of haustral folds and a small volume of residual endoluminal fluid.

a laborious and time-consuming process, requiring a great deal of user interaction for navigation through tortuous or poorly distended segments of bowel. Reading times of 30–60 minutes per study using such techniques are not uncommon, which is impractical in most busy clinical radiology centers (2).

Most centers now reserve limited 3D endoluminal views for problem solving in situations where pathology is suspected on the axial 2D views (3,16,20). This improves reader confidence in reporting subtle abnormalities and adds little in terms of interpretation times. However, it still requires some familiarity with 3D image manipulation and is unlikely to improve detection of larger polyps.

If CT colonography is to become a routine tool for examining the colon and is to be incorporated into standard radiology practice, it must be performed and interpreted in a manner that is fast, practical, and accessible to most radiologists. The method of lumen tracking using supine and prone 2D axial images alone can be rapidly learned and does not require additional software for complex image manipulation (Fig. 3). With experience, studies can be interpreted in 10 minutes or less, allowing CT colonography to become part of a radiologist's regular workload. This is a particularly important point in busy clinical practices where prompt interpretation of CT colonography studies is required, in order to identify patients who need to undergo conventional colonoscopy on the same day, thereby avoiding repeat bowel cleansing for the patient. In our own institution, it is now our policy to read CT colonography studies using only 2D axial images. Since the clinical importance of small polyps is questionable, our primary aim is to detect polyps larger than 5 mm in size, thereby deferring further colon examination for a number of years in patients with normal colons at CT colonography.

A range of more complex image-processing methods has been used in CT colonography including those that display the colonic lumen as a flat surface (21), but these have not been embraced in clinical practice primarily due to limited familiarity with such techniques. Automated computer-aided detection of colonic polyps is an exciting possibility and is undergoing active development (22–24).

Polyp Detection and Interpretation Pitfalls

Following an initial period of training with lumen tracking techniques and familiarization with the normal appearance of the air-distended colon, 2D axial CT images can be rapidly read with a high degree of confidence. Images should be reviewed both at lung and at soft tissue window settings. Lung windows provide maximum contrast resolution between the colonic

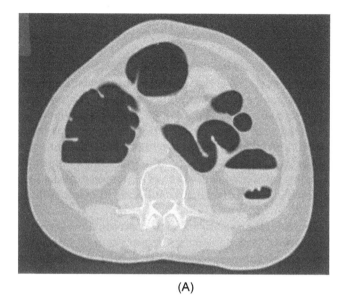

(A)

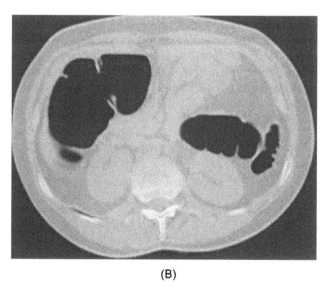

(B)

FIGURE 3 The value of dual positioning. (A) Residual fluid in the ascending and descending colon limits adequate visualization of the underlying colonic mucosa with the patient supine. (B) With the patient in the prone position, there is redistribution of fluid and air, allowing the same segments of colon to be clearly visualized.

mucosa and endoluminal air, while soft tissue settings provide additional information about the nature of bowel wall abnormalities and are necessary for evaluation of extracolonic structures.

Polyps are identified as focal polypoid or sessile protrusions from the colonic mucosa (Figs. 4,5). These can be distinguished from normal haustral folds, which appear as continuous bands of mucosa that are seen on several successive slices spiraling around the colonic lumen. Confusion sometimes arises between polyps and other structures such as residual fecal material, inverted diverticuli and impressions from adjacent extracolonic organs such as the liver, spleen, kidneys, or loops of small bowel. Use of soft tissue settings helps resolve such difficulties by demonstrating the presence of air in stool, fat in inverted diverticuli, and detail of extracolonic anatomy (Fig. 6).

Polyps are usually missed because of perceptual errors, exacerbated by technical factors such as poor distension or retained intraluminal fluid or stool. Polyps may be submerged by fluid or may be difficult to distinguish from haustral folds in partially collapsed segments of bowel; alternatively, unusually prominent or bulbous haustral folds can be mistaken for polyps. This is a particular problem in the sigmoid colon in patients with diverticular disease where folds may appear thickened and at the flexures where folds may be opposed. In most cases, errors can be avoided by comparing supine and prone images, where a shift in endoluminal contents or an improvement in distension can clarify the nature of lesions in question or reveal previously unsuspected pathology.

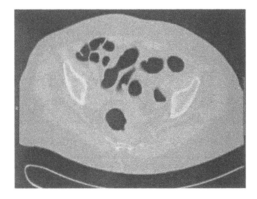

FIGURE 4 Axial 2D image demonstrating a 6 mm polyp in the sigmoid colon. Adequate colonic distension is required to help differentiate polyps from thickened or bulbous haustral folds particularly in the sigmoid colon.

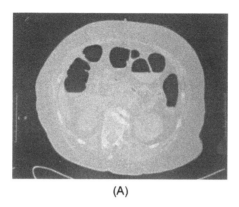

(A)

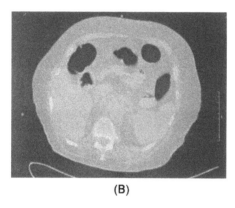

(B)

FIGURE 5   (A) A tiny polyp <5 mm in diameter can be identified near the hepatic flexure because of adequate colonic distension and a dry mucosal surface. (B) A significant volume of endoluminal fluid almost obscures a small polyp in the sigmoid colon. For this reason, bowel cleansing is better performed with phosph-soda preparations than with polyethylene glycol solutions such as Klean-Prep.

An unusually prominent ileocecal valve can also be mistaken for a cecal mass. However, by detecting the presence of fat in the valve or by recognizing the relationship of the valve to the terminal ileum, its true nature can usually be confidently determined.

The greatest difficulty arises in segments of colon affected by severe diverticular disease. In such patients, distension is usually poor, and it may be impossible to distinguish a diverticular stricture or marked bowel wall muscle thickening with spasm from an annular carcinoma. Where doubt exists and the issue cannot be resolved by CT colonography, patients should be referred for conventional endoscopy. CT colonography has also

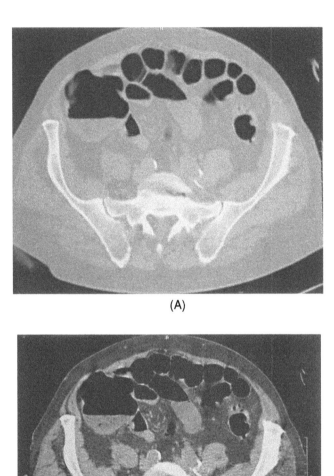

(A)

(B)

FIGURE 6   (A) Supine scan viewed at lung windows demonstrates a 5 mm polypoid lesion in the descending colon. (B) When viewed at soft tissue window settings, fat is identified within this polypoid lesion confirming that this represents an inverted diverticulum rather than a polyp.

been criticized for its poor sensitivity for flat polyps (25). There are reports that flat colonic lesions are more common than previously suspected, although this may apply more to Asian populations than in the West. Particular attention should be paid to any asymmetry in colonic wall thickness and to peri-colic fat stranding. Further research is required as to the exact prevalence of flat polyps in the population and ways of improving their detection.

CT COLONOGRAPHY AS A DIAGNOSTIC TEST

Reported sensitivity ranges of CT colonography for polyps > 9, 6–9, and < 6 mm are 70–100%, 47–82%, and 26–59%, respectively. Results from some of the larger studies are outlined in Table 1. Specificity rates are similar, ranging from 90 to 96%, 63 to 96%, and 80 to 92%, respectively. A more important index of clinical efficacy of CT colonography is its ability to accurately identify patients who have polyps and who require colonoscopy and biopsy or polypectomy (referred to as the per-patient performance). Reported per-patient sensitivities and specificities are generally higher than the per-polyp performance.

To date published results of CT colonography are from studies of patients at greater than average risk of colon cancer, performed in academic centers, and using a variety of methods for image interpretation. The actual performance of CT colonography in a mixed population of patients at varying risk of cancer as seen in routine clinical practice is therefore difficult to assess. Furthermore, there have been no published large-scale studies of CT colonography in an average risk screening population, although several such trials are in progress. It is therefore difficult to make definite recommendations about the role of CT colonography in existing diagnostic or screening algorithms.

TABLE 1   Diagnostic Accuracy of CT Colonography in Published Series

| No. patients | % sensitivity per polyp | | | % specificity per patient | | | Ref. |
	>10 mm	6–9 mm	<6 mm	>10 mm	6–9 mm	<6 mm	
70	70	63	26	90	63	80	2
100	91	82	55	96	92	N/A	4
200	100	65	33	90	96	92	28
180	75	47	N/A	93	72	N/A	5
300	90	80	59	N/A	N/A	N/A	6
165	92	82	50	N/A	N/A	N/A	7
105	93	70	12	N/A	N/A	N/A	16

No direct comparisons have been made between CT colonography and double contrast barium enema. However, the National Polyp Study group showed that the overall sensitivity of double contrast barium enema for polyps >1 cm is no higher than 48% (26). This would support the general opinion that CT colonography has a higher diagnostic accuracy compared with barium enema for polyp detection (Fig. 7). In certain situations, CT colonography has a clear advantage over either colonoscopy or barium enema. In the presence of a known obstructing colonic neoplasm where evaluation of the proximal colon is important to outrule synchronous tumors, CT colonography has been shown to be superior to either conventional colonoscopy or barium enema and should now be the test of choice in such cases (27–29) (Fig. 8).

In patients with known or a high probability of colon cancer, CT colonography has an advantage over other techniques in being able to image extracolonic disease. By administering IV contrast and scanning at a higher mA in these patients, CT colonography can simultaneously assess peri-colic tumor infiltration, the presence of nodal disease, and the presence of liver metastases, thereby avoiding a repeat CT staging examination (30,31).

CT COLONOGRAPHY AS A SCREENING TOOL

Colon cancer is the second leading cause of death in the United States. Current colon cancer screening recommendations include annual fecal occult blood testing, flexible sigmoidoscopy every 5 years, double contrast barium enema every 5–10 years, or conventional colonsoscopy every 10 years. Neither of the latter two strategies has undergone validation in large screening trials in average risk populations. Likewise, there have not yet been any published reports from large-scale, multi-institutional screening trials of CT colonography, although several are underway. The attraction of CT colonography appears to be its ability to non-invasively exclude the presence of clinically significant polyps with a high degree of accuracy, thereby deferring further colon examinations for a number of years. Furthermore, recent experience has shown that CT colonography can be performed at low radiation doses without significantly impairing diagnostic performance and, as such, deserves consideration for inclusion in any screening strategy (15,16).

Frequency and timing of referral for colonoscopy following an abnormal CT colonography study are important determinants of the success of any colon cancer screening program. For many patients, same-day referral to the endoscopy suite for removal or biopsy of polyps or

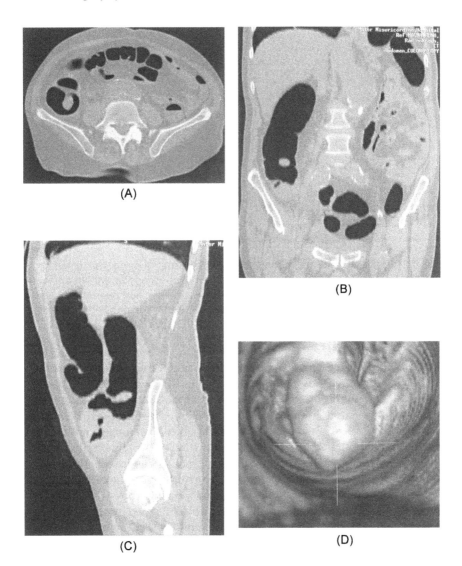

(A)

(B)

(C)

(D)

FIGURE 7 CT colonography images can be viewed in the axial plane, as 2D multiplanar images and as 3D perspective rendered views of the endolumen. (A–C) 2D multiplanar views of a 2 cm polyp in the ascending colon. (D) 3D surface-rendered view of the same polyp.

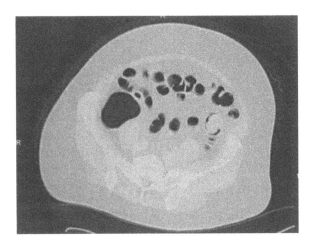

FIGURE 8 In patients with obstructing colonic neoplasms, the proximal colon can be difficult or impossible to evaluate using either colonoscopy or barium enema. Adequate air distension and visualization of the proximal colon can be achieved at CT colonography, as demonstrated in this patient with an obstructing carcinoma in the sigmoid colon.

masses detected at CT colonoscopy would be preferable, thereby avoiding the need for a second bowel preparation. This strategy, however, would require CT colonography studies to be read immediately and for patients to be accommodated for colonoscopy at very short notice. This has considerable implications for the organization of a screening program. On the other hand, with patients taking a more proactive role in their clinical management, there is currently a trend away from this approach. Increased patient advocacy means that clinicians may no longer be the sole arbitrators of what constitutes a significant polyp, and patients may wish to defer colonoscopy until they have had time to consider the significance of the results of their CT colonography study. It should be kept in mind that the clinical significance of polyps smaller than 5 mm is doubtful. Many of these polyps are hyperplastic rather than adenomatous, with no malignant potential, and the necessity and benefit of removing such polyps is clinically and economically questionable. Only 0.01% of polyps <5 mm have any malignant potential, and appropriately informed patients may well elect not to proceed to colonoscopy for their removal (32).

Because the specificity of CT colonography for polyps <5 mm is also poor, it can be argued that diminutive polyps should not be reported at CT colonography, thereby avoiding an excessive rate of referral for unnecessary colonoscopy (32). The primary aim of CT colonography, therefore, would be to detect polyps > 5 mm with a high degree of accuracy, thereby identifying patients who require colonoscopy without an unduly high false-positive rate. A high rate of referral for unnecessary colonoscopy has important implications both in terms of patient morbidity and the economic feasibility of a screening program.

Cost-effectiveness and patient compliance are major determinants when considering a feasible screening tool. Sonnenberg et al. calculated that for CT colonography to be a cost-effective screening tool at a postulated minimum sensitivity of 60%, it must be associated with a compliance rate of 15–20% greater than colonoscopy or a procedural cost of 54% less than colonoscopy (33). Currently, CT colonography is seen in a positive light by the general public as a noninvasive colon test, and further development of prepless CT colonography will greatly add to this appeal. By reviewing 2D axial images only without undue reliance on more complex 3D images, more radiologists will be willing to read CT colonography studies and in less time, which could be mirrored by a reduction in billing costs to levels approaching those of a conventional CT of abdomen and pelvis.

CONCLUSION

CT colonography is a safe, noninvasive, and accurate method of examining the colon that can be easily learned by any practicing radiologist. Current experience suggests that its sensitivity exceeds that of double contrast barium enema and approaches that of conventional colonoscopy, but it remains to be seen if these results can be reproduced in the general community outside of academic centers. For CT colonography to become a widespread tool for routine imaging of the colon, it must be fast, practical for any radiologist to perform following basic training, and easily incorporated into a busy clinical workload. The demand for CT colonography is likely to increase with greater patient awareness. Indeed, increasing patient advocacy may require a change in the way screening programs are designed and in the aims of colon screening. A true indication of the diagnostic performance of CT colonography in mixed and average risk populations will depend on the results of larger ongoing studies.

REFERENCES

1. Vining DJ, Gelfand DW. Noninvasive colonoscopy using helical CT scanning, 3D reconstruction, and virtual reality. Presented at the annual meeting of the Society of Gastrointestinal. Radiologists, February 13–18, 1994, Maui, HI.

2. Hara AK, Johnson CD, Reed JE, Ahlquist DA, Nelson H, MacCarty RL, Harmsen WS, Ilstrup DM. Detection of colorectal polyps with CT colography: initial assessment of sensitivity and specificity. Radiology 1997; 205:59–65.
3. Dachman AH, Kuniyoshi JK, Boyle CM, Samara Y, Hoffmann KR, Rubin DT, Hanan I. CT colonography with three-dimensional problem solving for detection of colonic polyps. AJR Am J Roentgenol 1998; 171:989–995.
4. Fenlon HM, Nunes DP, Schroy III PC, Barish MA, Clarke PD, Ferrucci JT. A comparison of virtual and conventional colonoscopy for the detection of colorectal polyps. N Engl J Med 1999; 341:1496–1503.
5. Fletcher JG, Johnson CD, Welch TJ, MacCarty RL, Ahlquist DA, Reed JE, Harmsen WS, Wilson LA. Optimization of CT colonography technique: prospective trial in 180 patients. Radiology 2000; 216:704–711.
6. Yee J, Akerbar GA, Hung RK, Steinauer-Gebauer AM, Wall SD, McQuaid KR. Characteristics of CT colonography for the detection of colorectal neoplasia in 300 patients. Radiology 2001; 219:685–692.
7. Laghi A, Iannaccone R, Carbone I, Catalano C, Di Giulio E, Schillaci A, Passariello R. Detection of colorectal lesions with virtual computed tomographic colonography. Am J Surg 2002; 183(2):124–131.
8. Callstrom MR, Johnson CD, Fletcher JG, Reed JE, Ahlquist DA, Harmsen WS, Tait K, Wilson LA, Corcoran KE. CT colonography without cathartic preparations: feasibility study. Radiology 2001; 219(3):693–699.
9. Lefere PA, Gryspeerdt SS, Dewyspelaere J, Baekelandt M, Van Holsbeeck BG. Dietary fecal tagging as a cleansing method before CT colonography: initial results polyp detection and patient acceptance. Radiology 2002; 224(2):393–403.
10. Yee J, Hung RK, Akerar GA, Wall SD. The usefulness of glucagon hydrochloride for colonic distension in CT colonography. AJR Am J Roentgenol 1999; 173:169–172.
11. Morrin MM, Farrel RJ, Keogan MT, Kruskal JB, Yam CS, Raptopoulos V. CT colonography: colonic distention improved by dual positioning but not intravenous glucagon. Eur Radiol 2002; 12(3):525–530.
12. Murray JP. Buscopan in diagnostic radiology of the alimentary tract. Br J Rad 1966; 93:102–111.
13. Rogalla P, Schmidt E, Korvea M, Hamm III BK. Optimal colon distension for virtual colonoscopy: room air versus CO_2 insufflation. Radiology 1999; 213(P):341.
14. Chen S, Lu DS, Hecht JR, Kadell BM. CT colonography: value of scanning in both the supine and prone positions. AJR Am J Roentgenol 1999; 172:595–599.
15. Hara AK, Johnson CD, Reed JE, Ahlquist DA, Nelson H, Ehman RL, Harmsen WS. Reducing data size and radiation dose for CT colonography. AJR Am J Roentgenol 1997; 168:1181–1184.
16. Macari M, Bini EJ, Xue X, Milano A, Katz SS, Resnick D, Chandarana H, Krinsky G, Klingenbeck K, Marshall CH, Megibow AJ. Colorectal neoplasms: prospective comparison of thin-section row CT colonography and conventional colonoscopy for detection. Radiology 2002; 224:383–392.

17. Hara AK, Johnson CD, McCarty RL, Welch TJ, McCollough CH, Harmsen WS. CT colonography: single- versus multi-detector row imaging. Radiology 2001; 219:461–465.
18. Hara AK, Johnson CD, Reed JE, Ehman RL, Ilstrup DM. Colorectal polyp detection with CT colography: two- versus three-dimensional techniques. Radiology 1996; 200:49–54.
19. Royster AP, Fenlon HM, Clarke PD, Nunes DP, Ferrucci JT. CT colonoscopy of colorectal neoplasms: two-dimensional and three-dimensional virtual-reality techniques with colonoscopic correlation. AJR Am J Roentgenol 1997; 169:1237–1242.
20. Macari M, Milano A, Lavelle M, Berman P, Megibow AJ. Comparison of time-efficient CT colonography with two- and three-dimensional colonic evaluation for detecting colorectal polyps. AJR Am J Roentgenol 2000: 1543–1549.
21. Paik DS, Beaulieu CF, Jeffrey Jr RB, Karadi CA, Napel S. Visualization modes for CT colonography using cylindrical and planar map projections. J Comput Assist Tomogr 2000; 20:179–188.
22. Yoshida H, Masutani Y, MacEneaney P, Rubin DT, Dachman AH. Computerized detection of colonic polyps at CT colonography on the basis of volumetric features: pilot study. Radiology 3003; 222(2):327–336.
23. Paik DS, Beaulieu CF, Jeffrey RB, Yee J, Steinauer-Gebauer AM, Napel S. Computer-aided detection of polyps in CT colonography: method and free-response ROC evaluation of performance. Presented at the 86th Scientific Assembly and Annual Meeting of the RSNA, 2000. Radiology 3000; 217(P):370.
24. Summers RM, Jerebko AK, Franaszek MK, Mally JD, Johnson CD. Colonic polyps: complementary role of computer-aided detection in CT colonography. Radiology 2002; 225:391–399.
25. Fidler JL, Johnson CD, MacCarty RL, Welch TJ, Hara AK, Harmsen WS. Detection of flat lesions in the colon with CT colonography. Abdom Imaging 2002; 27(3):292–300.
26. Winawer SJ, Stewart ET, Zauber AG, Bond JH, Ansel H, Waye JD, Hall D, Hamlin JA, Schapiro M, O'Brien MJ, Sternberg SS, Gottlieb LS. A comparison of colonoscopy and double-contrast barium enema for surveillance after polypectomy. National Polyp Study Work Group. N Engl J Med 2000; 342(24):1766–1772.
27. Fenlon HM, McAnaeny DB, Nunes DP. Occlusive colon carcinoma: virtual colonoscopy in the preoperative evaluation of the proximal colon. Radiology 1999; 210:423–428.
28. Morrin MM, Farrell RJ, Raptopoulos V, McGee JB, Bleday R, Kruskal JB. Role of virtual computed tomographic colonography in patients with colorectal cancers and obstructing colorectal lesions. Dis Colon Rectum 2000; 43:303–311.
29. Macari M, Megibow AJ, Barman P, Milano A, Dicker M. CT colography in patients with failed colonoscopy. AJR Am J Roentgenol 1999; 173: 561–564.

30. Neri E, Giusti P, Battolla L, Vagli P, Boraschi P, Lencioini R, Caramella D, Bartolozzi C. Colorectal cancer: role of CT colonography in preoperative evaluation after incomplete colonoscopy. Radiology 2002; 223:615–619.
31. Morrin MM, Farrell RJ, Kruskal JB, Reynolds K, McGee JB, Raptopoulos V. Utility of intravenously administered contrast material at CT colonography. Radiology 2000; 217:765–771.
32. Ferrucci JT. Colon cancer screening with virtual colonoscopy: promises, polyps, politics. Am J Roentgenol AJR 2001; 177:975–988.
33. Sonnenberg A, Delco F, Bauerfeind P. Is virtual colonscopy a cost-effective option to screen for colorectal cancer? Am J Gastroenterol 1999; 94: 2268–2274.

2

MR Colonography

**Thomas C. Lauenstein and
Jörg F. Debatin**
University Hospital Essen, Essen, Germany

BACKGROUND

Colorectal cancer remains associated with considerable morbidity and mortality. In the United States alone, more than 130,000 newly diagnosed patients and 50,000 deaths are attributed to colorectal cancer each year (1). The majority of colon cancers develop from nonmalignant colonic adenomas or polyps (2). Thus, cancer screening programs targeting precancerous colonic polyps with subsequent endoscopic polypectomy are designed to reduce the cancer mortality by more than 80%. Colorectal screening for polyps may therefore be considered one of the most promising preventive measures in medicine (3).

With regard to detection of precancerous lesions of the colon, conventional colonoscopy is considered the gold standard (4). However, even in countries with free access to this diagnostic modality, participation in cancer screening programs is inadequate. While various psychological factors inhibit the acceptance of cancer screening programs in general, efforts targeting the colon have been particularly unsuccessful. Non-invasive cancer screening programs such as testing of fecal occult blood are burdened with both a low sensitivity and specificity in the detection of precancerous as well as cancerous lesions (5). Endoscopic screening programs are characterized by high sensitivity and specificity but lack sufficient acceptance by the target populations (6). Among the causes for poor compliance, one issue relates to the discomfort associated with the preparation for the procedure (i.e., bowel cleansing and dietary restriction prior to colonoscopy). In addition, anticipation of an endoscopic study of the colon is associated by the majority of the population with an unpleasant expectation focusing on procedure-related pain, discomfort, and the risk of complications such as bowel perforation. Even if these expectations do not fully reflect reality, it is a matter of fact that colonoscopy is poorly utilized by the target population even if it is offered as a cancer screening procedure free of charge (6). Thus, the impact of colonoscopy on colonic cancer morbidity and mortality remains limited. This has motivated the development and evaluation of alternative strategies to assess the colon, including virtual colonography.

Virtual colonography (VC) is based on either computed tomography (CT) or magnetic resonance (MR) three-dimensional (3D) data sets. Based on cross-sectional images, this type of exam offers several advantages over conventional colonoscopy, the most significant of which relates to the lack of procedural pain and discomfort. In contrast to conventional colonoscopic analysis, VC is not limited to endoscopic viewing. Rather, the 3D data sets can be assessed interactively in the multiplanar reformation mode on a workstation, displaying the colonic morphology from any desired angle. This type of multiplanar reformation analysis depicts the colonic lumen and colonic wall in relation to the surrounding abdominal structures. Lesions in the colon can thus be more accurately localized (7). Even in the presence of stenotic tumors, the entire colon can be assessed, which often is not possible in conventional colonoscopy. A further advantage of virtual colonography based on CT or MRI is the simultaneous assessment of other abdominal organs. In the case of patients with suspected colorectal tumors, imaging of the liver must be considered a welcome addition.

Recent studies have shown CT and MR colonography to be effective regarding the detection of clinically relevant polyps exceeding 8 mm in size [8–12]. In contrast to conventional colonoscopy, neither CT nor MR colonography requires the administration of analgesics or sedatives (13). Both cross-sectional techniques are less painful than conventional colonoscopy. Angtuaco et al. demonstrated that more than 60% of potential patients preferred virtual colonography over conventional colonoscopy when both methods were offered (14).

Despite promising results, the future of CT colonography as a screening method is uncertain: the CT examination may expose patients to considerable doses of ionizing radiation. Since a screening examination of the colon should be repeated at regular intervals (every 3–5 years) , this radiation issue may even evolve into a public health concern. Hence the

European Commission on Radiation Safety has decreed that examinations based on the use of ionizing radiation should not be used for screening purposes (15). Therefore, it seems reasonable to focus on MRI for colorectal screening. The technique is not associated with any radiation exposure or other harmful side effects. Furthermore, contrast agents applied in conjunction with MRI exams are characterized by a more favorable safety profile than CT contrast agents as they lack any nephrotoxicity and are associated with far fewer anaphylactoid reactions (16,17).

TECHNICAL CONSIDERATIONS

Similar to contrast-enhanced 3D MR angiography, MR colonography (MRC) is based on the principles of ultrafast, T1-weighted 3D GRE acquisitions (9). Hence, an MR scanner equipped with high-performance gradients is required. The acquired 3D MR data set usually consist of 96 contiguous coronal sections, ranging in thickness between 1.5 and 2 mm. Acquisition time amounts to less than 25 seconds. The technique is based on the use of short repetition (TR 1.6–3.8 ms) and echo times (0.6–1.6 ms). The achievable minimum TR should be shorter than 5 ms; otherwise, the acquisition of a 3D data set cannot be collected within the confines of a breathhold. In conjunction with a field of view of 400×400 mm and an imaging matrix of 460×512, the spatial resolution involves an interpolated voxel size of nearly $1 \times 1 \times 1.6$ mm.

To permit homogeneous signal transmission and reception over the entire colon with high contrast-to-noise (CNR) values, a combination of

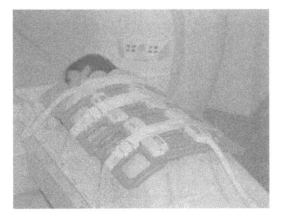

FIGURE 1   A combination of two phased-array coils is used for MRC. Thus, coverage of the entire colon in conjunction with homogenous signal reception is guaranteed.

two phased-array surface coils should be used covering the entire colon (Fig. 1). Since colonic lesions often cannot be differentiated from stool, the patient has to undergo bowel preparation in a manner similar to that required for conventional colonoscopy. To limit patient discomfort related to extended fasting, MRC should be performed in the morning. Prior to the examination, the patient should be screened for contraindications to MRI such as presence of metallic implants, cardiac pacemakers, or severe claustrophobia. The presence of hip prostheses, which normally is not regarded as a contraindication to MRI, impedes a complete analysis of the rectum and sigmoid colon. Therefore, these patients should not be examined by MRC.

To date, two distinct techniques are in clinical use for MRC. Based on the signal within the colonic lumen, they can be considered either as bright lumen or dark lumen MRC.

BRIGHT LUMEN MR COLONOGRAPHY

Applying this technique the colon is filled in the prone position via a rectal catheter (Fig. 2) with 2000–2500 mL of a water-based enema. The water is labeled 1:100 with a gadolinium containing contrast agent and administered using 100 cm of hydrostatic pressure (Fig. 3). To reduce bowel motion and alleviate colonic spasm, MRC mandates the intravenous administration of a spasmolytic agent (e.g., scopolamine or glucagon) just prior to bowel filling. In contrast to conventional colonoscopy, neither analgesic agents nor sedatives are required. After finishing the bowel filling process,

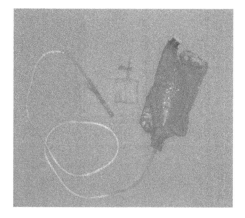

FIGURE 2   Set of enema bag and rectal catheter for MR colonography.

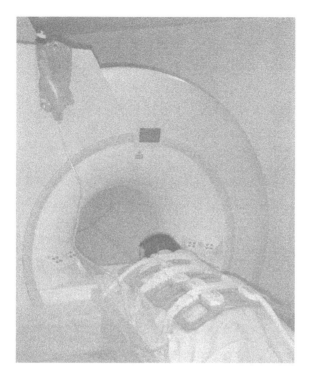

FIGURE 3   To ensure sufficient bowel distension, the liquid enema is applied using 100 cm of hydrostatic pressure.

a 3D data set of the abdomen encompassing the entire colon is acquired. To compensate for the presence of residual air exhibiting a signal void within the colon, the 3D acquisition needs to be performed in both the prone and supine positions. When the procedure is complete the enema bag is lowered to facilitate colon emptying, the rectal tube removed, and the patient can leave the scanner room.

On the 3D gradient echo data sets, only the colonic lumen that contains the enema material is bright, whereas all other tissues remain low in signal intensity (Fig. 4). The resulting contrast between the colonic lumen and surrounding structures is the basis for subsequent virtual colonographic viewing (Fig. 5). Differential diagnostic considerations for luminal filling defects within the bright colonic lumen include residual air, residual fecal material, or a polypoid colonic mass. Differentiating features of residual air and stool include their change in position from the prone to the supine data set. On the other hand, polyps remain largely unchanged in

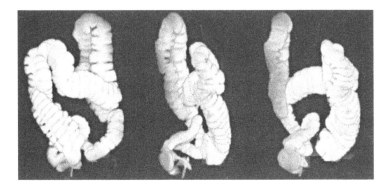

FIGURE 4 T1w GRE data sets of bright-lumen MRC displayed in maximum-intensity projection. Only the gadolinium containing colonic lumen is bright, whereas all other tissues show a low signal intensity. Due to the 3D property of the data, the colon can be analysed from different perspectives.

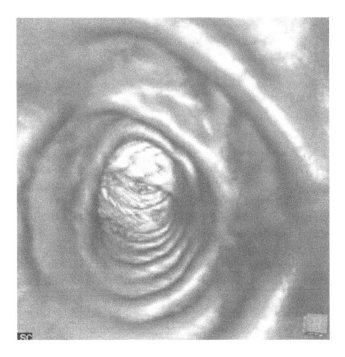

FIGURE 5 The high contrast between the colonic wall and colonic lumen is the basis for virtual colonographic viewing.

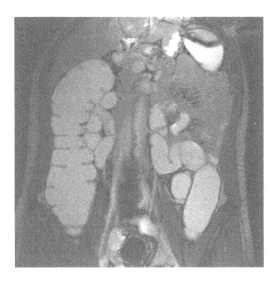

FIGURE 6 Bright lumen MRC in conjunction with TrueFISP imaging. This technique lacks the need of rectal or i.v. administration of paramagnetic contrast.

position in both prone and supine data sets. Based on lesion size and morphology, detected masses can further be characterized as either a polyp or carcinoma. Regardless, colonoscopy is indicated if a mass is identified. The MRC protocol can be further amplified by the acquisition of 2D gradient-echo data sets following the intravenous application of a gadolinium-containing contrast compound. This permits a more comprehensive assessment of extracolonic abdominal organs and enhances the ability to detect hepatic metastases.

A new technique for bright lumen MRC is based on the acquisition of TrueFISP sequences. Using a rectal water-enema, contrast is generated in a manner comparable to the use of a paramagnetic contrast enema and acquisition of T1w GRE sequences (Fig. 6). Since residual air exhibits no signal within the colon, the TrueFISP acquisition must also be performed in both prone and supine position (Fig. 7). Since the TrueFISP technique requires neither the administration of intravenous or rectal paramagnetic contrast medium, it is economically attractive. In addition, this sequence is rather insensitive to motion artifacts. However, initial study results indicate a considerable number of false-positive findings using this sequence due to difficulty differentiating residual stool from colorectal masses (Fig. 8).

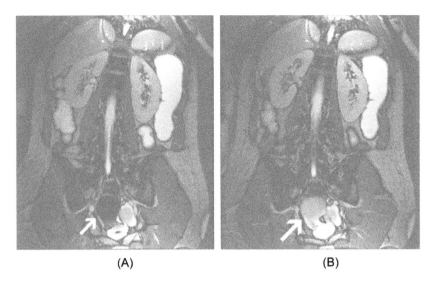

(A)   (B)

FIGURE 7 Bright lumen MRC needs to be performed both in prone (A) and supine position (B), because residual air inhibits the analysis of the entire colonic wall (arrow).

DARK LUMEN MR COLONOGRAPHY

The detection of colorectal lesions with bright lumen MRC relies on visualizing filling defects within the column of intraluminal contrast material. This technique has proven effective in most cases. However, it may be associated with both false-positive and false-negative results: polyps with a long stalk may move sufficiently to simulate residual stool, while stool adherent to the colonic wall may not move at all and thus be falsely reported as a polyp. Dark lumen MRC, however, is based on contrast being generated between a brightly enhancing colonic wall and a homogeneously dark colonic lumen (18). The technique differs from bright lumen MRC in several aspects:

1. Instead of using a gadolinium enema, only tap water is instilled rectally, rendering low-signal on T1-weighted 3D GRE acquisitions.
2. To obtain a bright colonic wall, a paramagnetic contrast compound is administered intravenously. 3D data sets are collected prior to IV contrast and after a 75-second delay.
3. Since residual air exhibits no signal in the colonic lumen, the examination needs to be performed in only one position (either supine or prone).

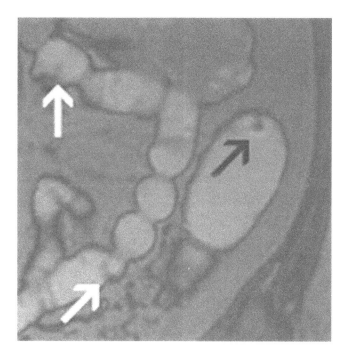

FIGURE 8 Bright lumen MRC in conjunction with TrueFISP imaging. Since colorectal polyps impress as filling defects (black arrow), it may be difficult to distinguish them from residual fecal material (white arrows).

Compared to bright lumen MRC, dark lumen MRC offers several advantages including reduced examination and postprocessing times because acquisition of only one 3D data set is required. Furthermore, the dark lumen technique copes with the problem of residual stool in an effective way: if the lesion enhances it is a polyp or carcinoma, if it does not enhance it represents stool (Figs. 9–11). Suspicious lesions are analyzed by comparing signal intensities on the pre- and postcontrast images. If analysis is limited to the post-contrast data set, bright stool could be misinterpreted as a polyp. Comparison with the pre-contrast images documents lack of contrast enhancement, which assures the correct diagnosis.

Enhancement of colorectal masses following administration of IV contrast material has been described in conjunction with both MRC (19) and CT colonography (20). The use of IV contrast material significantly improves reader confidence in the assessment of bowel wall conspicuity and the ability to depict medium-sized polyps in suboptimally prepared

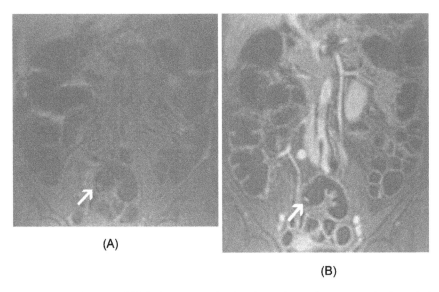

(A)

(B)

Figure 9   Dark lumen MRC. A colorectal polyp (arrow) can be accurately detected on the T1w GRE data sets due to a significant contrast uptake comparing the pre-contrast scan (A) with the postcontrast images (B).

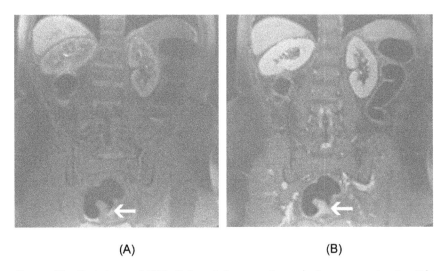

(A)   (B)

Figure 10   Dark lumen MRC. Colorectal cancer (arrow) shows a contrast uptake comparing precontrast scans (A) and postcontrast images (B).

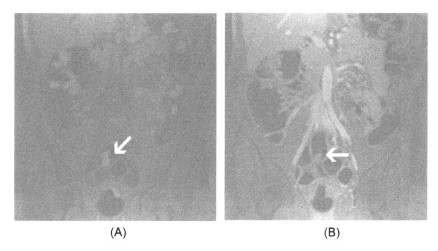

(A) (B)

FIGURE 11 Dark lumen MRC. In contrast to colorectal pathologies, residual stool is bright on both precontrast scans (A) and postcontrast scans (B).

colons. The enhancement observed within polyps exceeds that of the normal colonic wall. This may aid in differentiating even very small polyps from thickened haustral folds.

Dark lumen MRC also permits a direct analysis of the bowel wall. This facilitates evaluation of inflammatory changes in patients with inflammatory bowel disease such as ulcerative colitis or Crohn's disease (Fig. 12). Increased enhancement following contrast and bowel wall thickening demonstrated on contrast-enhanced T1-weighted images has been shown to correlate well with the degree of inflammation in the small bowel (21). Hence, the dark lumen approach may expand the list of indications for MRC to include inflammatory bowel disease in the future.

Use of IV paramagnetic contrast agents also provides a more reliable assessment of extracolonic abdominal organs contained within the field of view. By combining pre- and postcontrast T1-weighted imaging, the liver can be accurately evaluated for the presence and nature of coexisting pathology. Furthermore, dark lumen MRC offers further possibilities concerning agents used for large bowel distention. Although the administration of water as a rectal enema does not adversely effect patient comfort in most cases, a modified strategy could be based on the use of gases like CO_2 (22) or room air (23). These gases are signaless and provide high contrast compared with the contrast-enhanced colonic wall and masses. This approach has been shown to be feasible in preliminary studies.

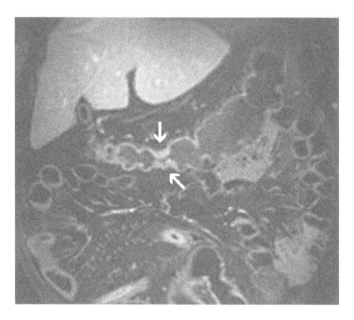

FIGURE 12 Dark lumen MRC in patient with Crohn's disease. This techniques permits the detection of inflammatory changes due to the direct analysis of the colonic wall. A thickened bowel wall and an increased contrast uptake (arrows) on the postcontrast scans can be observed.

IMAGE INTERPRETATION

An MRC examination can be completed within 20 minutes, including the time for patient positioning, image planning, and data acquisition. The acquired 3D data sets are postprocessed using commercially available software and hardware. A complete analysis of an MRC examination still requires nearly 15 minutes of interactive image viewing on a high-performance workstation. Initially an MRC examination should be viewed in the multiplanar reformation mode, scrolling through the prone 3D data set in all three orthogonal planes. For bright lumen MRC, this assessment needs to be supplemented by viewing the supine data set. The data should then be assessed based on virtual endoscopic renderings displaying the inside of the colonic lumen. A virtual endoscopic fly-through allows the observer to focus on the colon facilitating detection of small lesions protruding into the colonic lumen. Furthermore, the three-dimensional depth perception allows the assessment of haustral fold morphology, thereby enhancing the observer's ability to distinguish polyps from haustra. To assure complete visualization of both sides of haustral folds, the virtual fly-through should

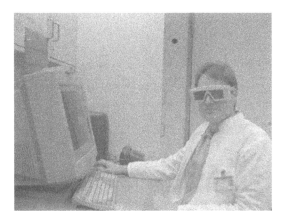

FIGURE 13   A three-dimensional plastic effect can be produced at the workstation by using a special software and shutter-glasses (stereo viewing).

be performed in an antegrade as well as retrograde direction. Regarding the detection of polyps at MRC, virtual endoscopic viewing renders improved sensitivity and specificity values compared with inspection of the individual cross-sectional images alone (24). In addition, a three-dimensional plastic effect can be produced on the monitor using shutter-glasses and specialized stereo-viewing software (Fig. 13).

MR COLONOGRAPHY: DIAGNOSTIC ACCURACY

The diagnostic performance of bright lumen MRC has been assessed in several studies using conventional colonoscopy as the standard of reference (8,10,25). While most mass lesions < 5 mm in size were missed, almost all lesions >10 mm were correctly identified. In a study by Pappalardo et al. (10), MRC detected a greater number of polyps >10 mm in size than conventional colonoscopy (Fig. 14) by identifying additional polyps in regions of the colon not reached by colonoscopy.

Direct observational data on growth rates indicate that polyps < 10 mm in size remain fairly constant in size over 3–5 years and are not prone to malignant degeneration (26,27). Therefore, it seems reasonable to concentrate on lesions larger than 10 mm. Hence, one could argue that MRC is almost as reliable as conventional colonoscopy with regard to the assessment of colonic lesions at risk for malignant degeneration. Nevertheless, attempts are underway to increase the spatial resolution of the 3D data sets and so improve the diagnostic accuracy of MRC for lesions between 5 and 10 mm in size. Technique refinements encompass the use of even

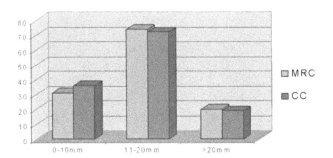

FIGURE 14   Diagnostic accuracy of bright lumen-MRC depending on the size of colorectal lesions. A considerable number of polyps smaller than 10 mm are missed by MRC. However, the total number of detected colorectal lesions >10 mm is similar for MRC and conventional colonoscopy (CC). (Modified from 10.)

shorter repetition times in conjunction with zero filling routines and the implementation of parallel imaging techniques (28). Regardless of these efforts, it is likely that very small lesions will continue to be missed in the future. Furthermore, MRC will continue to have difficulty demonstrating flat lesions, which recently have been shown to be more prevalent than previously believed (29).

BOWEL CLEANSING

Since colorectal lesions often cannot be accurately differentiated from stool, virtual colonography requires bowel purgation in a manner similar to conventional colonoscopy. Various oral agents for bowel cleansing are used in practice. Although some substances have been found to evoke fewer side effects (30,31), bowel preparation in general negatively impacts on patient acceptance. Patients complain of symptoms ranging from "feeling unwell" to "inability to sleep" (32). Thomeer et al. examined 124 patients undergoing virtual colonography with prior bowel cleansing (33). When asked about discomfort associated with the examination, the majority of patients rated bowel cleansing as the most unpleasant part of the examination (Fig. 15). If colonic cleansing could be avoided, patient acceptance of virtual endoscopy should be considerably enhanced. Hence, virtual colonography should be combined with "virtual bowel cleansing."

Virtual bowel cleansing can be achieved in conjunction with MRC by fecal tagging, a method that results in a change in the signal characteristics of feces to assimilate those of the applied rectal enema. The latter is

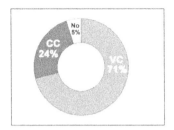

FIGURE 15   Preference of patients for both virtual and conventional colonoscopy. The majority of patients rated virtual colonography as more pleasant. (Modified From Ref. 33.)

required for adequate colonic distension. Thus, stool becomes virtually invisible with fecal tagging as it is indistinguishable from the rectal enema on MR images. To accomplish fecal tagging, patients have to ingest a contrast agent within a certain time range prior to the examination. The contrast agent adheres to the foodstuff modulating the MRI signal characteristics of the bowel contents. An ideal tagging agent should be cheap, nontoxic when applied orally, and, of course, it should not negatively affect patients' acceptance and compliance. Different models based on different contrast mechanisms have been evaluated.

At first, the principle of fecal tagging was demonstrated on the basis of bright-lumen MRC (34). For fecal tagging, the signal intensity of stool has to be augmented to simulate the bright rectal enema. By adding a T1-shortening, gadolinium-based MR contrast agent to regular meals prior to the MR examination, better harmonization of signal properties between fecal material and the Gd-based enema can be achieved. MR imaging following the administration of a gadolinium-containing enema provides a homogeneously bright colonic lumen. Gadolinium includes some properties required for a tagging agent: the oral administration of a paramagnetic MR contrast agent has been shown to be safe (35). Furthermore, there is no absorption through mucosal surfaces, the agent is stable over a wide range of pH values (36), and the ingestion of gadolinium is well accepted by patients as it is flavorless and odorless (37). However, the clinical implementation of bright fecal tagging is hindered by the high cost of the gadolinium-based paramagnetic contrast agent. The use of less expensive tagging agents such as chocolate or fruit juices (38) does not result in a sufficiently high increase in signal intensity in the colonic content.

A second strategy for fecal tagging is based on rendering the colonic lumen dark (39,40). For this form of fecal tagging, 200 mL of a highly

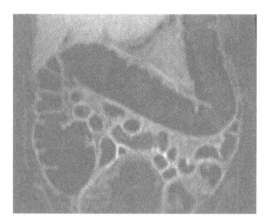

FIGURE 16   Dark lumen MRC in conjunction with barium-based fecal tagging. Signal characteristics of fecal material are modified by the ingestion of barium sulfate prior to MRC. Thus, stool can hardly be distinguished from the rectal enema.

concentrated barium sulfate contrast agent (Micropaque; Guerbet, Sulzbach, Germany) (1 g barium sulfate/mL) is taken with each of four to five main meals prior to MRC. Patients are instructed to avoid all fiber-rich foodstuff and nourishments with high concentration of manganese such as chocolate or fruits during this period, because manganese leads to an increased signal intensity in T1w sequences. Barium-based fecal tagging is combined with dark lumen MRC (Fig. 16): the colon is distended with a rectally administered water enema or gas, and paramagnetic contrast is administered intravenously to render the colonic wall and colorectal mass lesions bright.

Barium sulfate is a well-known diagnostic contrast compound, still in common use as an oral agent for esophageal, gastric, and small bowel radiography. Compared to Gd-based contrast compounds, it is far less expensive and characterized by an even better safety profile. Anaphylactoid reactions or other adverse side effects are hardly known. Barium is not absorbed and mixes well with stool. Thus, it fulfills all the requirements of an ideal oral tagging agent for MRC.

The barium-based fecal tagging concept has been evaluated in a pilot patient study (40). Dark lumen MRC in conjunction with barium-based fecal tagging detected all polyps larger than 8 mm in a population of 24 patients with known or suspected colorectal tumors. Overall sensitivity of MRC amounted to 89.3% for the detection of colorectal masses, and specificity was 100%. Although further work is required to confirm these results, it seems that barium-tagged MRC has tremendous potential to emerge as the examination strategy of choice for the detection of polyps in asymptomatic subjects. The technique appears to combine excellent diagnostic accuracy with high patient acceptance based on a painless examination with no need for colonic cleansing.

FUTURE DIRECTIONS

Future work will focus on improving the spatial resolution of the T1-weighted 3D data sets. Parallel imaging strategies, promising to double spatial resolution without increasing data collection times, will be implemented. This should improve the detection of polyps between 5 and 10 mm in size. Other work will center on improving the barium-based fecal tagging concept in conjunction with dark lumen MRC, assuring homogeneously dark signal of colonic contents. Administration of the barium agent will be optimized with regard to volume, concentration, and timing. Furthermore, the effect of adding other signal reducing agents and their incorporation into premixed meals will be examined.

REFERENCES

1. Landis SH, Murray T, Bodden S, Wingo PA. Cancer statistics, 1998. CA Cancer J Clin 1998; 48:6–29.
2. O'Brien MJ, Winawer SJ, Zauber AG, Gottlieb LS, Sternberg SS, Diaz B, Dickersin GR, Ewing S, Geller S, Kasimian D. The National Polyp Study. Patient and polyp characteristics associated with high-grade dysplasia in colorectal adenomas. Gastroenterology 1990; 98:371–379.
3. Winawer SJ, Zauber AG, Ho MN, O'Brien MJ, Gottlieb LS, Sternberg SS, Waye JD, Schapiro M, Bond JH, Panish JF. Prevention of colorectal cancer by colonoscopic polypectomy. The National Polyp Study Workgroup N Engl J Med 1993; 329(27):1977–1981.
4. Liebermann DA, Smith FW. Screening for colon malignancy with colonoscopy. Am J Gastroenterol 1991; 86:946–951.
5. Ahlquist DA, Wieland HS, Moertel CG et al. Accuracy of fecal occult blood screening for colorectal neoplasia. A prospective study using Hemoccult and HemoQuant tests. JAMA 1993; 269:1262–1267.
6. Rex DK, Rahmani EY, Haseman JH, Lemmel GT, Kaster S, Buckley JS. Relative sensitivity of colonoscopy and barium enema for detection of colorectal cancer in clinical practice. Gastroenterology 1997; 112:17–23.
7. McFarland EG, Brink JA, Pilgram TK, Heiken JP, Balfe DM, Hirselj DA, Weinstock L, Littenberg B. Spiral CT colonography: reader agreement and diagnostic performance with two- and three-dimensional image-display techniques. Radiology 2001; 218:375–383.

8. Luboldt W, Bauerfeind P, Wildermuth S, Marincek B, Fried M, Debatin JF. Colonic masses: detection with MR colonography. Radiology 2000; 216: 383–388.
9. Luboldt W, Bauerfeind P, Steiner P, Fried M, Krestin GP, Debatin JF. Preliminary assessment of three-dimensional magnetic resonance imaging for various colonic disorders. Lancet 1997; 349(9061):1288–1291.
10. Pappalardo G, Polettini E, Frattaroli FM, Casciani E, D'Orta C, D'Amato M, Gualdi GF. Magnetic resonance colonography versus conventional colonoscopy for the detection of colonic endoluminal lesions. Gastroenterology 2000; 119(2):300–304.
11. Luboldt W, Debatin JF. Virtual endoscopic colonography based on 3D MRI. Abdom Imaging 1998; 23(6):568–572.
12. Fletcher JG, Johnson CD, Welch TJ, MacCarty RL, Ahlquist DA, Reed JE, Harmsen WS, Wilson LA. Optimization of CT colonography technique: prospective trial in 180 patients. Radiology 2000; 216(3):704–711.
13. Bauerfeind P, Luboldt W, Debatin JF. Virtual colonography. Baillieres Best Pract Res Clin Gastroenterol 1999; 13(1):59–65.
14. Angtuaco TL, Banaad-Omiotek GD, Howden CW. Differing attitudes toward virtual and conventional colonoscopy for colorectal cancer screening: surveys among primary care physicians and potential patients. Am J Gastroenterol 2001; 96:887–893.
15. Debatin JF, Luboldt W, Bauerfeind P. Virtual colonoscopy in 1999: computed tomography or magnetic resonance imaging? Endoscopy 1999; 31(2):174–179.
16. Murphy KJ, Brunberg JA, Cohan RH. Adverse reactions to gadolinium contrast media: a review of 36 cases. AJR 1996; 167:847–849.
17. Prince MR, Arnoldus C, Frisoli JK. Nephrotoxicity of high-dose gadolinium compared with iodinated contrast. J Magn Reson Imaging 1996; 6:162–166.
18. Lauenstein TC, Herborn CU, Vogt FM, et al. Dark-lumen MR-colonography: initial experience. Rofo Fortschr Geb Rontgenstr Neuen Bildgeb Verfahr 2001; 173:785–789.
19. Luboldt W, Steiner P, Bauerfeind P, Pelkonen P, Debatin JF. Detection of mass lesions with MR colonography. Radiology 1998; 207:59–65.
20. Morrin MM, Farrell RJ, Kruskal JB, Reynolds K, McGee JB, Raptopoulos V. Utility of intravenously administered contrast material at CT colonography. Radiology 2000; 217:765–771.
21. Marcos HB, Semelka RC. Evaluation of Crohn's disease using half-Fourier RARE and gadolinium-enhanced SGE sequences: initial results. Magn Reson Imaging 2000; 18:263–268.
22. Lomas DJ, Sood RR, Graves MJ, Miller R, Hall NR, Dixon AK. Colon carcinoma: MR imaging with CO_2 enema. Radiology 2001; 219:558–562.
23. Morrin MM, Hochman MG, Farrell RJ, Marquesuzaa H, Rosenberg S, Edelman RR. MR Colonography using colonic distention with air as the contrast material. AJR 2001; 176:144–146.
24. Schoenenberger AW, Bauerfeind P, Steiner P, et al: Virtual colonoscopy with magnetic resonance imaging: in vitro evaluation of a new concept. Gastroenterology 1997; 112:1863–1870.

25. Saar B, Heverhagen JT, Obst T, et al. Magnetic resonance colonography and virtual magnetic resonance colonoscopy with the 1.0-T system: a feasibility study. Invest Radiol 2000; 35:521–526.

26. Villavicencio RT, Rex DX. Colonic adenomas: prevalence and incidence rates, growth rates, and miss rates at colonoscopy. Semin Gastrointest Dis 2000; 11:185–193.

27. Hofstad B, Vatn MH, Andersen SN, et al. Growth of colorectal polyps: redetection and evaluation of unresected polyps for a period of three years. Gut 1996; 39:449–456.

28. Griswold MA, Jakob PM, Nittka M, Goldfarb JW, Haase A. Partially parallel imaging with localized sensitivities (PILS). Magn Reson Med 2000; 44: 602–609.

29. Bond JH. Colon polyps and cancer. Endoscopy 2001; 33:46–54.

30. Lee J, McCallion K, Acheson AG, et al. A prospective randomised study comparing polyethylene glycol and sodium phosphate bowel cleansing solutions for colonoscopy. Ulster Med J 1999; 68:68–72.

31. Lai AK, Kwok PC, Man SW, et al. A blinded clinical trial comparing conventional cleansing enema, Pico-salax and Golytely for barium enema bowel preparation. Clin Radiol 1996; 51:566–569.

32. Elwood JM, Ali G, Schlup MM, et al. Flexible sigmoidoscopy or colonoscopy for colorectal screening: a randomized trial of performance and acceptability. Cancer Detect Prev 1995; 19:337–347.

33. Thomeer M, Bielen D, Vanbeckevoort D, et al. Patient acceptance for CT colonography: what is the real issue? Eur Radiol 2002; 12:1410–1415.

34. Weishaupt D, Patak MA, Froehlich J, et al. Faecal tagging to avoid colonic cleansing before MRI colonography. Lancet 1999; 354:835–836.

35. Runge VM, Clanton JA, Foster MA, et al. Paramagnetic NMR contrast agents. Development and evaluation. Invest Radiol 1984; 19:408–415.

36. Schwizer W, Maecke H, Siebold K, et al: Gd-DOTA as gastrointestinal contrast agent for gastric emptying with MRI. Magn Reson Med 1994; 31:388–393.

37. Squillaci E, Crecco M, Cecconi L, et al. Gadolinium-DTPA dimeglumine administered orally for the study of the abdomen with magnetic resonance. Clinical evaluation and tolerance. Radiol Med 1993; 86:284–293.

38. Hiraishi K, Narabayashi I, Fujita O, et al. Blueberry juice: preliminary evaluation as an oral contrast agent in gastrointestinal MR imaging. Radiology 1995; 194:119–123.

39. Lauenstein T, Holtmann G, Schoenfelder D, et al. MR colonography without colonic cleansing: a new strategy to improve patient acceptance. AJR Am J Roentgenol 2001; 177:823–827.

40. Lauenstein TC, Goehde SC, Ruehm SG, et al. MR colonography with barium-based fecal tagging: initial clinical experience. Radiology 2002; 223:248–254.

3

MR Imaging of the Liver

**Koenraad J. Mortelé, Hope Peters,
Hoon Ji, and Matthew Barish**
Brigham & Women's Hospital, Harvard Medical School,
   Boston, Massachusetts, U.S.A.

INTRODUCTION

As the body's largest solid organ, the liver remains the primary focus of the gastrointestinal radiologist interested in magnetic resonance imaging (MRI) or computed tomography (CT). The liver is susceptible to a wide variety of neoplastic and nonneoplastic conditions of major clinical importance. While up to now MR imaging of the liver has been restricted to a role of "problem solver," only applied when dynamic bolus contrast-enhanced CT was inconclusive or in cases where iodinated contrast material is contraindicated, recent refinements in MR technology have advanced MR imaging as a primary hepatic imaging tool. Over the last decade, MRI has continued to evolve and mature with the development of new improved hardware, imaging sequences, and tissue-specific contrast agents. Advances in MR pulse sequences, phased array body coils, imaging speed, and gradient architecture have made MRI the optimal modality for the detection and characterization of focal and diffuse liver pathology.

This chapter will focus on the techniques of MR imaging of the liver and highlight the characteristic MR appearance of a vast array of pathological entities involving the liver.

TECHNIQUES

Magnetic resonance imaging is capable of providing superior soft tissue contrast when compared to other hepatic imaging methods. This versatile and variable soft tissue contrast can be manipulated to focus on either improving detection or characterization of hepatic disease entities. Imaging strategies for the liver should focus on maximizing these two goals while minimizing imaging time and artifacts. The use of multiple pulse sequences providing complementary information is usually required. In general, a combination of T1- and T2-weighted sequences is obtained to gather sufficient data. Contrast agents should be routinely administered to increase both lesion detection and characterization. In the ideal MR imaging sequence, the spatial resolution is maximized within a short acquisition time, while the signal-to-noise ratio is kept sufficiently high. Recent advances in both MR imaging hardware and software allow for a complete evaluation of the hepatic parenchyma, vasculature, and biliary tree in a reasonable amount of time without substantial artifacts. In fact, most of the newer techniques are capable of reducing imaging artifacts related to motion because of the substantial reduction in imaging time allowing for breath-hold imaging.

Artifact Reduction

Respiratory motion artifact is one of the more difficult challenges in abdominal imaging. Faster pulse sequences have been developed to reduce imaging time and to decrease artifacts related to motion (Fig. 1). With the introduction of high-performance gradient systems and fast pulse

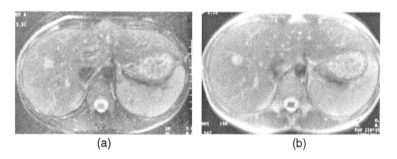

(a)   (b)

FIGURE 1   Breath-hold imaging. (a) Turbo spin-echo T2-weighted image of the liver (acquisition time: 3 minutes). Due to the presence of motion and respiratory artifacts, the small hemangioma (arrow) in the right lobe of the liver is not well defined. (b) Axial half-Fourier single-shot turbo spin-echo T2-weighted HASTE image (acquisition time: 18 seconds) in the same patient shows absence of motion artifacts. Note sharp delineation of hepatic hemangioma (arrow).

sequences, breath-hold imaging is now possible for both T1- and T2-weighted protocols. Reductions in imaging time, however, are usually accompanied by a decrease in signal-to-noise ratio. Phased array surface coils are available to counteract the reduction in signal and improve overall image quality (1), allowing for production of diagnostic breath-hold T2-weighed sequences (2–4). Advantages of the phased-array technology are improved signal-to-noise ratios allowing a smaller field of view and thus higher resolution images compared with use of the whole-volume body coil (5,6). As a consequence, a significant improvement in the lesion-to-liver contrast and a better lesion detection ratio is obtained (5). One of the disadvantages of using surface coils is the resultant high signal intensity that results from the close proximity of the coil to subcutaneous fat. This high signal can result in increased respiratory motion artifact by increasing the intensity of the ghosting artifact. Minimization of this artifact can be achieved by using postprocessing filters available within the pulse sequences, by reducing scan time sufficiently to accomplish imaging during a single breath-hold, or by the addition of fat suppression techniques (4,7). An alternative to fat suppression is the use of spatial presaturation bands placed over the subcutaneous tissues.

Pulse Sequences

Standard liver MRI begins with a survey image. Depending on the individual MR manufacturer, the options for the survey sequence may be limited. Ideally, one would choose a multiplanar (axial, sagittal, coronal) survey that provides spatial information in all three planes allowing for localization of the liver borders and biliary tree. These sequences provide little additional information other than spatial localization. Alternatively, a thick section coronal breath-hold T2-weighted sequence can be used providing both anatomical localization and gross lesion detection.

Routine hepatic imaging should include sequences that provide excellent anatomical localization, hepatic lesion detection, hepatic lesion characterization, and disease staging. This requires a combination of T1, T2, and contrast enhanced sequences.

T1-Weighted Sequences

The normal liver demonstrates a higher or similar signal intensity compared to muscle or T1-weighted images due to the presence of a larger amount of free water binding protein within hepatocytes (8) (Fig. 2). Most focal hepatic lesions (metastases, cysts, and hemangioma) have a longer T1 and thus have lower signal intensity compared with surrounding normal hepatic tissue (Fig. 3). However, lesions arising from hepatocellular tissue including

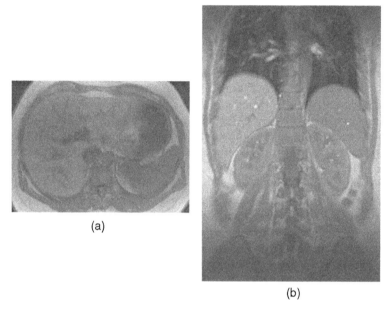

(a)

(b)

Figure 2   T1-weighted sequences. (a) Axial and (b) coronal spoiled gradient echo T1-weighted FLASH images illustrate the appearance of the normal liver: it demonstrates a higher signal intensity compared to muscle and spleen due to the presence of a larger amount of free water binding protein within hepatocytes.

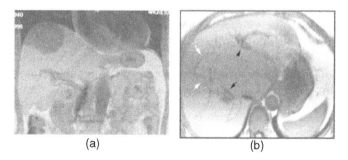

(a)   (b)

Figure 3   Focal hepatic lesions on T1-weighted images. (a) Coronal spoiled gradient echo T1-weighted FLASH image of the liver in a patient with colon cancer shows well-defined metastatic lesion (arrow) with lower signal intensity when compared to normal hepatic tissue. (b) Axial spoiled gradient echo T1-weighted FLASH image of the liver in another patient with focal nodular hyperplasia shows a well-defined lesion (black arrows) that is isointense, due to its hepatocellular origin, compared to normal hepatic tissue. Note intrahepatic venous collateral due to mass effect of the lesion on the hepatic veins (white arrows).

adenoma, focal nodular hyperplasia (FNH), regenerative nodule, and well-differentiated hepatocellular carcinoma (HCC) are isointense or even hyperintense compared with liver parenchyma (9). This hyperintense signal intensity (as a result of increased glycogen content or fatty change) within a liver mass is suggestive, but not specific, for a lesion of hepatocellular origin. Rarely, other lesions can contain high signal from fat. These include intrahepatic lipoma, angiomyelolipoma, and metastases of liposarcoma and teratocarcinoma (10). Melanoma (due to the paramagnetic effects of melanin) and hemorrhagic lesions such as hepatic adenoma, biliary cyst, and hepatocellular carcinoma (due to the paramagnetic effect of methemoglobin) can also present as hyperintense masses (11,12) (Fig. 4).

Unenhanced T1-weighted imaging is best performed using a breathhold gradient echo sequence with a short TR and short TE (13,14). These sequences (FLASH—Siemens, Erlangen, Germany; SPGR—GE Medical systems, Milwaukee, WI) generate an echo by gradient reversal rather than by a 180° refocusing pulse. The TR is chosen sufficient to scan the liver in a multislice acquisition, and a short TE (<5 ms) and a high flip angle ($>60°$) are mandatory for T1-weighting (15). This technique allows examination of the liver in 16–30 seconds with 11–15 sections (16). In one of the sequences used, the TE should be chosen to ensure that fat and water are

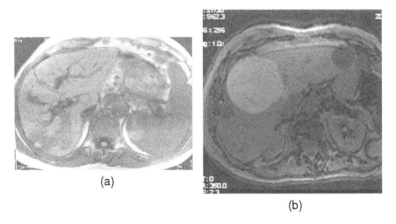

(a)

(b)

FIGURE 4 Focal hepatic lesions on T1-weighted images. (a) Axial spoiled gradient echo T1-weighted FLASH image of the liver in a patient with metastatic melanoma shows an ill-defined lesion in the right hepatic lobe. Areas of high signal intensity within the lesion are due to the paramagnetic effect of melanin. (b) Axial spoiled gradient echo T1-weighted image shows large hyperintense lesion, consistent with a hemorrhagic cyst, in this patient with AD hepatorenal polycystic disease. The high signal intensity is due to the paramagnetic effect of methemoglobin.

in-phase (4.6 ms at 1.5 T), which increases the background signal of liver. The higher background signal for liver increases lesion conspicuity since most lesions are hypointense to liver parenchyma. Out-of-phase imaging (TE equal to 2.3 ms at 1.5 T) should also be performed in order to detect microscopic lipid within focal fatty change or lesions of hepatocellular origin such as HCC (14,17,18) (Fig. 5).

Ultra-fast, subsecond T1-weighted imaging is also possible using magnetization prepared (inversion-recovery) gradient-echo sequences [turbo fast low-angle shot (TurboFLASH), Siemens; turbo-field-echo (TFE), Philips] (2,19,20). These sequences produce images with strong T1-weighting, negligible artifacts related to motion, and minimal phase-encoding artifacts from flowing blood. These sequences are, however, very sensitive to choices of parameters and the order of raw data collection (20). Because the spatial resolution is inferior, these techniques are not recommended to replace spoiled gradient echo imaging except when the motion artifacts require ultra-fast imaging (2).

Contrast-enhanced gradient echo T1-weighted imaging following the injection of gadolinium-based contrast agents have become key sequences for both the characterization and detection of liver lesions (21,22) as well as the evaluation of the vascular supply (23). The ability to acquire images in a short period of time allows for multiphasic imaging in the arterial, portal, and equilibrium phases. The pattern of enhancement within the various phases of imaging has a very important role in lesion

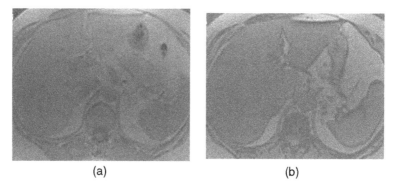

(a)   (b)

FIGURE 5 In- and-out-of-phase T1-weighted imaging. (a) In-phase breath-hold T1-weighted gradient-echo image shows the liver to be brighter in signal intensity than the spleen and paraspinal muscles. (b) Out-of-phase image demonstrates a significant drop in signal intensity of the liver. This low signal intensity is characteristic of diffuse fatty change. Note the typical "India ink" artifact where the abdominal organs interface the retroperitoneal fat (arrows).

characterization since many different enhancement and washout patterns are characteristic for a variety of focal liver lesions, thus frequently allowing a specific diagnosis (24,25). The details of these enhancement patterns are presented elsewhere in this chapter.

T2-Weighted Imaging

T2-weighted sequences, especially newer breath-hold techniques, remain important in the detection of focal liver lesions and in differentiating benign from malignant conditions 4,26–29. Because most hepatic neoplasms have a longer T2 relaxation time than liver, they demonstrate high signal intensity on T2-weighted images. T2-weighted imaging is performed with a longer TR (>2000 ms) and TE (>100 ms) compared with the T1-weighted sequences. Images obtained with conventional SE pulse sequences require an acquisition time of greater than 10 minutes and are usually compromised by motion artifacts. For these reasons, various modifications of fast spin-echo sequences have completely replaced conventional T2-weighted sequences.

Fast SE (FSE) or turbo SE (TSE) imaging can be performed in signifi-cantly less time, namely 3–4 minutes versus the 12–16 minutes necessary for conventional T2-weighted sequences. This decrease in acquisition time with FSE and TSE sequences is possible because multiple (8–256) lines of K-space are sampled within each TR interval as opposed to standard SE, where only one line is sampled for each TR. There is continuing evidence regarding the superiority of FSE techniques over conventional SE sequences, with several studies showing that FSE sequences compare favorably to conventional SE sequences for focal liver lesion detection and characterization (27,28). The most important differences in image appearance between FSE and conventional SE images are a decrease of the magnetic susceptibility effect of iron and other metals and an increase of the signal intensity of fat on FSE images (30,31). The routine use of fat suppression for fast T2-weighted imaging improves lesion conspicuity and reduces ghost artifact from motion of the abdominal wall (4,27).

Respiratory motion artifacts can be reduced or eliminated by the use of respiratory triggering or breath-hold imaging. Respiratory-triggering allows the acquisition to be timed to the respiratory cycle such that mea-surement occurs during the quiet phase of breathing. Breath-hold imaging requires faster sequences and can be used to obtain T2-weighted images of the entire liver in one or two breath-holds. With the HASTE sequence (half-Fourier acquisition single-shot turbo spin-echo), individual images can be obtained in about one second since only half of K-space (half Fourier imaging) is sampled (32). Kanematsu et al. (27) reported that fat-sup-pressed respiratory-triggered fast spin-echo was the preferred sequence for the detection of liver lesions when compared to conventional SE, breath-hold FSE, and echo-planar imaging. However, Augui et al. (29) reported the use of a fast-recovery fast SE sequence (FRFSE) with improved signal-to-noise and contrast-to-noise ratios compared with both breath-hold half-Fourier and non–breath-hold respiratory-triggered imaging. The FRFSE sequence uses a fast-recovery modification (180° pulse followed by a $-90°$ pulse) in order to force the residual magnetization into the longitudinal axis instead of allowing it to recover with T1 processes (29). Although future investigations are needed to confirm the preliminary data, studies suggest that ultra-fast imaging sequences can replace other T2-weighted imaging techniques (4,29,33).

Biliary Imaging (MR Cholangiography)

The basic principle underlying all MR cholangiography (MRC) techniques is that the T2 relaxation time of bile is extremely long, approximately 20 times longer than surrounding fat and parenchymal tissues. Therefore, on heavily T2-weighted sequences, fluid within the biliary tree remains of relatively high signal while the background tissues are suppressed (34). Background suppression can be further enhanced with the use of fat suppression. MRC is usually performed using one of the hybrid rapid acquisitions with relaxation enhancement (RARE) sequences or its derivatives (35,35). Early techniques used primarily 2D fast spin-echo (FSE) (36) and 3D FSE (37) acquired in the coronal plane, which were then postprocessed using the maximum intensity pixel projection (MIP) algorithm. Long acquisition times and motion artifacts limited these sequences.

The introduction of single shot RARE (38–40) techniques and single shot HASTE (41,42) imaging has reduced imaging times to within a single breath-hold. The tradeoff associated with these more rapid sequences is a loss of spatial resolution. Soto et al. (43) compared the performance of three pulse sequences (3D FSE, single slab HASTE, and multislice HASTE) commonly used for MRC and found the three MRC sequences had similarly high sensitivities and specificities for the detection of choledocholithiasis. The breath-hold techniques are best applied in two forms: a single thick coronal (or axial) slab and a multislice thin coronal sequence (34). Because of the short imaging times. it seems prudent to combine both single-slab and multislice breath-hold sequences to capitalize on the relative advantages of each (34,43).

The thick slab sequence produces an image in less than 2 seconds providing a rapid overview of the biliary tree without the need for postprocessing (Fig. 6). The slab thickness varies between 30 and 80 mm and

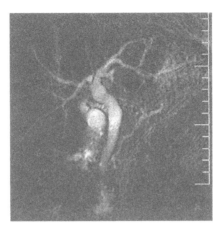

FIGURE 6 MR cholangiography. Oblique coronal projective MR cholangiographic image in a patient with abnormal liver function tests shows mild dilation of the biliary tree due to sphincter of Oddi dysfunction.

should be repeated in various degrees of obliquity to avoid overlapping fluid structures. One potential pitfall of the single slab technique is that bright fluid surrounding a filling defect can potentially obscure visualization.

The multislice sequence can be acquired in approximately 10–35 seconds and allows the acquisition of multiple thin contiguous slices. Slice thickness is usually set to the minimum value that still provides adequate signal-to-noise ratio (SNR). The multiple slices can be postprocessed into a projectional view using the MIP algorithm. However, these "raw data" slices should be carefully reviewed to detect subtle filling defects or structures that could be overlooked in the MIP image or thick slab image (34).

MR CONTRAST AGENTS

Several types of contrast agents have been clinically investigated for MR imaging of the liver. According to their biodistribution pattern, four major categories can be recognized: (a) extracellular agents, (b) reticuloendothelial agents, (c) hepatocyte-specific agents, and (d) intravascular contrast agents (44,45). Regarding magnetic activity, contrast agents can also be classified into two groups pending the predominant effect on relaxation times. Paramagnetic contrast agents with extracellular or hepatobiliary distribution contain gadolinium or manganese and especially shorten T1 and, thus, increase the signal intensity of the liver on

T1-weighted images (T1 agents). Superparamagnetic iron oxides (SPIO) or reticuloendothelial contrast agents, on the other hand, especially shorten T2 (45), and consequently the liver signal intensity is decreased on T2-weighted images (T2 agents). Finally, the intravascular contrast agents or ultrasmall superparamagnetic iron oxide (USPI0) can be used either as a T1 agent on T1-weighted images or as a T2 agent on T2-weighted images due to a balanced relaxivity profile (45).

Extracellular Contrast Agents

Gadolinium (Gd) chelates, the first contrast agents available for clinical use, are initially distributed in the intravascular space but then rapidly filtered into the extracellular or interstitial space of normal and abnormal tissues. Because of this rapid equilibration, utilization of imaging techniques with high temporal resolution (as are breath-hold GRE T1-weighted sequences) after bolus injection of the gadolinium chelate is mandatory to capture the rapid changes in contrast distribution (46). The extremely narrow imaging window also explains the limited role of gadolinium-enhanced T1-weighted imaging in lesion detection. With the exemption of extremely hypo- or hypervascular masses, many lesions may be missed due to the similarity between lesion enhancement and enhancement of the surrounding liver. For example, some studies showed that dynamic-gadolinium enhanced images do not detect more liver metastases than an unenhanced MR imaging examination (47,48).

Extracellular gadolinium-containing contrast agents play a very important role in tissue characterization as different enhancement and washout patterns exist corresponding to differences in the intravascular and extracellular spaces of a variety of focal liver lesions, frequently allowing a specific diagnosis to be made (49,50) (Fig. 7). The details of these enhancement patterns are presented elsewhere in this chapter.

Reticuloendothelial Cell-Specific Contrast Agents

When injected into the bloodstream, superparamagnetic crystalline-coated iron oxides particles (SPIO) or ferumoxides (Feridex IV and Endorem) are specifically taken up by the endothelial and Kupffer cells of the liver. Because of osmolarity constraints, ferumoxides are administered slowly as a drip infusion over 30 minutes after dilution. Most focal hepatic lesions, especially metastases, are devoid of reticuloendothelial cells and contrast sharply with the adjacent normal liver parenchyma, which is darkened by iron oxide phagocytosis on T2-weighted images. As a result, there is a significant increase in contrast-to-noise ratio, lesion's signal-to-noise ratio, and consequently better lesion demarcation and lesion detection. Many

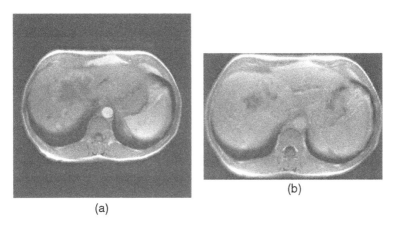

(b)

(a)

FIGURE 7   Extracellular contrast agents (gadolinium-chelates). (a) Axial arterial-phase gadolinum-enhanced T1-weighted gradient-echo image shows a well-defined lesion in segments 4 and 8 of the liver. The lesion shows peripheral rim-like enhancement. (b) Delayed-phase gadolinum-enhanced T1-weighted gradient-echo image shows persistent enhancement of the lesion compared to the surrounding liver. This enhacement pattern is characteristic for intrahepatic cholangiocarcinoma.

studies have shown an improvement in lesion detection on SPIO-enhanced T2-weighted images compared with spiral CT and unenhanced T2-weighted images (51,52). Although, as mentioned before, the predominant effect of SPIO agents is T2 shortening, shortening of T1 can also be observed, especially in the early phase following intravenous administration of low concentrations.

Pulse sequences especially sensitive to the presence of iron oxide are T2*-weighted gradient echo images, due to their high sensitivity for magnetic field heterogeneity (53). There is no consensus yet concerning the optimal T2* GRE sequence to be used. Some authors have demonstrated that even relatively T1-weighted GRE images (flip angle 75°) are superior for lesion detection when compared with breath-hold T2-weighted FSE sequences following the injection of ferumoxides (54) (Fig. 8).

SPIO-enhanced imaging can also be helpful in lesion characterization. Most FNHs and some adenomas and well-differentiated HCC accumulate ferumoxides due to the presence of Kupffer cells, with a corresponding decrease in signal intensity on post-contrast T2-weighted images (55) (Fig. 9). Also, in lesions in which blood pooling occurs, as in hemangiomas, a decrease in signal intensity on T2-weighed images is reported (56).

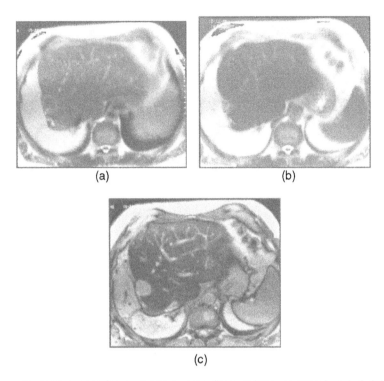

(a)   (b)

(c)

FIGURE 8   Hepatospecific contrast agents (iron oxides particles). (a) Axial unenhanced T2-weighted HASTE image in a patient with colon cancer and status
post right hepatectomy shows the presence of a 2-cm liver metastasis in the left
hepatic lobe next to the resection margin. (b) Axial T2-weighted HASTE image
obtained after IV administration of SPIO shows darkening of liver and spleen but
no significant increased conspicuity of the lesion. (c) Axial T2*-weighted GRE
image shows increased conspicuity of the lesion due to the increased susceptibility
of this sequence for iron.

Hepatobiliary Contrast Agents

Hepatobiliary contrast agents are a heterogeneous group of soluble paramagnetic molecules predominantly affecting T1 contrast. They are taken
up by the hepatocytes by either organic anion transporters (Gd-BOPTA,
Gd-EOB-DPTA) or the similarity between the contrast agent and vitamin
B_6 (Mn-DPDP) and are finally exceted in bile (45). In contrast to extracellular contrast agents, hepatobiliary molecules cause prolonged liver
enhancement and, therefore, provide a wide imaging window of several
hours. Due to the specificity for hepatic tissue, T1-weighted images show

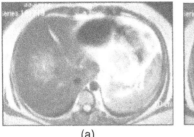 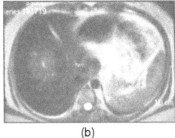

(a)   (b)

FIGURE 9   Hepatospecific contrast agents (iron oxides particles). (a) Axial un-enhanced fast-spin-echo T2-weighted image shows the presence of a 4-cm FNH. (b) Axial T2-weighted fast-spin-echo image obtained after IV administration of SPIO shows darkening of liver and spleen and significant decreased signal intensity of the lesion.

increased signal in normal liver tissue without enhancement of nonhepatocellular lesions (metastases, lymphoma, intrahepatic cholangiocarcinoma) and, therefore, increase lesion-to-liver contrast and lesion detection on T1-weighted images (44) (Fig. 10). HCC, hepatic adenoma, FNH, and regenerative nodules enhance with hepatobiliary contrast agents since they are composed of hepatocytes. HCC enhancement patterns are complex and nonuniform with greater enhancement characteristic of well-differentiated lesions (57).

Compared with Mn-DPDP, the gadolinium chelates with hepatobiliary retention (Gd-BOPTA, Gd-EOB-DTPA) have the advantage that they can be administered as a bolus to perform dynamic studies and thus add diagnostic information based on the differences in enhancement pattern. The specific biliary excretion of hepatobiliary contrast agents has the potential for improving the delineation of the biliary tree, which may be helpful in the diagnosis of biliary infiltration by hepatic liver lesions and to increase the diagnostic accurracy in patients with associated biliary diseases (58).

Intravascular (Blood Pool) Agents

In contrast to all other contrast agents discussed above, dextran-coated ultrasmall superparamagnetic iron oxide particles or USPIO (e.g., AMI-227) are molecules with a long half-time in blood (appoximately 200 min) and thus are very suitable for use as intravascular (bloodpool) contrast agents (59). Because of the differences in blood volume per unit weight between normal liver and solid hepatic tumors, improved detection of focal liver lesions can be achieved. Furthermore, since USPIO particles generate

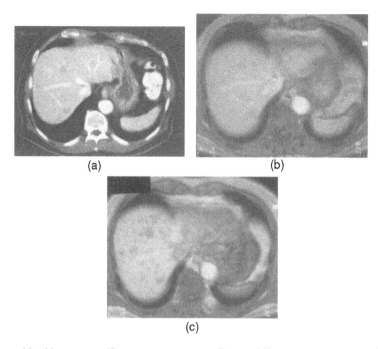

(a)   (b)

(c)

FIGURE 10   Hepatospecific contrast agents (hepatobiliary contrast agents). (a) Axial contrast-enhanced CT image in a patient with metastatic colon cancer shows faint hypodense focal liver lesions suggestive for liver metastases. (b) Axial early-phase contrast-enhanced T1-weighted image obtained after intravenous admininstration of gadolinium-EOB shows hypovascular character of the lesions. (c) Contrast-enhanced T1-weighted image obtained 20 minutes after contrast administration shows intense uptake of contrast by normal liver parenchyma, which increases the conspicuity of the liver metastases.

a relatively strong T1 and T2 relaxivity, these contrast agents can be used either as a negative agent (on T2-weighted images) or as a positive agent (on T1-weighted images) (59).

FOCAL LIVER LESIONS

Benign Liver Lesions

Hepatic (Biliary) Cyst

Hepatic biliary cysts are common and reported to be present in 1–14% of people in autopsy series (60). Although they are almost always asympto-matic, large cysts (>10 cm) may become symptomatic from extrinsic compression on adjacent structures and cause abdominal fullness, nausea, vomiting, or obstructive jaundice (61). Typically, liver function tests are normal, because the overall functioning volume of hepatic parenchyma is adequate. Hepatic cysts are either solitary or multiple as part of autosomal dominant (adults) or recessive (children) polycystic liver disease. Although hepatic cysts are found in 40% of cases with autosomal dominant polycystic disease involving the kidneys, they may be seen without radiological evidence of renal involvement (10%)

Histopathologically, a simple hepatic cyst is defined as a single, unilocular cyst lined by a single layer of cuboidal, bile duct epithelium. The wall is a thin layer of fibrous tissue and the adjacent liver is normal. Grossly, the wall is 1 mm or less in thickness (62,63).

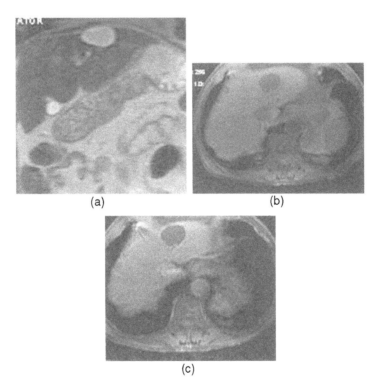

(a)   (b)

(c)

FIGURE 11   Hepatic cyst. (a) Coronal heavily T2-weighted image shows well-defined homogenous lesion in the lateral segment of the left hepatic lobe. (b) Corresponding axial unenhanced T1-weighted image shows homogenous appearance. (c) Axial contrast-enhanced T1-weighted image shows no enhancement.

Due to their fluid content, hepatic cysts are homogeneous and show no enhancement following administration of contrast material (60,61,64). They are typically round or ovoid shaped, well delineated, and have thin, smooth walls, without septations (64). Hepatic cysts reveal very low signal intensity on T1-weighted and very high signal intensity on T2-weighted images, respectively (65) (Fig. 11). The signal typically increases on so-called heavily T2-weighted images (65). In case of intracystic hemorrhage, a rare complication, when mixed blood products are present, the lesion's signal intensity is high on both T1- and T2-weighted images with a fluid-fluid level frequently seen (66).

Hemangioma

Cavernous hemangioma is the most common benign hepatic tumor and the second most common tumor seen in the liver after metastases (67). The incidence of hemangiomas in the general population has been estimated to range from 1% to approximately 20% (67). Hemangioma is more common in women than in men (ratio 5:1) and can be seen in any age group (67). They are usually asymptomatic (85%) and incidentally detected (67,68). They can, however, produce symptoms of abdominal pain, nausea, or vomiting as a result of extrinsic compression of adjacent structures, rupture, hemorrhage, or thrombosis. A hemangioma is usually solitary (80%), typically measures less than 4 cm in diameter, and is most often peripherally located. With the exception of hemangiomas in pregnant females, where enlargement secondary to the estrogen effect may occur, stability of the lesions is an important hallmark (69). A giant hemangioma is defined as greater than 10 cm in diameter and often contains a central cleftlike area of fibrosis or cystic degeneration (67).

Pathologically, hemangiomas consist of large well-defined areas of blood-filled spaces lined by a single layer of endothelium and separated by fibrous septae. Areas of cystic degeneration, fibrosis, thrombosis, and occasional calcifications may be present (62,63).

MR imaging findings in hemangiomas reflect the vascular nature of the lesion (70–74). On T1- and T2-weighted images, respectively, the lesions show decreased and markedly increased homogeneous signal intensity compared to normal liver tissue (71–74). Atypically, a heterogeneous appearance may be present in case of intratumoral fibrosis, hemorrhage, or thrombosis (75). Because of their high water content and subsequent prolonged T2 relaxation time, hemangiomas classically show an increase in signal intensity on heavily T2-weighted images (70–74). The use of heavily T2-weighted images in the work-up of focal liver lesions has been associated with a sensitivity of 100%, accuracy of 97%, and specificity of 92% for the diagnosis of hemangioma (70–74) (Fig. 12).

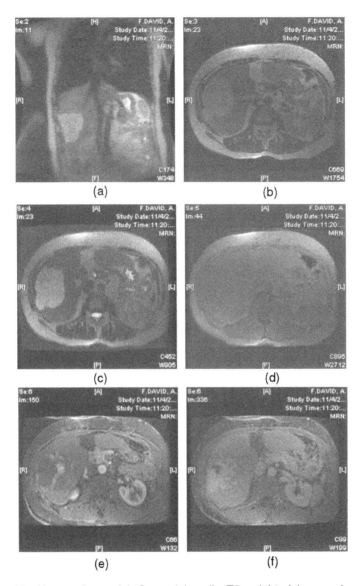

(a)

(b)

(c)

(d)

(e)

(f)

FIGURE 12 Hemangioma. (a) Coronal heavily T2-weighted image shows well-defined homogenous lesion in the right hepatic lobe. Note associated capsular retraction. Corresponding (b) axial T2-weighted, (c) heavily T2-weighted, and (d) unenhanced T1-weighted image shows homogenous appearance of the lesion. (e) Axial early-phase contrast-enhanced T1-weighted image shows peripheral incomplete nodular enhancement. (f) Axial delayed-phase contrast-enhanced T1-weighted image shows fill-in with persistent enhancement of the lesion.

Dynamic T1-weighted imaging following intravenous administration of gadolinium chelate classically shows a peripheral, nodular, centripetal enhancement pattern progressing to homogeneity (70–74). Immediate and complete enhancement is usually seen in small lesions, while in 94% of giant hemangiomas a persistent hypointense center is present on the delayed images, the latter due to variable degree of fibrosis and cystic degeneration (70). Hemangiomas do not show uptake of SPIO or Mn-DPDP because they do not contain Kupffer cells or normal hepatocytes. However, following administration of ultrasmall superparamagnetic iron oxide (USPIO), a specific enhancement pattern is noticed (76). On T1-weighted images, hemangiomas enhance immediately due to their vascularity and become isointense with normal liver (76). On T2-weighted images, hemangiomas demonstrate decreased signal intensity and may become isointense to the liver at higher doses of USPIO (76).

Focal Nodular Hyperplasia

Focal nodular hyperplasia (FNH) is a benign tumor-like condition that is predominantly (80–95%) diagnosed in females during their 3rd to 5th decade of life, although it has been described in other age groups and males as well (77,78). FNH accounts for approximately 8% of all primary hepatic tumors and is the second most common benign liver tumor after hemangioma (77,78). FNH is usually discovered incidentally in asymptomatic patients. In less than one third of patients, clinical symptoms, such as right upper quadrant or epigastric pain, lead to their discovery. To date, the etiology and pathogenesis of FNH is not well understood: a congenital vascular malformation or vascular injury has been suggested as the underlying mechanism for secondary hepatocellular hyperplasia (77). Although oral contraceptive use has been linked to the growth of FNH, its exact influence remains controversial. Data from a recent large study suggested that neither size, number of lesions, nor growth of FNH is influenced by oral contraceptives (79). Typically, the growth of FNH remains proportional to its blood supply, and, therefore, necrosis or hemorrhage is extremely unusual.

Histopathologically, FNH is a well-circumscribed, nonencapsulated, usually solitary mass composed of nodules of hyperplastic hepatocytes and Kupffer's cells surrounding a central vascular scar, the latter typically containing prominent vessels, bile ductules, and inflammatory cells, all embedded in a loose myxomatous fibrous stroma (62,63). The size of the lesions may range between 1 and 15 cm, but most lesions are smaller than 5 cm, with a mean diameter of 3–4 cm at the time of diagnosis (78).

Typical MRI features of FNH include iso- or hypointensity on T1-weighted images (94–100%), mild hyperintensity or isointensity on T2-weighted (94–100%) images, homogeneity (96%), and the presence of a central scar which appears hypointense on T-1 and hyperintense on T2-weighted images (84%) (80,81) (Fig. 13). The latter is due to the presence of vascular channels, bile ductules, and increased edema within the myxomatous tissue. Following administration of gadolinium, the enhancement profile is identical to that seen on contrast-enhanced CT images: dramatic enhancement in the arterial phase, followed by isointensity of the lesion during the portal venous phase (80). On delayed phase imaging, the central scar shows high signal intensity, due to the accumulation of contrast material (80,81). Recently, the use of reticuloendothelial MR contrast agents, such as SPIO particles, has markedly expanded the role of MRI in the characterization of FNH (84). Since FNH contains Kupffer cells, it will show

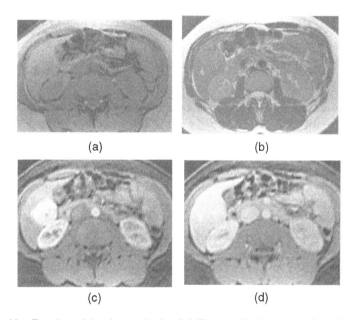

(a)   (b)

(c)   (d)

FIGURE 13   Focal nodular hyperplasia. (a) T1-weighted image of a 44-year-old woman shows a nearly isointense lesion in the right lobe of the liver. (b) On T2-weighted image this same lesion is mildly hyperintense with a hyperintense scar. (c) Axial arterial-phase contrast-enhanced MR image shows early and homogeneous enhancement of the lesion (except central scar). (d) Axial delayed-phase contrast-enhanced MR image shows enhancement of the central scar and wash-out of the lesion.

loss of signal on T2-weighted images due to contrast uptake. Furthermore, the degree of signal loss seen in FNH on SPIO-enhanced T2-weighted images is significantly greater than for other focal liver lesions. Hepatobiliary MR contrast agents, such as Mn-DPDP and Gd-EOB-DTPA, are also helpful in characterizing FNH (84). Since FNH consists of hepatocytes, it will show uptake of the contrast agent, resulting in hyper- or isointensity of the lesion relative to the liver on T1-weighted images (84).

Although atypical imaging features are the exception rather than the rule, differentiation of FNH that lack characteristic findings from other primary and secondary hepatic lesions is sometimes difficult (85). Atypically, FNH may present as a large lesion, sometimes multiple, and may demonstrate internal necrosis, hemorrhagic foci, and fatty infiltration (85). Other rare imaging features include nonvisualization of the central scar, nonenhancement of the central scar, pseudocapsular enhancement on delayed imaging, and hypointensity of the scar on T2-weighted images. The latter, presumably due to obliteration or absence of vascular channels within the scar, is important to recognize since it may mimic the collageneous scar seen in fibrolamellar carcinoma, HCC, or intrahepatic cholangiocarcinoma (85).

Hepatocellular Adenoma

Hepatocellular adenoma (HCA) is a rare, benign liver neoplasm strongly associated with oral contraceptive and androgen steroid use (86,87). Generally, it is estimated to occur in 1 of 1,000,000 people. HCA is most commonly discovered in women of child-bearing age who have a history of prolonged use of oral contraceptives (86,87). In this subgroup, its incidence is increased to 3 per 100,000 people. HCA can also occur spontaneously or be associated with underlying metabolic diseases, such as type I glycogen storage disease and diabetes mellitus (88). Identification of hepatic adenomas is important because of the associated risk of life-threatening hemorrhage (89). This results from the fact that HCA, in contrast to FNH, has the propensity to outgrow its arterial vascular supply, resulting in hemorrhage, necrosis, and occasionally rupture. Withdrawal of estrogen medication may result in regression of the tumor, although it may require a period of several months (90).

Usually solitary (80%), hepatic adenoma consists histopathologically of an encapsulated proliferation of normal or nearly normal hepatocytes lacking well-defined bile ducts, portal venous tracts, and terminal hepatic veins (62,63). Intracellular fat and glycogen, intratumoral necrosis, hemorrhage, peliosis, or large subcapsular vessels are common features detected on gross examination (62,63).

MR imaging classically shows a heterogeneous (93%) mass, with predominantly hyperintense signal intensity on T2-weighted images (47–75%), and variable signal intensity on T1-weighted images, according to the presence of fatty change and hemorrhage (increased signal), or necrosis (decreased signal) (Fig. 14) (91–93). Approximately 30% of HCA have a peripheral rim, hypointense on both T1-and T2-weighted images, corresponding to a fibrous capsule. On dynamic gadolinium-enhanced T1-weighted images, 86% of adenomas show early arterial enhancement, secondary to their hepatic arterial blood supply. Adenomas in some cases may take up SPIO, resulting in a decreased signal on T2-weighted images (82).

Hepatic adenomatosis is a rare entity characterized by the presence of multiple (more than 10) HCAs in an otherwise normal liver and is considered a distinct entity because of different clinico-pathological features (94,95). First, hepatic adenomatosis is unrelated to oral contraceptive use. Second, it affects men and women equally. Finally, an increase in serum alkaline phosphatase and gamma-glutamyl transpeptidase is common in adenomatosis. The imaging and histopathological features of individual adenomatous lesions are similar to those reported in young women who are taking oral contraceptives (96). The MR features of hepatic adenomatosis include evidence of hypervascularity (63%), intratumoral fat (80% at MR), and decreased conspicuity at portal venous and delayed-

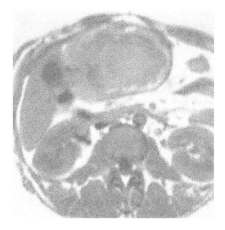

FIGURE 14 Hepatocellular adenoma. Axial unenhanced T1-weighted MR image shows a large heterogeneous mass arising from segment 4 of the liver. The high signal intensity areas are consistent with presence of methemoglobin. Note also low signal intensity fibrous capsule bordering the mass.

phase imaging (96). Fifty percent of patients also have congenital or acquired hepatic vascular abnormalities.

Biliary Hamartoma (von Meyenburg Complex)

Bile duct hamartomas or von Meyenburg complexes develop when embryonic bile ducts fail to involute (97). They are usually encountered as an incidental finding at laparatomy, autopsy, or imaging studies (98). An estimated incidence of 1–3% has been reported in autopsy series (97,98). The association between biliary hamartomas and other ductal plate abnormalities, such as hepatic fibrosis and polycystic liver disease, has been described. Although biliary hamartomas have no clinical manifestations and are in general defined as benign lesions, association with malignancies has been reported in literature (99). Usually, they are stable and without significant growth over time. On gross pathology, they present as greyish-white nodular lesions scattered throughout the liver parenchyma, typically measuring between 0.1 and 0.5 cm in diameter (100).

On MRI, biliary hamartoma is usually hypointense compared to liver parenchyma on T1-weighted images and strongly hyperintense on T2-weighted images (101–104) (Fig. 15). On heavily T2-weighted images, the signal intensity increases further reaching almost the intensity of fluid. Biliary hamartoma does not exhibit a characteristic pattern of enhancement after intravenous administration of gadolinium. Some authors have reported homogeneous enchancement of these lesions, while others could not find any enchancement following gadolinium administration. Recently, a thin rim of enhancement, correlating pathologically with the compressed liver parenchyma that surrounds these lesions, has been described in some cases.

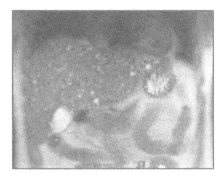

FIGURE 15   Biliary hamartoma. Coronal T2-weighted MR image shows numerous subcentimenter hyperintense lesions scattered throughout the liver.

Biliary Cystadenoma

Biliary cystadenomas are rare, usually slow-growing, multilocular cystic tumors, comprising less than 5% of intrahepatic cystic masses of biliary origin (105,106). Although generally intrahepatic, extrahepatic locations have been described. They occur predominantly in middle-aged women (mean age: 38 years) and are considered premalignant lesions.

Biliary cystadenomas range in size from 1.5 to 35 cm and are characterized by the presence of a cystic mass with a well-defined thick fibrous capsule, mural nodules, and rarely capsular calcification (62,63). The fluid within the tumor can be proteinaceous, mucinous, and occasionaly gelatinous, purulent, or hemorrhagic due to trauma. Polypoid, pedunculated excrescences are seen more commonly in biliary cystadenocarcinoma than in cystadenomas, although papillary areas and polypoid projections have been described in cystadenoma without frank malignancy.

Although the MRI descriptions of hepatic biliary cystadenoma are limited, the characteristics of an uncomplicated biliary cystadenoma correlate well with the pathological features: a fluid-containing multiloculated mass, revealing homogeneous low-signal and high-signal intensities on the T1- and T2-weighted images, respectively (Fig. 16) (107,108). Variable signal intensities on both T1- and T2-weighted images depend on the presence of solid components, hemorrhage, and high protein content (107). The septations are evident on T2-weighted images as low signal intensity bands separating the high signal intensity locules (108).

Biliary cystadenomas cannot be distinguished from cystadenocarcinoma by imaging characteristics alone. This distinction is not essential, since surgical resection is the treatment of choice for both.

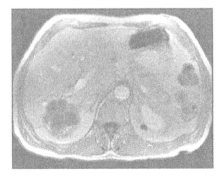

FIGURE 16   Biliary cystadenoma/carcinoma. Axial contrast-enhanced MR image shows exophytically located multiloculated cystic mass arising from the right lobe of the liver. Subsequent resection revealed biliary cystadenocarcinoma.

Angiomyolipoma

Angiomyolipomas are lesions composed of angiomyomatous and fatty components (109). In the abdomen, angiomyolipomas typically occur in the kidney, with hepatic involvement being very unusual (110). There is a higher incidence of angiomyolipoma in patients with tuberous sclerosis, an autosomal dominant phakomatosis clinically characterized by mental retardation, seizures, and skin lesions (adenoma sebaceum) (111).

MRI imaging clearly demonstrates the presence of the fatty component in angiomyolipomas (Fig. 17) (112–115). Angiomyolipomas are highly hyperintense on T1- and FSE T2-weighted images. On MRI, angiomyolipoma consists of two parts: an angiomyomatous component and a fatty component. In contrast to the absence of enhancement with contrast material seen in hepatic lipoma, enhancement of a part of the lesion following gadolinium administration is suggestive of the presence an angiomatous component. These angiomatous parts have been characterized to have a "macroaneurysmal" appearance by angiography, which is also apparent on MRI.

Mesenchymal Hamartoma

Mesenchymal hamartoma of the liver (MHL) is a rare developmental cystic tumor, most likely to occur between 15 and 24 months of age with a male-to-female ratio of 2:1 (116,117). It usually involves the right lobe and can grow to large sizes (16 cm being an average tumor size). Clinically, slow, progressive, painless abdominal enlargement is seen. Sometimes rapid enlargement may occur because of rapid accumulation of fluid in the cyst,

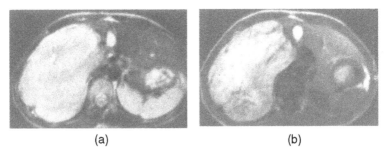

(a)   (b)

Figure 17 Angiomyolipoma. (a) Axial T2-weighted MR image in a patient with tuberous sclerosis shows the presence of a large hyperintense mass in the right lobe of the liver. (b) Corresponding axial unenhanced T1-weighted MR image shows the mass to be hyperintense due to its fatty nature.

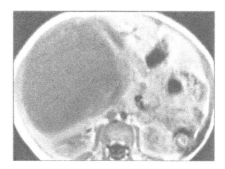

FIGURE 18 Mesenchymal hamartoma. Axial unenhanced T1-weighted MR image in a 3-year-old boy shows the presence of a large cystic mass in the right lobe of the liver.

and this may occasionally cause respiratory distress and edema of the lower extremities.

Histopathologically, the lesion is composed of immature mesen chymal cells, bile ducts, and hepatocytes. Grossly the tumor reveals a mass consisting of solid and cystic components of variable size, without a capsule.

The MRI features usually reflect the predominantly cystic nature of this tumor (Fig. 18) (117). MHL typically demonstrates low signal intensity on T1-weighted images with high signal intensity on T2-weighted images. Varying signal intensities due to varying concentration of protein contained in the cysts can be present.

Infantile Hemangioendothelioma

Infantile hemangioendothelioma (IHE) is the most common benign vascular tumor of infancy (116). Usually the masses are made up of multiple spongy nodules, with a solitary nodule being uncommon (62,63). The majority of patients with IHE present as young infants between 1 and 6 months of age, with less than 5% of cases detected beyond 1 year of age (116). IHE is predominantly seen in girls, with a female-to-male ratio of 2:1. Albeit benign, the condition can be manifested by congestive heart failure, platelet sequestration, disseminated intravascular coagulopathy, spontaneous rupture with resultant hemoperitoneum, and more rarely malignant transformation (118).

Microscopically, IHE consists of a proliferation of multiple anatomosing vascular spaces with an endothelial cell lining (62,63). Areas of hemorrhagic necrosis, dystrophic calcification, thrombosis, or fibrosis are common.

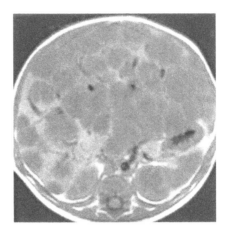

FIGURE 19   Infantile hemangioendothelioma. Axial unenhanced T1-weighted MR image in a 7-month-old boy with cardiac failure shows the presence of multiple low signal intensity masses scattered throughout all liver segments.

On noncontrast MRI, IHE is been described to be heterogeneous on both T1- and T2-weighted images because of the presence of hemorrhage, necrosis, and fibrosis (Fig. 19) (118,119). The vascular nature of the lesion is established by various degrees of high signal intensity on T2-weighted images similar to that of an adult hemangioma. Dynamic gadolinium-enhanced MRI features also correlate well with those of an adult giant hemangioma and are characterized by an early dense peripheral nodular enhancement of the tumor followed by variable delayed central enhancement.

Rare Benign Tumors

Some uncommon benign tumors of the liver are mentioned here for completeness. They are of limited radiological importance, and their MR imaging findings have been described primarily in small series.

Inflammatory pseudotumor (IPT) is a rare benign entity patho-logically characterized by proliferating fibrovascular tissue and infiltrating chronic inflammatory cells (120). Many causative hypotheses, such as vascular and infectious etiologies, have been suggested, but the exact pathogenesis remains unclear (120). Usually, IPT presents as a solitary mass with a slight male predominance. Hepatic IPT has been described in all age groups although the highest incidence occurs in young adults (120). Clinical manifestations of IPT include fever, malaise, weight loss, and right upper quadrant pain. Laboratory data often reveal evidence of an inflammatory process indicated by leukocytosis, an elevated erythrocyte sedimentation rate, and a positive C-reactive protein (120). The prognosis of IPT is usually good with either spontaneous recovery or recovery following conservative therapy (steroids, antibiotics, nonsteroidal anti-inflammatory drugs) or surgery. Reports illustrating the MRI features of IPT are exceedingly rare. Signal intensity characteristics on both noncontrast T1- and T2-weighted images vary from hypointense to hyperintense (120). The most common finding on unenhanced MRI is, however, hyperintensity on T2-weighted images. Following administration of gadolinium chelates, two different enhancement patterns have been described: a hypovascular mass with peripheral rim-like enhancement or an irregular and intensely enhancing lesion with rapid contrast washout (120).

Lipomas are exceedingly rare benign mesenchymal tumors, with only a few reports in the radiological literature (121). Because these lesions remain asymptomatic, they are usually incidentally detected. Intrahepatic lipomas appear on MRI as masses with high signal intensity on T1-weighted images with only a minimal signal decrease on T2-weighted sequences (121).

Lymphangioma is defined as a mass or multiple masses (lymphangiomatosis) composed of prominent lymphatic channels that compress the normal hepatic parenchyma (122). Lymphangiomatosis is usually part of a systemic syndrome in which other organs, including the spleen, skeleton, soft tissues, lung, and/or brain, are also involved. Imaging features include the presence of cystic, well-delineated lesions without enhancement following gadolinium administration.

Leiomyoma, a well-circumscribed smooth muscle tumor, is an extremely rare lesion in the liver and has no specific radiological characteristics (123). Several cases of leiomyoma have been described in patients infected with HIV, suggesting that there may be a clinical association between these two entities. On MRI, leiomyomas are hypointense and hyperintense relative to the liver on T1- and T2-weighted images, respectively.

Malignant Liver Lesions

Hepatocellular Carcinoma

Hepatocellular carcinoma (HCC), a malignant neoplasm derived from hepatocytes, is the most common primary epithelial neoplasm of the liver (63,124). The cause and incidence vary greatly throughout the world. Generally, the pathogenesis of HCC occurs by two separate and distinct pathways (125). In low-incidence areas (western Europe and North America), underlying cirrhosis from either alcoholism, hemochromatosis, or hepatitis is the most common causative factor (125). Development of HCC in chronic liver disease is more common in men than in women, and HCC is usually diagnosed in patients between 60 and 80 years of age (124). In high-incidence regions (Japan, China, Africa) development of HCC is predominantly a response to hepatitis B and aflatoxin ingestion (63). In these areas patients present usually at a younger age (30–50 years) (124).

Histopathologically, most HCC present as one or more focal masses, with diffuse hepatic involvement being exceptional. Tumor encapsulation, internal necrosis and hemorrhage, and vascular or biliary invasion are frequently seen. Less common features are fatty or cystic metamorphosis, or scar formation.

Hepatocellular carcinoma has a variable appearance on MR imaging. On T2-weighted images, typical cases of HCC demonstrate a mild hyper-intensity relative to normal liver (Fig. 20). The variable signal intensity seen on T1-weighted images depends on the presence or absence of steatosis or

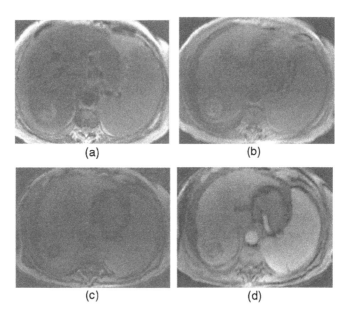

(a)   (b)

(c)   (d)

FIGURE 20 Hepatocellular carcinoma. (a) Axial T2-weighted MR image in a patient with cirrhosis shows the presence of a well-defined hyperintense mass in the right lobe of the liver. (b) In-phase breath-hold T1-weighted gradient-echo image shows the lesion to be hyperintense. (c) Out-of-phase T1-weighted image demonstrates a significant drop in signal intensity of the lesion consistent with fatty metamor-phosis. (d) Axial arterial-phase contrast-enhanced MR image shows central enhancement of the lesion.

hemorrhage (126,127). High signal intensity on T2-weighted images is especially useful in the setting of underlying cirrhosis to help differentiate HCC from regenerating nodules. The latter typically have a low intensity on T2-weighted images due to accumulation of iron (63). In tumors with encapsulation, a low-signal intensity rim representing fibrous tissue is detectable on the T1-weighted images. On T2-weighted images, this fibrous capsule appears as a double layer: the inner low signal intensity layer represents fibrous tissue, while the outer high signal intensity rim is thought to be due to compressed vessels and bile ducts (126). Following intravenous administration of gadolinium, smaller lesions tend to be hypervascular (with important early enhancement). Larger lesions are more hypovascular and reveal a mosaic-like enhancement pattern. Signs of vascular invasion and arterial-portal shunting are frequently present (124).

Fibrolamellar Hepatocellular Carcinoma

Fibrolamellar carcinoma is an uncommon slowly growing variant of hepatocellular carcinoma that has distinct clinical, histological, and radiological features (128). It is found in younger patients, is less frequently associated with underlying liver disease (0–22%), and has a better prognosis (128).

Pathologically, fibrolamellar carcinoma is characterized by lamellar bands of fibrous connective tissue surrounding malignant hepatocytes with granular eosinophylic cytoplasm. In contrast to HCC, hemorrhage and necrosis are unusual (128).

On MRI, fibrolamellar carcinoma is classically a large (10–20 cm), well-defined lobulated mass with central scar (80%) and dystrophic calcification (55%) (Fig. 21) (63,128). Although usually solitary, satellite

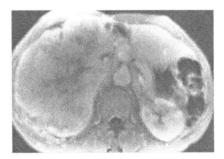

FIGURE 21   Fibrolamellar carcinoma. Axial contrast-enhanced MR image shows large mass occupying the right lobe of the liver with a large non-enhancing fibrotic central scar.

nodules may be present (124). Intrahepatic ductal dilatation and portal vein invasion may be seen. On T1- and T2-weighted images, the lesion is usually isointense to normal liver. Some reports describe a slightly hyperintense or hypointense appearance of fibrolamellar carcinoma on T2-weighted images (63). The central scar, if present, is classically hypointense on both T1- and T2-weighted images, which may help distinguish this entity from FNH (63,125). Some reports, however, indicate that the central scar in fibrolamellar carcinoma may occasionally be bright on T2-weighted images, making the distinction with FNH impossible (129). Dynamic gadolinium-enhanced images show early diffuse heterogeneous enhancement with return to homogeneous, isointense signal intensity in the delayed phase (124).

Intrahepatic (Peripheral) Cholangiocarcinoma

Intrahepatic cholangiocarcinoma is a primary adenocarcinoma originating in small and distal bile ducts. Although a relatively uncommon tumor, it represents 5–30% of primary malignant liver tumors and is the second most common hepatic malignant neoplasm after HCC (130–133). It accounts for 10% of all cholangiocarcinomas, most of which involve the common bile duct and hilum (131,132). A variety of underlying liver diseases, including Caroli's disease, sclerosing cholangitis, hepatolithiasis, and Thorotrast deposition, may predicpose to the development of intrahepatic cholangiocarcinoma (131,132). In addition, association between peripheral cholangiocarcinoma and clonorchiasis has also been reported. The average age of the patients with intrahepatic cholangiocarcinoma ranges from 50 to 60 years, with no strong gender differences (130). Because of its peripheral location relative to the main hepatic ducts, jaundice is seldom present at presentation (134).

Tumors are homogeneously hypointensive relative to liver paranchyma on T1-weighted spin-echo images (100%) and heterogeneous but generally high in signal on T2-weighted spin-echo images (Fig. 22) (130–133). Comparison with pathological examination reveals that lesion signal intensity of T2-weighted images is due mostly to the amount of fibrosis, necrosis, and mucous secretion within the lesion (131,133). On dynamic MR studies, tumors characteristically have minimal or moderate rim enhancement with progressive and concentric filling (75%), which can be homogeneous and complete, inhomogeneous and complete, or incomplete (130–134). Homogeneous complete enhancement is seen mainly in small tumors (2–4 cm) (133) and is probably due to a smaller amount of nonenhancing fibrous stroma component (133).

Other MRI features of intrahepatic cholangiocarcinoma are invasion of the portal veins, usually without evidence of tumor thrombus (25–75%),

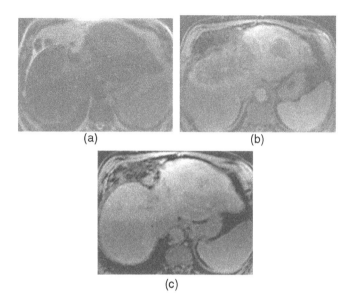

(a)   (b)

(c)

FIGURE 22   Intrahepatic cholangiocarcinoma. Axial T2-weighted image shows large slightly hyperintese mass in the left lobe of the liver. Note associated capsular retraction, mild biliary ductal dilatation, and central hypointensity in the mass indicating fibrosis. (b) Axial arterial-phase contrast-enhanced MR image shows enhancement of the periphery of the mass. (c) Axial delayed-phase contrast-enhanced MR image shows persistent enhancement of the central portions of the mass due to the fibrosis.

focal liver atrophy (43%), dilatation of intrahepatic bile ducts (29%), capsular retraction (21%), and small central calcifications (131–133). Some authors report the presence of a thin hypointense rim in the outermost periphery of the tumors in some patients on delayed-phase contrast-enhanced MR images. The presence of this hypointense rim is thought to be due to minimal relative hypervascularity of the tumor periphery, resulting in early washout of contrast medium from the more peripheral portion of the tumor on delayed phase images.

Undifferentiated Embryonal Sarcoma

Undifferentiated embryonal sarcoma (UES) is a rare malignant hepatic tumor, which occurs predominantly in older children and adolescents (mean age: 12 years), although it can present in young adults as well (135,136). It is the fourth most common hepatic neoplasm in children

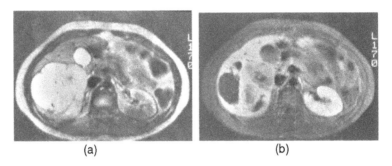

(a)   (b)

Figure 23 Undifferentiated embryonal sarcoma. Axial T2-weighted image obtained in a 27-year-old female shows well-defined hyperintense lesion in the posterior aspect of the right lobe of the liver. (b) Axial contrast-enhanced MR image shows enhancement of the solid portions of the mass.

after hepatoblastoma, infantile hemangioendothelioma (IHE), and hepatocellular carcinoma (HCC) (135,136).

On cross-sectional imaging the tumor is seen as a large (10–25 cm), solitary, predominantly cystic mass with well-defined borders, occasionally having a pseudocapsule that separates the mass from normal liver (135,136). Calcification has been reported in only one case. Although at gross examination UES appears predominantly solid (83%), MRI images usually display a discordant cystic appearance, due to the high water content of the myxoid stroma typical of UES (135,136). Therefore, on MR imaging, large portions of the mass are hypointense on T1-weighted images and have high signal intensity on T2-weighted images (Fig. 23) (135,136). The presence of streaky areas of high signal intensity of T1-weighted images and low signal intensity on T2-weighted images represent intratumoral hemorrhage (135,136). On postcontrast enhanced MR images, heterogeneous enhancement is present in the solid, usually peripheral portions of the mass, especially on delayed images (135,136).

Thorotrast-Induced Angiosarcoma

Thorotrast is a 25% aqueous colloidal suspension of thorium dioxide, a mixture of 11 radioisotopes, which emits 90% of its energy as alpha-particles (137,138). Following intravascular administration, thorotrast, which has a biological half-life of more than 400 years, is phagocytized by reticuloendothelial cells including Kupffer cells in the liver and spleen (137,138). Thorotrast was introduced as a radiographic contrast agent in 1928, predominantly used for cerebral angiography and hepatolienography (137,138). Early in the 1950s it became apparent that a number of pathological conditions could be associated with the previous use of Thorotrast (137). Reported findings are local granulomas at the site of injection, development of hepatic fibrosis usually 15 years after exposure, and development of a myriad of malignant tumors 20–30 years after Thorotrast administration (137). Hepatic neoplasms are, next to blood dyscrasias, the most significant long-term complications of Thorotrast (137). The most common neoplasm induced by Thorotrast is angiosarcoma, a malignant tumor of the reticuloendothelial system (138). Angiosarcoma represents approximately 25% of the liver tumors in patients with proven thorium exposure, whereas in general population angiosarcoma accounts for only 1.8% of all primary hepatic neoplasma (137). Differential diagnosis of a hepatic mass in the presence of Thorotrast exposure should include hepatocellular carcinoma and intrahepatic cholangiocarcinoma (137).

Previous Thorotrast administration reveals a characteristic CT appearance of the liver, spleen, and abdominal lymph nodes, producing a reticular to homogeneous high attenuating radiopacity of the organs mentioned above (138). In most cases described, the unopacified tumor is easily identified by its displacement of the remainder opacified liver parenchyma (138). On dynamic contrast-enhanced CT images, angiosarcoma shows an enhancement pattern similar to that of a giant hemangioma with early intense peripheral enhancement and centripetal fill-in of the lesion (137). Smaller lesions, however, can show a homogeneous enhancement. MRI is inferior to CT in demonstrating evidence of previous Thorotrast exposure. MRI features of hepatic angiosarcoma are non-specific showing low signal intensity and high signal intensity on T1- and T2-weighted images, respectively (139).

Epithelioid Hemangioendothelioma

Epithelioid hemangioendothelioma (EHE) is a rare vascular tumor of intermediate malignancy usually discovered in adults (mean age: 39–45 years) (140,141). It is described as arising in soft tissues, lung, bone, liver and spleen (140). Histopathologically, the tumor is composed of epithelioid and dentritic cells within a tumor matrix that may become sclerotic, hyalinized, and calcified (140). Intratumoral necrosis and hemorrhage are common findings (140). In the liver, the tumor typically consists of multiple peripherally located coalescencing nodules, measuring 1–10 cm (140,141). In contrast to almost all other primary liver neoplasms, except intrahepatic cholangiocarcinoma, these tumors do not cause bulging of the hepatic capsule, but retract the hepatic surface inwards (140).

On MRI, viable tumor peripheries are moderately hyperintense on T2-weighted images (Fig. 24). The central area of the tumor shows a

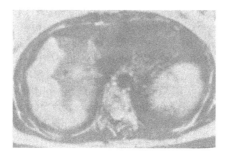

FIGURE 24 Epithelioid hemangioendothelioma (EHE). Axial T2-weighted image shows multiple peripherally located hyperintense lesions (suggesting hypervascularity) with associated capsular retraction in this 17-year-old boy. Combination of imaging features and clinicodemographic data is consistent with EHE.

variable signal intensity, depending upon the presence of edematous connective tissue (hyperintense signal) or hemorrhage and calcification (hypointense signal) (140). Post–gadolinium-enhanced T1-weighted images classically show a peripheral moderate enhancement and a delayed central enhancement. MRI can also depict invasion of intrahepatic branches of the portal vein or tributaries of the hepatic veins (140).

Metastases

Metastases to the liver are the most common malignant hepatic lesions encountered in clinical practice but often have a nonspecific appearance. In general, metastatic disease of the liver has components that are isointense to the spleen on both T1- and T2-weighted images (142). Thus, liver metastates usually demonstrate lower signal intensity than liver on T1-weighted images and higher signal intensity on T2-weighted images. Patterns of enhancement after administration of gadolinium include rim-enhancement, heterogeneous diffuse enhancement, and peripheral washout on equilibrium phase images (142) (Fig. 25).

Liver metastases may have a cystic appearance. These "cystic" metastases may be seen with adenocarcinomas such as mucinous carcinoma of the colon (142). Metastatic tumors having rapid growth leading to necrosis and cystic degeneration include carcinoid, sarcoma, melanoma, and lung carcinoma. In these patients, contrast-enhanced studies should be performed since these metastases can simulate a hemangioma or cyst on heavily T2-weighted images (142) (Fig. 26).

Hypervascular metastases include metastatic deposits from breast, islet cell, and renal cell neoplasms, as well as sarcoma, melanoma, and lymphoma (142). According to their hypervascularity and predominant

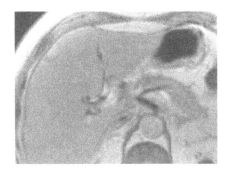

Figure 25   Liver metastasis. Delayed-phase axial contrast-enhanced MR image shows peripheral wash-out of the contrast in this patient with metastatic colon cancer. The peripheral wash-out is suggestive for a malignant lesion.

arterial blood supply, these lesions enhance rapidly and intensively compared with liver on postcontrast MRI images obtained during the arterial phase of hepatic enhancement. Generally, hypervascular metastases demonstrate irregular rim or central enhancement (143). A study performed by Leslie et al. (143) showed that the majority (92%) of hypervascular metastases in their series was characterized by nonglobular enhancement, and none of the metastases showed an isodense enhancement in relation to the aorta, a feature detected in 62% of the hemangiomas (143). Other studies also confirmed the ability of MRI to differentiate hypervascular metastases from hemangiomas (144).

Ovarian metastases commonly spread by peritoneal seeding rather than hematogeneously (145). They will, therefore, appear on cross-sectional images as cystic serosal implants on both the visceral peritoneal surface of the liver and the parietal peritoneum of the diaphragm (145). This is in contradistinction to most other cystic hepatic lesions, which are intraparenchymal. Metastases to the peritoneal surface of the liver and intraparenchymal liver metastases have been reported to occur in about 10% of patients with ovarian carcinoma (145).

DIFFUSE LIVER DISEASES

Cirrhosis

Cirrhosis is a diffuse, progressive process of liver fibrosis, pathologically characterized by architectural distortion and nodular regenerative change (146). The spectrum of nodules may range from benign regenerative nodules (RN) to HCC, and the regeneration pattern can be cathegorized as

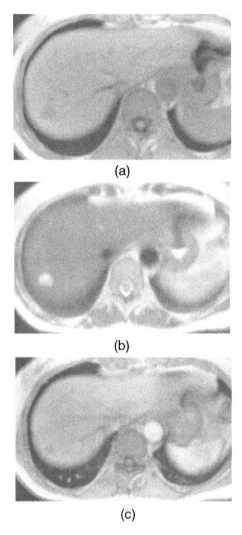

(a)

(b)

(c)

FIGURE 26   Cystic liver metastasis. (a) T1-weighted MR image shows hypointense metastasis in the right lobe of the liver. (b) Corresponding T2-weighted image shows the metastasis to be hyperintense. (c) Axial contrast-enhanced MR image shows hypovascular aspect of the central portion of the metastasis.

either micronodular (nodules <3 mm in size), macronodular (nodules >3 mm in size), or mixed (146,147). Alcohol-related liver disease and hemochromatosis typically results in micronodular cirrhosis, whereas viral hepatitis usually presents as macronodular regenerative change (147).

Universally, all types of progressive fibrosis evoke hepatic failure, portal hypertension, and the complications associated with the latter, such as varices and hemorrhage.

Because of the small size of regenerative nodules, cross-sectional imaging usually does not allow reliable distinction between micronodular and macronodular cirrhosis (148). However, when nodularity is detectable by imaging, especially by MR imaging, it is most likely to result from underlying macronodular disease. The presence of other intra- and extrahepatic imaging findings of cirrhosis (e.g., surface nodularity, hepatic morphological, changes, splenomegaly, ascites, portosystemic collaterals) depends on the severity of the underlying chronic liver disorder (149). Enlargement of the hilar periportal space, in the absence of other conventional signs, has been described as a helpful sign in the diagnosis of early cirrhosis (150). This enlargement of the hilar periportal space results from atrophy of the medical segment of the left hepatic lobe, presumably caused by selective reduced portal venous inflow (150). More pronounced lobar or segmental changes of hepatic morphology are seen in advanced cirrhosis. These include atrophy of the right hepatic lobe and left medial segment, enlargement of the caudate lobe and left lateral segment, and the expanded gallbladder fossa sign (151). Although a caudate–to–right lobe ratio equal to or greater than 0.65 is 90% specific for the presence of advanced cirrhosis, this ratio does not help in identifing the presence of early cirrhosis (149). Morphological changes usually occur in all types of cirrhosis, but certain features are seen more commonly with certain etiologies: enlargement of the lateral segment of the left lobe in combination with atrophy of the right lobe and medial segment of the left lobe is usually associated with viral-induced disease, whereas caudate lobe enlargement is primarily caused by alcoholic cirrhosis or primary sclerosing cholangitis (149). The expanded gallbladder fossa sign, caused by one or more of the above morphological changes, has been described as one of the most specific indicators of cirrhosis, with a specificity and positive prodictive value of 98% (152).

Accurate identification of different types of hepatocellular nodules arising in the cirrhotic liver in crucial. Unlike regenerative nodules, dysplastic nodules are considered premaligant and precursors of HCC, and, therefore, their presence may indicate more advanced disease or preclude treatment options (e.g., liver transplantation) (148). Nowadays, MR imaging is by far the most specific imaging technique for differentiating the different types of nodules based on characteristic features, such as signal intensity and enhancement pattern. Regenerative nodules, like normal liver, invariably have a portal venous blood supply with minimal contribution from the hepatic artery (153,154). As a consequence, they are usually isointense with other background nodules on both T1- and T2-weighted images, and they show no predominant enhancement pattern following gadolinum administration (Fig. 27). Since, although less commonly, regenerative nodules may be hyperintense on T1-weighted images (due to increased glycogen or fat) or hypointense on T1- and T2-weighted images (due to iron deposition), regenerative nodules may not always be distinghuished from dysplastic nodules (148,155). Fortunately, however, unlike the majority of HCC, regenerative nodules are almost never hyperintense on T2-weighted images.

Dysplastic nodules (DN) are neoplastic premalignant nodules found in approximately 25% of cirrhotic livers. Usually, they can be distinguished pathologically from ordinary regeneration nodules based on their size (usually >8 mm), color, or texture (153,154). Low-grade dysplastic nodules are characterized by cell dysplasia without atypia, whereas high-grade dysplastic nodules may have cytologic atypia (148). The latter may also contain focal areas of HCC, the so-called dysplastic nodule with subfocus of HCC (156). Like regeneration nodules, the main blood supply to dysplastic nodules is from the portal venous system. However, many investigators have demonstrated that a minority, especially with high-grade dysplasia, may also be fed by hepatic arteries, and therefore, present as hypervascular lesions on contrast-enhanced CT and MRI studies (148). The signal intensity characteristics of dysplastic nodules slightly overlap with both RN and HCC, although some common patterns exist. A DN is typically homogeneously hyperintense on T1-weighted images, hypointense on T2-weighted images, shows portal-venous phase enhancement, is smaller than 3 cm, and has no capsule (Fig. 28) (148). In cases of DNs with foci of HCC, the classic appearnce is that of a "nodule within a nodule," consisting of a high signal intensity focus of HCC within a low signal intensity dysplastic nodule on T2-weighted images (Fig. 29) (156).

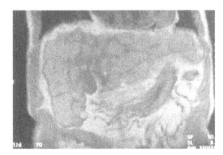

FIGURE 27   Cirrhosis. Coronal T1-weighted image shows multiple isointense regenerative nodules in the liver separated by low signal intensity fibrosis. Note small hyperintense dysplastic nodule.

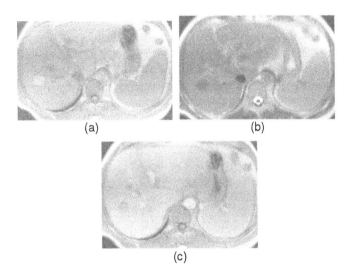

(a)   (b)

(c)

FIGURE 28 Dysplastic nodule. (a) T1-weighted MR image shows hyperintense dysplastic nodule in the right lobe of the liver. (b) Corresponding T2-weighted image shows the DN to be low signal intensity. (c) Axial contrast-enhanced MR image shows hypovascular aspect of the DN.

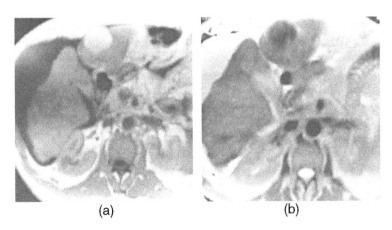

(a)   (b)

FIGURE 29 Dysplastic nodule (DN) with early HCC. (a) T1-weighted MR image shows hyperintense dysplastic nodule in the left lobe of the liver. Note low signal intensity nodule in the inferior aspect of the DN. (b) Corresponding T2-weighted image shows the DN to be low signal intensity and the area corresponding with early HCC to be hyperintense.

Extrahepatic signs of cirrhosis include features of portal hypertension, such as splenomegaly and the formation of portosystemic collateral vessels, and findings related to hepatocellular dysfunction (ascites, small bowel edema, gallbladder wall thickening) (146). Nowadays, MR angiography provides useful information regarding the presence, location, and flow pattern in porto-systemic shunts. These findings are useful for diagnostic purposes (e.g., detection of bleeding varices) and for treatment planning (e.g., prior to TIPS placement, shunt surgery).

Other Metabolic and Storage Disorders

Steatosis

Hepatic steatosis results from a variety of abnormal processes including increased production or mobilization of fatty acids (e.g., obesity, steroid use) or decreased hepatic clearance of fatty acids due to hepatocellular injury (e.g., alcoholic liver disease, viral hepatitis) (157). Histopathologically, the hallmark of all forms of fatty liver is the accumulation of fat globules within the hepatocytes. The distribution of steatosis can be variable, ranging from focal, to regional, to diffuse. Diffuse steatosis is common and estimated to occur in approximately 30% of obese patients (158). Patients with steatosis are usually asymptomatic, although some individuals may present with right upper quadrant pain due to hepatomegaly or abnormal liver function parameters (159).

Undoubtedly the most sensitive technique to detect microscopic fatty change of the liver is the use of gradient echo MR pulse sequences (160). With these sequences, by varying the echo time to image water and fat in and out phase, chemical shift between water and lipid protons can be demonstrated (161). With in-phase imaging the water and lipid protons are in phase and their intravoxel signal intensities are additive, whereas with out-of-phase imaging the intravoxel signal intensities of water and fat are out of phase and cancel each other out (160,161). As a consequence, on out-of-phase images, areas with a significant amount of intracellular fat will show a lower signal intensity than on the corresponding in-phase images, and this loss of signal intensity between the two types of images allows to establish the diagnosis of fatty change of the liver (160,161). Characteristically, out-of-phase images are identifiable by the presence of a thick black rim, also called "India ink," or "boundary" artifact, at the boundary of tissues that contain both water and fat protons (Fig. 30) (161).

Hepatic fatty change is, however, not always uniform but can present as a focal area of steatosis in an otherwise normal liver (focal steatosis) or as subtotal fatty change with sparing of certain areas (focal sparing) (162–165). Both abnormalities may cause considerable diagnostic confusion, especially

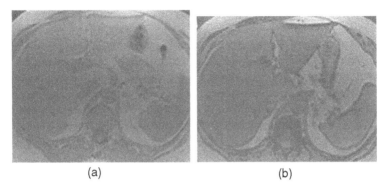

(a)	(b)

FIGURE 30   Steatosis. (a) In-phase breath-hold T1-weighted gradient-echo image shows the liver to be brighter in signal intensity than the spleen and paraspinal muscles. (b) Out-of-phase image demonstrates a significant drop in signal intensity of the liver consistent with diffuse fatty change.

in the work-up of focal liver lesions. In patients with focal fatty sparing, it is assumed that the spared regions do not have a normal portal blood supply and, therefore, do not receive lipid-rich blood from the gut (164). Because of their underlying vascular aberrance, most of these spared areas have a typical location (162). Characteristic examples include focal fatty sparing of the medial segment of the left liver lobe, which results from blood supply through the gastric veins, and sparing around the falciform ligament due to aberrant blood supply from the internal thoracic artery (162,164). Other typical locations include areas adjacent to the gallbladder fossa, the subcapsular region, or adjacent to the porta hepatis. The etiology of focal fatty change is more controversial (163). It is hypothesized that decreased delivery of unknown substances from the portal vein or relative ischemia

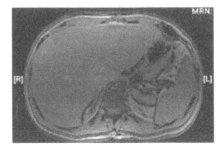

FIGURE 31   Focal fatty change. Out-of-phase T1-weighted MR image shows segmental decreased signal intensity in the left liver lobe due to focal fatty change.

from the paucity of portal blood supply are the main causative factors (Fig. 31).

On MR imaging, several features enable correct identification of focal fatty change or focal spared areas: (1) the typical periligamentous and periportal location, (2) lack of mass effect, (3) sharply angulated boundaries of the area, (4) nonspherical shape, (5) absence of vascular displacement or distorsion, (6) lobar or segmental distribution, and (7) using chemical-shift imaging with its high specificity for tissue characterization (163).

Iron Overload

Iron overload states are categorized as hemochromatosis, where the iron accumulates preferentially within the hepatocytes, and hemosiderosis, where it is deposited in the reticuloendothelial or Kupffer cells (166).

Primary hemochromatosis. Hereditary or primary hemochromatosis is an autosomal recessive disorder of iron metabolism characterized by abnormal absorption of iron from the gut with subsequent excessive deposition of iron into the hepatocytes, pancreatic acinar cells, myocardium, joints, endocrine glands, and skin (167). In addition, the reticuloendothelial system (RES) cells in patients with primary hemochromatosis are abnormal and unable to store processed iron effectively (166,167). As a consequence, patients with primary hemochromatosis will not accumulate iron in the RES. Advanced primary hemochromatosis leads to hepatic cell death, fibrosis and eventually micronodular cirrhosis. Clinical findings of cirrhosis and its complications (portal hypertension, development of HCC) usually predominate in patients with long-lasting disease (168). Although the diagnosis of hemochromatosis is usually made by chromosomal analysis, imaging, and especially MRI, is still valuable in quantifying the iron deposition and in the follow-up of the patients.

MRI is far more specific than any other imaging modality for the characterization of iron overload due to the unique magnetic susceptibility effect of iron (169,170). The superparamagnetic effect of accumulated iron in the hepatocytes results in significant reduction of signal intensity of the liver parenchyma on T2-weighted images (Fig. 32) (170). T2*-weighted gradient-echo sequences are the most sensitive sequences to magnetic susceptibility effects of ferritin and hemosiderin because of their lack of a 180 degree refocusing pulse (170). Comparison of the signal intensity of liver with that of paraspinal muscles, which are normally less intense than liver and not prone to excessive iron accumulation, provides an useful internal control: if the signal intensity of liver is less (on all sequences) than that of paraspinal muscle, it should be considered abnormal (170). HCC, complicating 35% of untreated patients with advanced hemochromatosis, are

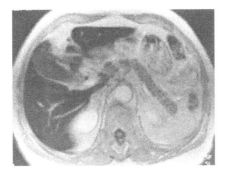

FIGURE 32 Hemochromatosis. Axial contrast-enhanced MR image shows decreased signal intensity of liver and pancreas, and normal signal intensity of the spleen and bone marrow in this patient with primary hemochromatosis.

usually easily detected on both T1- and T2-weighted images due to the decreased signal intensity of the background liver parenchyma.

Hemosiderosis. In patients with hemosiderosis or siderosis, either due to transfusional iron overload states or dyserythropoiesis (e.g., thalassemia major, sideroblastic anemia, pyruvate kinase deficiency, chronic liver disease), the excessive iron is processed and accumulates in organs containing reticuloendothelial cells, including liver, spleen, and bone marrow (Fig. 33) (171). As a result, although the distribution of iron in patients with siderosis is demonstrated in the liver as diffuse low signal intensity changes similar to those seen in primary hemochromatosis, extrahepatic signal intensity changes in the spleen and bone marrow enable MR imaging

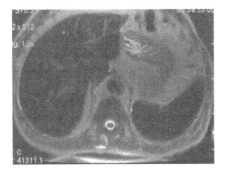

FIGURE 33 Hemosiderosis. Axial T2-weighted image shows decreased signal intensity of both liver and splenn, as also bone marrow, in this patient with transfusional iron overload.

to distinguish primary hemochromatrosis from hemosiderosis (171). Although in general the clinical significance of transfusional iron overload states is negligible, patients with chronic tranfusional needs can develop, due to saturation of the RE system, so-called secondary hemochromatosis, which can have symptoms similar to those of the primary form (171).

Wilson's Disease

Wilson's disease, also known as hepatolenticular degeneration, is a rare autosomal recessive abnormality of copper metabolism characterized by accumulation of toxic levels of copper in the brain, cornea (Kayser-Fleischer rings), and liver, the latter due to impaired biliary excretion (172). Wilson's disease is predominantly seen in young people, and biochemically, "free" serum and hepatic copper levels are increased whereas serum levels of ceruloplasmin, the copper-binding protein, are typically decreased (172). Hepatic deposition of copper, predominantly seen in periportal areas and along the hepatic sinusoids, evokes an inflammatory reaction resulting in acute hepatitis with fatty change (48). Subsequently, chronic active hepatitis finally resulting in liver fibrosis and eventually macronodular cirrhosis develops.

During the early stage of the disease, before severe cirrhosis has evolved, and due to the paramagnetism of ionic copper, MR imaging can be valuable by demonstrating focal copper depositions as multiple nodular lesions, typically appearing hyperintense and hypointense on T1- and T2- weighted images, respectively (173,174).

Diffuse Neoplastic Diseases

Metastatic Disease

Neoplastic infiltration due to diffuse metastatic disease can occur with many primary tumors. Melanoma, malignant islet cell tumors, pancreatic adenocarcinoma, breast carcinoma, and colonic adenocarcinoma are some of the more commonly encountered causes of diffuse hepatic metastatic disease (175).

At MRI, lesions are typically hyperintense on T2-weighted images, hypointense on T1-weighted images, and appear hypo-or hyperintense following gadolinium administration, depending on their vascularity (Fig. 34). Hypovascular lesions, such as metastases from colorectal adenocarcinoma, are best detected on portal venous phase contrast-enhanced images (176). Hypervasuclar metastases, including islet cell tumors, melanoma, sarcoma, renal cell carcinoma, and certain subtypes of breast and lung carcinoma, enhance more rapidly than normal liver and require arter-

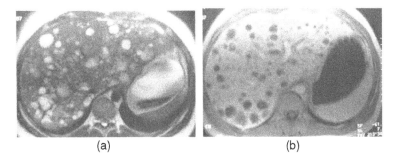

(a)   (b)

FIGURE 34   Diffuse cystic metastasis solid and papillary pancreatic tumor (SPT). (a) Axial T2-weighted image shows numerous hyperintense nodules scattered throughout the liver consistent with cystic metastases in a patient with SPT. (b) Axial contrast-enhanced MR image shows lack of enhancement of the central portion of the lesions due to their cystic nature.

ial phase enhanced imaging for accurate depiction (176). Infrequently, diffuse metastatic involvement is very discrete and only detectable through indirect features, such as diffuse parenchymal heterogeneity, vascular and architectural distortion, or alterations of the liver contour (177). The latter, seen particularly in patients with treated breast cancer metastases, has been reported as the "pseudocirrhosis" sign (177). Superparamagnetic iron oxides particles are extremely useful in the detection of hepatic metastatic disease, since no Kuppfer cells are present in metastases and, therefore, lack of uptake of contrast medium in the lesions increases significantly the tumor conspicuity (51).

Lymphoma

Lymphoma can involve the liver both as a primary and secondary tumor. Primary lymphoma of the liver is, however, exceedingly rare and classically manifests as a focal mass (178). The liver is more often secondarily involved in both Hodgkin's and non-Hodgkin's lymphoma (178). Typically, the liver parenchyma is diffusely infiltrated with microscopic nests of neoplastic cells without significant architectural distortion, and, therefore, lymphomateous involvement is difficult to detect by means of imaging along (178).

Reported MR imaging features of hepatic lymphoma are nonspecific (179). Diffuse infiltration may reveal a slight increase of liver parenchyma signal intensity on T2-weighted images, whereas focal masses appear relatively hypo- and hyperintense relative to background liver on T1- and T2-weighted images, respectively (179). The presence of associated abnormalities, such as splenomegaly and lymphadenopathy, may be a useful aid in narrowing the differential diagnosis.

Diffuse Hepatic Vascular Diseases

Budd-Chiari Syndrome

Budd-Chiari syndrome is characterized by hepatic venous outflow obstruction, resulting in progressive hepatic failure, ascites, and portal hypertension (180). Characteristic clinical manifestations are hepatomegaly from liver congestion, ascites developing due to liver dysfunction, and abdominal pain from hepatomegaly (180). A variety of etiologies may cause the Budd-Chiari syndrome including, in decreasing order of frequently, idiopathic causes, hematologic disorders, myeloprofliferative diseases, other hypercoagulable states (oral contraceptives, pregnancy, or postpartum states), tumoral conditions (HCC, renal carcinoma, and metastatic disease), infectious, traumatic, and congenital causes (membraneous webs or diaphragms), the latter referring to the so called "primary" Budd-Chiari syndrome (180). Several investigators classified the entity also by the location of the venous outflow obstruction. Type I patients have obstruction or occlusion at the level of the IVC with or without secondary hepatic vein occlusion, whereas Type II Budd-Chiari syndrome refers to primarily occluded hepatic veins (180). Type III involves obstruction at the level of the small centrilobular venules and has been considered a different entity, hepatic veno-occlusive disease, by many authors (180).

MR imaging findings associated with Budd-Chiari syndrome include direct findings of hepatic venous obstruction, secondary morphological changes of the liver parenchyma, and extrahepatic features. Direct findings of venous occlusion include visualization of intraluminal material (web, thrombus, tumor) within the hepatic veins (Fig. 35) (180). Absence of hepatic vein flow or localized flow disturbances caused by incomplete venous obstruction on MR venography are also useful findings (180). Additional direct features supporting the diagnosis are the presence of intraparenchymal collaterals between the hepatic veins and the portal veins or IVC, formed in an attempt to bypass the obstructed flow, and narrowing or nonvisualization of the hepatic veins or IVC (Fig. 36) (180). In cases with obstruction or stricture of the IVC, dilation of the azygos system is another important imaging finding. The hepatic venous outflow obstruction and resulting venous back pressure effect usually have striking impact on liver morphology. In an acute setting, the areas normally drained by the obstructed veins appear swollen due to congestion (180). Enhancement in these portions is typically heterogenous, mottled and delayed on contrast-enhanced MR images since blood is prohibited from diffusing readily throughout the liver (181–183). Since the caudate lobe has a separate venous drainage directly into the IVC, it exhibits compensatory enlargement and

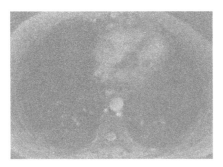

FIGURE 35   Budd-Chiari Syndrome. Axial contrast-enhanced MR image shows low signal intensity clot in the suprahepatic portion of the inferior vena cava.

has an increased enhancement compared with the rest of the liver (182). In chronic stages, the affected areas become fibrosed and shrink in size (31). Extrahepatic imaging findings in patients with acute Budd-Chiari syndrome include ascites, pleural fluid and gallbladder wall edema, and in more chronic cases, because of the development of portal hypertension, the presence of portosystemic collaterals and splenomegaly (180).

Hepatic veno-occlusive disease is another cause of hepatic venous outflow obstruction but differs from Budd-Chiari syndrome since, as mentioned above, the disease involves diffuse inflammation and obliteration of the postsinusoidal venules whereas the major hepatic veins and inferior vena cava remain patent (184). It is usually associated with the use of radiation and chemotherapy (182). To date, the MRI findings in patients with hepatic veno-occlusive disease have only been described sporadically (185). MRI may demonstrate some important features in

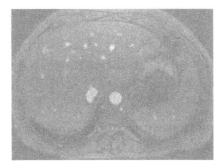

FIGURE 36   Budd-Chiari Syndrome. Axial unenhanced GRASS image shows multiple intrahepatic collaterals (white dots) that try to shunt the blood between the thrombosed sushepatic veins.

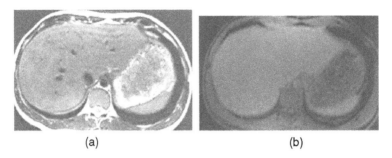

(a)   (b)

FIGURE 37   Veno-occlusive disease (VOD). (a) Axial T2-weighted image shows mild heterogeneity of the liver parenchyma, especially in the peripheral portion. Aslo, note increased signal intensity of the liver due to congestion. (b) Axial delayed phase contrast-enhanced MR image shows peripheral heterogeneous enhancement of the liver due to obstruction of the postsinusoidal venules in this patient with VOD due to herbal tea consumption.

differentiating hepatic veno-occlusive disease from Budd-Chiari syndrome: (1) the IVC and major hepatic veins remain patent, and (2) no predominant enlargement or heterogenous enhancement of the caudate lobe is seen (Fig. 37).

Passive Hepatic Congestion

Severe right-sided heart failure due to severe congestive heart failure or pericardial tamponade may result in passive hepatic congestion. On contrast-enhanced cross-sectional imaging studies, passive hepatic congestion can be recognized as a heterogeneous mosaiclike enhancement with reflux of contrast from the right atrium into the IVC or hepatic veins (182). Thus, in contrast to Budd-Chiari syndrome the hepatic veins are distended and enlarged rather than obstructed or compressed.

CONCLUSION

Because of the refinement of breath-hold pulse sequences and the introduction of liver-specific contrast agents, MR imaging of the liver has exceeded its preliminary role of a problem-solving modality in the evaluation of focal and diffuse liver pathology.

In this chapter we have reviewed the currently available MR pulse sequences and liver-specific contrast agents. In a practical approach, we have also tried to delineate the characteristic MRI findings of a gamut of usual and unusual focal liver lesions and diffuse hepatic abnormalities. Recognition and familiarity with the most relevant MRI features of each disorder allows the differential diagnosis to be narrowed substantially.

REFERENCES

1. Hayes CE, Dietz MJ, King BF, et al. Pelvic imaging with phased-array coils: quantitative assessment of signal-to-noise ratio improvement. J Magn Reson Imaging 1992; 2:321.

2. Keogan M, Edelman R. Technologic advances in abdominal MR imaging. Radiology 2001; 220:310–320.

3. Rydberg JN, Lomas DJ, Coakley KJ, Hough DM, Ehman RL, Riederer SJ. Comparison of breath-hold fat spin-echo and conventional spin-echo pulse sequences for T2-weighted MR imaging of liver lesions. Radiology 1995; 194:431–437.

4. Gaa J, Hatabu H, Jenkins RL, et al. Liver masses: replacement of conventional T2-weighted spin echo MR imaging with breath-hold MR imaging. Radiology 1996; 200:459–464.

5. Campeau NG, Johnson CD, Felmlee JP, et al. MR imaging of the abdomen with a phased-array multicoil: prospective clinical evaluation. Radiology 1995; 195:769.

6. Gauger J, Holzknecht NG, Lackenbauer CA, et al. Breathold imaging of the upper abdomen using a circular polarized-array coil: comparison with standard body coil imaging. Magma 1996; 4:93.

7. Kanematsu M, Hoshi H, Itoh K, Murakami T, Hori M, Kondo H, Yokoyama R, Nakamura H. Focal hepatic lesion detection: comparison of four fat suppressed T2-weighted MR imaging pulse sequences. Radiology 1999; 211: 363–371.

8. Cameron IL, Ord VA, Fullerton GD. Characterization of proton NMR relation times in normal and pathological tissues by correlation with other tissue parameters. Magn Reson Imaging 1984; 2:97.

9. Mitchell DG, Palazzo J, Hann HW, et al. Hepatocellular tumors with high signal on T1-weighted MR images: chemical shift MR imaging and histologic correlation. J Comput Assist Tomogr 1991; 15:762.

10. Ros PR. Hepatic angiomyolipoma: is fat in the liver friend or foe? (comment) Abdom Imaging 1994; 19:552.

11. Lewis KH, Chezmar JL. Hepatic metastases. Magn Reson Imaging Clin North Am 1997; 5:319.

12. Premkumar A, Marincola F, Taubenberger J, et al. Metastatic melanoma: correlation of MRI chacteristics and histopathology. J Magn Reson Imaging 1996; 6:190.

13. Yamashita Y, Yamamoto H, Tomohiro N, et al. Phased-array breath-hold versus non-breath-hold MR imaging of focal liver lesions: a prospective comparative study. J Magn Reson Imaging 1997; 7:292.

14. Martin J, Sentis M, Puig J, et al. Comparison of in-phase and opposed-phase GRE and conventional SE MR pulse sequences in T1-weighted imaging of liver lesions. J Comput Assist Tomogr 1996; 20:890.

15. Siegelman ES, Outwater EK. MR imaging techniques of the liver. Radiol Clin North Am 1998; 36:263.

16. Soyer P, Bluemke DA, Rymer R. MR imaging of the liver: technique. Magn Reson Imaging Clin North AM 1997; 5:205.
17. Kreft BP, Tanimoto P, Baba Y, et al. Diagnosis of fatty liver with MR imaging. J Magn Reson Imaging 1992; 2:463–471.
18. Levenson H, Greensite F, Hoefs J, et al. Fatty infiltration of the liver: quantification with phase-contrast MR imaging at 1.5T vs. biopsy. Am J Roentgenol 1991; 156:307–312.
19. Matthaei D, Haase A, Henrich D, Duhmke E. Fast inversion recovery T1 contrast and chemical shift contrast in high resolution snapshot F1ASH MR images. Magn Reson Imaging 1992; 10:1–6.
20. Brown MA, Semelka RC. MR imaging abbreviations, definition and descriptions: a review. Radiology 1999; 213:647–662.
21. Hamm B, Mahfouz AE, Taupitz M, et al. Liver metastases: improved detection with dynamic gadolinium-enhanced MR imaging? Radiology 1997; 202:677–682.
22. Coulam CH, Chan FP, Li KC. Can a multiphasic contrast-enhanced three-dimensional fast spoiled gradient-recalled echo sequence be sufficient for liver MR imaging? Am J Roentgenol 2002; 178:335–341.
23. Lavelle MT, Lee VS, Rofsky NM, Krinsky GA, Weinreb JC. Dynamic contrast-enhanced three-dimensional MR imaging of liver parenchyma: source images and angiographic reconstructions to define hepatic arterial anatomy. Radiology 2001; 218:389–394.
24. Hamm B, Thoeni RF, Gould RG, et al. Focal liver lesions: characterization with nonenhanced and dynamic contrast material-enhanced MR imaging. Radiology 1994; 190:417.
25. Mahfouz A-E, Hamm B, Wolf KJ. Peripheral washout: a sign of malignancy on dynamic gadolinium-enhanced MR images of focal liver lesions. Radiology 1994; 190:49.
26. Li KC, Glazer GM, Quint LE, et al. Distinction of hepatic cavernous hemangioma from hepatic metastases with MR imaging. Radiology 1988; 169:409.
27. Kanematsu M, Hoshi H, Murakami T, Hori M, et al. Focal hepatic lesion detection: Comparison of four fat-suppressed T2-weighted MR imaging pulse sequences. Radiology 1999; 211:363–371.
28. Hori M, Murakami T, Kim T, Kanematsu M, et al. Single breath-hold T2-weighted MR imaging of the liver: value of single-shot fast spin-echo and multishot spin-echo echoplanar imaging. Am J Roentgenol 2000; 174:1423–1431.
29. Augui J, Vignaux O, Aggaud C, Coste J, Gouya H, Legmann P. Liver: T2-weighted MR imaging with breath-hold fast-recovery optimized fast-spin-echo compared with breath-hold half-Fourier and non-breath-hold respiratory-triggered fast spin-echo pulse sequences. Radiology 2002; 223:853–859.
30. Tartaglino LM, Flanders AE, Vinistski S, et al. Metallic artifacts on MR images of the postoperative spine: reduction with fast-spin echo techniques. Radiology 1994; 190:565.

31. Henkelman RM, Hardy PA, Bishop JE, et al. Why fat is bright in RARE and fast spin-echo imaging. JMRI 1992; 2:533–540.

32. Tang Y, Yamashita Y, Namimoto T, et al. Liver T2-weighted MR imaging: comparison of fast and conventional half-Fourier single-shot turbo spin-echo, breath-hold turbo spin-echo, and respiratory-triggered turbo spin-echo sequences. Radiology 1997; 203:766.

33. Gaa J, Fisher H, Laub G, et al. Breath-hold MR imaging of focal liver lesions: comparison of fast and ultrafast techniques. Eur Radiol 1996; 6:838.

34. Hartman EM, Barish MA. MR cholangiography. Magn Reson Imaging Clin North Am 2001; 4:841–855.

35. Jara H, Barish MA. MR cholangiopancreatography techniques. Semin Ultrasound CT MR 1999; 20:281–293.

36. Reinhold C, Guibaud L, Genin G, Bret PM. MR cholangiopancreatography: comparison between two-dimensional fast spin-echo and three-dimensional gradient-echo pulse sequences. J Magn Reson Imaging 1995; 5:379.

37. Barish MA, Yucel EK, Soto JA, et al. MR cholangiopancreatography: efficacy of three-dimensional turbo spin-echo technique. AJR Am J Roentgenol 1995; 165:295–300.

38. Laubenberger J, Buchert M, Schneider B, Blum U, Hennig J, Langer M. Breath-hold projection magnetic resonance cholangio-pancreaticography (MRCP): a new method for the examination of the bile and pancreatic ducts. Magn Reson Med 1995; 33:18–23.

39. Schwartz LH, Coakley FV, Sun Y, Blumgart LH, Fong Y, Panicek DM. Neoplastic pancreaticobiliary duct obstruction: evaluation with breath-hold MR cholangiopancreatography. AJR Am J Roentgenol 1998; 170:1491–1495.

40. Reuther G, Kiefer B, Tuchmann A. Cholangiography before biliary surgery: single-shot MR cholangiography versus intravenous cholangiography. Radiology 1996; 198:561–566.

41. Miyazaki T, Yamashita Y, Tsuchigame T, Yamamoto H, Urata J, Takahashi M. MR cholangiopancreatography using HASTE (half-Fourier acquisition single-shot turbo spin-echo) sequences. AJR Am J Roentgenol 1996; 166: 1297–1303.

42. Regan F, Fradin J, Khazan R, Bohlman M, Magnuson T. Choledocholithiasis: evaluation with MR cholangiography. AJR Am J Roentgenol 1996; 167:1441–1445.

43. Soto JA, Barish MA, Alvarez O, Medina S. Detection of choledocholithiasis with MR cholangiography: comparison of three-dimensional fast spin-echo and single- and multisection half-Fourier rapid acquisition with relaxation enhancement sequences. Radiology 2000; 215:737–745.

44. Hahn PF, Saini S. Liver-specific MR imaging contrast agents. Radiol Clin North Am 1998; 36:287.

45. Mahfouz A-E, Hamm B. Contrast agents. Magn Reson Imaging Clin North Am 1997; 5:223.

46. Hamm B, Wolf KJ, Felix R. Conventional and rapid MR imaging of the liver with Gd-DTPA. Radiology 1987; 164:313.

47. Hamm B, Mahfouz A-E, Taupitz M, et al. Liver metastases: improved detection with dynamic gadolinium-enhanced MR imaging. Radiology 1997; 202:677.

48. Peterson MS, Baron RL, Murakami T. Hepatic malignancies: usefulness of acquisition of multiple arterial and portal venous phase images at dynamic gadolinium-enhanced MR imaging. Radiology 1996; 201:337.

49. Hamm B, Thoeni RF, Gould RG, et al. Focal liver lesions: characterization with nonenhanced and dynamic contrast material-enhanced MR imaging. Radiology 1994; 190:417.

50. Mahfouz A-E, Hamm B, Wolf KJ. Peripheral washout: a sign of malignancy on dynamic gadolinium-enhanced MR images of focal liver lesions. Radiology 1994; 190:49.

51. Ros PR, Freeny PC, Harms SE, et al. Hepatic MR imaging with ferumoxides: a multicenter clinical trial of the safety and efficacy in the detection of focal hepatic lesions. Radiology 1995; 196:481.

52. Hagspiel KD, Neidl KF, Eichenberger AC, et al. Detection of liver metastases: comparison of superparamagnetic iron-oxide-enhanced and unenhanced MR imaging at 1.5 T with dynamic CT, intraoperative US, and percutaneous US. Radiology 1995; 196:471.

53. Senéterre E, Taourel P, Bouvier Y, et al. Detection of hepatic metastases: ferumoxides-enhanced Mr imaging versus unenhanced Mr imaging and CT during arterial portography. Radiology 1996; 200:785.

54. Fretz CJ, Elizondo G, Weissleder R, et al. Superparamagnetic iron oxide-enhanced MR imaging: pulse sequence optimization for detection of liver cancer. Radiology 1989; 172:393.

55. Oudkerk M, Heuvel AG, Wielopolski PA, et al. Hepatic lesions: detection with ferumoxide-enhanced Tl-weighted MR imaging. Radiology 1997; 203:449.

56. Grandin C, Van Beers BE, Robert A, et al. Benign hepatocellular tumors: MRI after superparamagnetic iron oxide administration. J Comput Assist Tomogr 1995; 19:412.

57. Ji H, Ros PR. Magnetic resonance imaging: liver-specific contrast agents. Clin Liver Dis 2002; 6:73–90.

58. Chezmar JL, Redvanly RD, Sewell CW. Uptake of mangafodir trisodium (Mn-DPDP) by hepatocellular carcinoma: correlation with unenhanced imaging findings and histopathologic features. Acad Radiol 1996; 3:413.

59. Saini S, Edelman RR, Sharma P, et al. Blood-pool MR contrast material for detection and characterization of focal hepatic lesions: initial clinical experience with ultrasmall superparamagnetic iron oxide (AMI-227). AJR 1995; 164:1147.

60. Itai Y, Ebihara R, Eguchi N, et al. Hepatobiliary cysts in patients with autosomal dominant polycystic kidney disease: prevalence and CT findings. AJR 1995; 164:339–342.

61. Stevens W, Harford W, Lee E. Obstructive jaundice due to multiple hepatic peribiliary cysts. Am J Gastroenterol 1996; 91:155–157.

62. Buetow PC, Buck JL, Pantongrag-Brown L, et al. Biliary cystadenoma and cystadenocarcinoma: clinical-imaging-pathologic correlations with emphasis on the importance of ovarian stroma. Radiology 1995; 196:805–810.

63. Powers C, Ros PR, Stoupis C, et al. Primary liver neoplasms: MR imaging with pathologic correlation. Radio Graphics 1994; 14:459–482.

64. Mortele KJ, Ros PR. Cystic focal liver lesions in the adult: differential CT and MR imaging features. Radio Graphics 2001; 21:895–910.

65. Jung G, Benz-Bohm G, Kugel H, et al. MR cholangiography in children with autosomal recessive polycystic kidney disease. Pediatr Radiol 1999; 29:463–466.

66. Mathieu D, Paret M, Mahfouz AE, et al. Hyperintense benign liver lesions on spin-echo T1-weighted MR images: pathologic correlations. Abdom Imaging 1997; 22:410–417.

67. Semelka RC, Sofka CM. Hepatic hemangiomas. Magn Reson Imaging Clin North Am 1997; 5:241–253.

68. Gandolfi L, Leo P, Solmi L, et al. Natural history of hepatic hemangiomas: clinical and ultrasound study. Gut 1991; 32:677–680.

69. Gibney RG, Hendin AP, Cooperberg PL. Sonographically detected hepatic hemangiomas: absence of change over time. AJR 1987; 149:953–957.

70. Bennett GL, Petersein A, Mayo-Smith WW, et al. Addition of gadolinium chelates to heavily T2-weighted MR imaging: limited role in differentiating hepatic hemangiomas from metastases. AJR 2000; 174:477–485.

71. Kim TK, Choi BI, Han J, et al. Optimal MR protocol for hepatic hemangiomas. Comparison of conventional spin-echo sequences with T2-weighted turbo spin-echo and serial gradient-echo (FLASH) sequences with gadolinium enhancement. Acta Radiol 1997; 38:565–571.

72. Olcott EW, Li KC, Wright GA, et al. Differentiation of hepatic malignancies from hemangiomas and cysts by T2 relaxation times: early experience with multiply refocused four-echo imaging at 1.5 T. J Magn Reson Imaging 1999; 9:81–86.

73. Outwater EK, Ito K, Siegelman E, et al. Rapidly enhancing hepatic hemangiomas at MRI: distinction from malignancies with T2-weighted images. J Magn Reson Imaging 1997; 7:1033–1039.

74. Soyer P, Dufresne AC, Somveille E, et al. Differentiation between hepatic cavernous hemangioma and malignant tumor with T2-weighted MRI: comparison of fast spin-echo and breathhold fast spin-echo pulse sequences. Clin Imaging 1988; 22:200–210.

75. Vilgrain V, Boulos L, Vullierme MP, et al. Imaging of atypical hemangio-
     mas of the liver with pathologic correlation. Radiographics 2000; 20:
     379–397.
76. Saini S, Sharma R, Baron RL, et al. Multicentre dose-ranging study on the
     efficacy of USPIO ferumoxtran-10 for liver MR imaging. Clin Radiol 2000;
     55:690–695.
77. Kondo F. Focal nodular hyperplasia of the liver: controversy over etiology.
     J Gastroenterol Hepatol 2000; 15:1229–1231.
78. Nguyen BN, Flejou JF, Terris B, et al. Focal nodular hyperplasia of the liver:
     a comprehensive pathologic study of 305 lesions and recognition of new
     histologic forms. Am J Surg Pathol 1999; 23:1441–1454.
79. Mathieu D, Kobeiter H, Maison P, et al. Oral contraceptive use and focal
     nodular hyperplasia of the liver. Gastroenterology 2000; 118:560–564.
80. Mortele KJ, Praet M, Van Vlierberghe H, de Hemptine B, Zou K,
     Ros PR. Focal nodular hyperplasia of the liver: assessment with
     dual-phase gadolinium-enhanced fast MR imaging. Abdom Imaging 2002;
     27:700–707.
81. Vilgrain V, Flejou JF, Arrive L, et al. Focal nodular hyperplasia of the liver:
     MR imaging and pathologic correlation in 37 patients. Radiology 1992;
     184:699–703.
82. Paley MR, Mergo PJ, Torres GM, et al. Characterization of focal hepatic
     lesions with ferumoxides-enhanced T2-weighted MR imaging. AJR Am
     J Roentgenol 2000; 175:159–163.
83. Precetti-Morel S, Bellin MF, Ghebontni L, et al. Focal nodular hyperplasia of
     the liver on ferumoxides-enhanced MR imaging: features on conventional
     spin-echo, fast spin-echo and gradient-echo pulse sequences. Eur Radiol
     1999; 9:1535–1542.
84. Kacl GM, Hagspiel KD, Marincek B. Focal nodular hyperplasia of the liver:
     serial MRI with Gd-DOTA, superparamagnetic iron oxide, and Gd-EOB-
     DTPA. Abdom Imaging 1997; 22:264–267.
85. Mortele KJ, Praet M, Van Vlierberghe et al. CT and MR imaging findings in
     focal nodular hyperplasia of the liver: radiologic-pathologic correlation.
     AJR Am J Roentgenol 2000; 175:687–692.
86. Carrasco D, Prieto M, Pallardo L, et al. Multiple hepatic adenomas after
     long-term therapy with testosterone enanthate. Review of the literature.
     J. Hepatol 1985; 1:573–578.
87. Rabe T, Feldmann K, Gurnwald K, Runnebaum B. Liver tumors in women on
     oral contraceptives. Lancet 1994; 3:1568–1569.
88. Labrune P, Trioche P, Duvaltier I, et al. Hepatocellular adenomas in
     glycogen storage disease type I and III: a series of 43 patients and review of
     the literature. J Pediatr Gastroenterol Nutr 1997; 24:276–279.
89. Meissner K. Hemorrhage caused by ruptured liver cell adenoma following
     long-term oral contraceptives: a case report. Hepatogastroenterology 1998;
     45:224–225.

90. Kawakatsu M, Vilgrain V, Erlinger S, et al. Disappearance of liver cell adenoma: CT and MR imaging. Abdom Imaging 1997; 22:274–276.

91. Chung KY, Mayo-Smith WW, Saini S, et al. Hepatocellular adenoma: MR imaging features with pathologic correlation. AJR 1995; 165:303–308.

92. Miyazaki T, Yamashita Y, Yamamoto H, et al. Dynamic MR imaging of hepatic adenomas with pathologic correlation. Comput Med Imaging Graph 1994; 18:373–380.

93. Paulson EK, McClellan JS, Washington K, et al. Hepatic adenoma: MR characteristics and correlation with pathologic findings. AJR 1994; 163:113–116.

94. Arsenault TM, Johnson CD, Gorman B, et al. Hepatic adenomatosis. Mayo Clin Proc 1996; 71:478–480.

95. Chiche L, Dao T, Salame E, et al. Liver adenomatosis: reappraisal, diagnosis, and surgical management: eight new cases and review of the literature. Ann Surg 2000; 231:74–81.

96. Grazioli L, Federle MP, Ichikawa T, et al. Liver adenomatosis: clinical, histopathologic, and imaging findings in 15 patients. Radiology 2000; 216: 395–402.

97. Desmet VJ. Ludwig symposium on biliary disorders—part I. Pathogenesis of ductal plate abnormalities. Mayo Clin Proc 1998; 73:80–89.

98. Principe A, Lugaresi ML, Lords RC, et al. Bile duct hamartomas: diagnostic problems and treatment. Hepatogastroenterology 1997; 44:994–997.

99. Burns CD, Kuhns JG, Wieman TJ. Cholangiocarcinoma in association with multiple biliary microhamartomas. Arch Pathol Lab Med 1990; 114: 1287–1289.

100. Lev-Toaff AS, Bach AM, Wechsler RJ, et al. The radiologic and pathologic spectrum of biliary hamartomas. AJR Am J Roentgenol 1995; 165:309–313.

101. Mortele B, Mortele KJ, Seynaeve P, et al. Hepatic bile duct hamartomass (von Meyenburg complexes): MR and MR cholangiography imaging findings. JCAT 2002; 26:438–443.

102. Cheung YC, Tan CF, Wan YL, et al. MRI of multiple biliary hamartomas. Br J Radiol 1997; 70:527–529.

103. Slone HW, Bennett WF, Bova JG. MR findings of multiple biliary hamartomas. AJR 1993; 161:581–583.

104. Semelka RC, Hussain SM, Marcos HB, et al. Biliary hamartomas: solitary and multiple lesions shown on current MR techniques including gadolinium enhancement. J Magn Reson Imaging 1999; 10:196–201.

105. Ishak KG, Willis GW, Cummins SD, et al. Biliary cystadenoma and cystadenocarcinoma: report of 14 cases and review of the literature. Cancer 1977; 39:322–338.

106. Marcial MA, Hauser SC, Cibas ES, et al. Intrahepatic biliary cystadenoma. Clinical, radiological, and pathological findings. Dig Dis Sci 1986; 31:884–888.

107. Gabata T, Kadoya M, Matsui O, et al. Biliary cystadenoma with mesenchymal stroma of the liver: correlation between unusual MR appearance and pathologic findings. J Magn Reson Imaging 1998; 8:503–504.

108. Stoupis C, Ros PR, Dolson DJ. Recurrent biliary cystadenoma: MR imaging appearance. J Magn Reson Imaging 1994; 4:99–101.
109. Goodman ZD, Ishak KG. Angiomyolipomas of the liver. Am J Surg Pathol 1984; 8:745–750.
110. Nonomura A, Mizukami Y, Kadoya M. Angiomyolipoma of the liver: a collective review. J Gastroenterol 1994; 29:95–105.
111. Carmody E, Yeung E, McLoughlin M. Angiomyolipomas of the liver in tuberous sclerosis. Abdom Imaging 1994; 19:537–539.
112. Ascenti G, Gaeta M, Zimbaro G, et al. US power Doppler of hepatic angiomyolipoma with low fat content. Eur Radiol 2000; 10:935–937.
113. Hooper LD, Mergo PJ, Ros PR. Multiple hepatorenal angiomyolipomas: diagnosis with fat suppression, gadolinium-enhanced MRI. Abdom Imaging 1994; 19:549–551.
114. Ros PR. Hepatic angiomyolipoma: is fat in the liver friend or foe? Abdom Imaging 1994; 19:552–553.
115. Yeh HC, Klion FM, Thung SN, et al. Angiomyolipoma: ultrasonographic signs of lipomatous hepatic tumors. J Ultrasound Med 1996; 15:337–342.
116. Horton KM, Bluemke DA, Hruban RH, et al. CT and MR imaging of benign hepatic and biliary tumors. Radiographics 1999; 19:431–451.
117. Ros PR, Goodman ZD, Ishak KG, et al. Mesenchymal hamartoma of the liver: radiologic-pathologic correlation. Radiology 1986; 158:619–624.
118. Mortele KJ, Mergo PJ, Urrutia M, et al. Dynamic gadolinium-enhanced MR findings in infantile hepatic hemangioendothelioma. J Comput Assist Tomogr 1998; 22:714–717.
119. Mortele KJ, Vanzieleghem B, Mortele B, Benoit Y, Ros PR. Gadolinium-enhanced MR imaging of infantile hemangioendothelioma: atypical features. Eur Radiol 2002; 12:862–865.
120. Mortele KJ, Wiesner W, Elewaut A, et al. Hepatic inflammatory pseudotumor: Gadolinium-enhanced, Ferrumoxides-enhanced, and Mangofodipir trisodium-enhanced MR Imaging findings. Eur Radiol 2002; 12:304–308.
121. Reading CC, Charboneau JW. Case of the day. Ultrasound. Hepatic lipoma. Radio Graphics 1990; 10:511–512.
122. O'Sullivan DA, Torres VE, de Groen PC, et al. Hepatic lymphangiomatosis mimicking polycystic liver disease. Mayo Clin Proc 1998; 73:1188–1192.
123. Reinertson TE, Fortune JB, Peters JC. Primary leiomyoma of the liver. A case report and review of the literature. Dig Dis Sci 1992; 37:622–627.
124. Buetow PC, Midkiff RB. Primary malignant neoplasms in the adult. Magn Reson Imaging Clin North Am 1997; 5:289.
125. Winter III TC, Takayasu K, Muramatsu Y, et al. Early advanced hepatocellular carcinoma: evaluation of CT and MR appearance with pathologic correlation. Radiology 1994; 192:379.
126. Kadoya M, Matsui O, Tak ashima T, Nonomura A. Hepatocellular carcinoma: correlation of MR imaging and histopathologic findings. Radiology 1992; 183:819.

127. Ishigushi T, Shimanmoto K, Fukatsu H, Yamakawa K, Ishigaki T. Radiologic diagnosis of hepatocellular carcinoma. Sem Surg Oncol 1996; 12:164.

128. Stevens WR, Johnson CD, Stephens DH, et al. Fibrolamellar hepatocellular carcinoma: stage at presentation and results of aggressive surgical management. AJR 1995; 164:1153.

129. Hamrick-Tumer JE, Shipk ey FH, Cranston PE. Fibrolamellar hepato-cellular carcinoma: MR appearance mimicking focal nodular hyperplasia. J Comput Assist Tomogr 1994; 18:301.

130. Hamrick-Tumer J, Abbit PL, Ros PR. Intrahepatic cholangiocarcinoma: MR appearance. AJR 1992; 158:77.

131. Vilgrain V, Van Beers BE, Flejou JF. Intrahepatic cholangiocarcinoma: MRI and pathologic correlation in 14 patients. J Comput Assist Tomogr 1997; 21.

132. Soyer P, Bluemke DA, Reichle R, et al. Imaging of intrahepatic cholangio-carcinoma: 1. Peripheral cholangiocarcinoma. AJR 1995; 165:1427.

133. Adjei ON, Tamura S, Sugimura H, et al. Contrast-enhanced MR imaging of intrahepatic cholangiocarcinoma. Clin Radiol 1995; 50:6.

134. Fan ZM, Yamashita Y, Harada M, et al. Intrahepatic cholangiocarcinoma: spin-echo and contrast-enhanced dynamic MR imaging. AJR 1993; 161:313.

135. Yoon W, Kim JK, Kang HK. Hepatic undifferentiated embryonal sarcoma. MR findings. J Comput Assist Tomogr 1997; 21:100.

136. Buetow PC, Buck JL, Pantongrag-Brown L, et al. Undifferentiated (embryonal) sarcoma of the liver: pathologic basis of imaging findings in 28 cases. Radiology 1997; 203:779.

137. Azodo MV, Gutierrez OH, Greer T. Thorothrast-induced ruptured hepatic angiosarcoma. Abdom Imaging 1993; 18:78.

138. Silverman PM, Ram PC, Korobkin M. CT appearance of abdominal thorotrast deposition and thorotrast-induced angiosarcoma of the liver. J Comput Assist Tomogr 1983; 7:655.

139. Marichy C, Dumontet C, Bastion Y et al. Hepatic angiosarcoma in a patient with essential thrombocytaemia and Budd-Chiari syndrome. Eur J Cancer 1995; 1:423.

140. Van Beers B, Roche A, Mathieu D, et al. Epithelioid hemangioendothelioma of the liver: MR and CT findings. J Comput Assist Tomogr 1992; 16:420.

141. Miller JW, Dodd GD, Federle MP. Epithelioid hemangioendothelioma of the liver: imaging findings with pathologic correlation. AJR 1992; 159:53.

142. Lewis KH, Chezmar JL. Hepatic metastases. Magn Reson Imaging Clin North Am 1997; 5:319.

143. Leslie DF, Johnson CD, Maccarty RL, et al. Single-pass CT of hepatic tumors: value of globular enhancement in distinguishing hemangiomas from hypervascular metastases. AJR 1995; 165:1403.

144. Yamashita Y, Hatanaka Y, Yamamoto H, et al. Differential diagnosis of focal liver lesions: role of spin-echo and contrast-enhanced dynamic MR imaging. Radiology 1994; 193:59.

145. Lundstedt C, Holmin T, Thorvinger B. Peritoneal ovarian metastases simulating liver parenchymal masses. Gastrointest Radiol 1992; 17:250.

146.   Brown JJ, Naylor MJ, Yagan N. Imaging of hepatic cirrhosis. Radiology
        1997; 202:1–16.
147.   Hytiroglou P, Theise ND. Differential diagnosis of hepatocellular nodular
        lesions. Semin Diagn Pathol 1998; 15:285–299.
148.   Krinsky GA, Lee VS. MR imaging of cirrhotic nodules. Abdom Imaging
        2000; 25:471–482.
149.   Ito K, Mitchell DG. Hepatic morphologic changes in cirrhosis: MR imaging
        findings. Abdom Imaging 2000; 25:456–461.
150.   Ito K, Mitchell DG, Gabata T. Enlargement of hilar periportal space: a sign
        of early cirrhosis at MR imaging. J Magan Reson Imaging 2000; 11:136–140.
151.   Harbin WP, Robert NJ, Ferrucci JT, Jr. Diagnosis of cirrhosis based on
        regional changes in hepatic morphology: a radiological and pathological
        analysis. Radiology 1980; 135:273–283.
152.   Ito K, Mitchell DG, Gabata, et al. Expanded gallbladder fossa: simple MR
        imaging sign of cirrhosis. Radiology 1999; 211:723–726.
153.   Mortele KJ, Ros PR. MR imaging of cirrhosis and chronic hepatitis. Sem in
        US, CT, and MRI 2002; 23:79–100.
154.   Ohtomo K, Itai K, Ohtomo Y, et al. Regenerating nodules of liver cirrhosis:
        MR imaging with pathologic correlation. AJR 1990; 154:505–507.
155.   Ito K, Mitchell DG, Gabata, et al. Hepatocellular carcinoma: association
        with increased iron deposition in the cirrhotic liver at MR imaging.
        Radiology 1999; 212:235–240.
156.   Mitchell DG, Rubin R, Siegelman ES, et al. Hepatocellular carcinoma within
        siderotic regenerative nodules: appearance as a nodule within a nodule on
        MR images. Radiology 1991; 178:101–103.
157.   El-Hassan AY, Ibrahim EM, al-Mulhim FA, et al. Fatty infiltration of the
        liver: analysis of prevalence, radiological and clinical features and influence
        of patient management. Br J Radiol 1992; 65:774–778.
158.   Wanless IR, Lentz JS. Fatty liver hepatitis (steatohepatitis) and obesity:
        an autopsy study with analysis of risk factors. Hepatology 1990; 12:
        1106–1110.
159.   Van Steenbergen W, Lanckmans S. Liver disturbances in obesity and
        diabetes mellitus. Int J Obes Rel Metab Disord 1995; 19:S27–S36.
160.   Siegelman ES, Outwater EK, Vinitski S, et al. Fat suppression by
        saturation/opposed phase hybrid techniaue: Spin echo versus gradient-ech
        imaging. Magn Reson Imaging 1995; 13:545.
161.   Rofsky NMK, Weinreb JC, Ambrosino MM, et al. Comparison between
        in-phase and opposed-phase Tl-weighted breath-hold FLASH seauences for
        hepatic imaging. J Comput Assist Tomogr 1996; 20:230–235.
162.   Arai K, Matsui O, Takashima T, et al. Focal spared areas in fatty liver caused
        by regional decreased portal flow. AJR 1988; 151:300–302.
163.   Kawamori Y, Matsui O, Takahashi S, et al. Focal hepatic infiltration in the
        posterior edge of the medial segment associated with aberrant gastric venous
        drainage: CT, US, and MR findings. J Comput Assist Tomogr 1996; 17:
        590–595.

164. Matsui O, Kadoya M, Takahashi S, et al. Focal sparing of segmenet IV in fatty livers shown by sonography and CT: correlation with aberrant gastric venous drainage. AJR 1995; 164:1137–1140.

165. Ohashi I, Ina H, Gomi N, et al. Hepatic pseudolesion in the left lobe around the falciform ligament at helical CT. Radiology 1995; 196:245–249.

166. Lee R. Storage and metabolic disorders. In: Diagnostic Liver Pathology. St Louis, MO: Mosby, 1994:237–280.

167. Conrad ME, Umbreit JN, Moore EG, et al. Hereditary hemochromatosis: A prevalent disorder of iron metabolism with an elusive etiology. Am J Hematol 1994; 47:218–224.

168. Deugnier YM, Guyader D, Crantock L, et al. Primary liver cancer in genetic hemochromatosis: A clinical, pathological, and pathogenetic study of 54 cases. Gastroenterology 1993; 104:228–234.

169. Siegelman ES, Mitchell DG, Semelka RC. Abdominal iron deposition: metabolism, MR findings, and clinical importance. Radiology (1996) 1996; 199:13–22.

170. Siegelman ES. MR imaging of diffuse liver disease (hepatic fat and iron). MRI Clin North Am 1997; 5:347–365.

171. Siegelman ES, Mitchell DG, Rubin R, et al. Parenchymal versus reticuloendothelial iron overload in the liver: distinction with MR imaging. Radiology 1991; 179:361.

172. Schilsky ML, Tavill AS. Wilson disease. In: Schiff ER, Sorrell MF, Maddrey WC, eds. Diseases of the Liver. Philadelphia: JB Lippincott, 1999: 1091–1106.

173. Ko S, Lee T, Ng S, Lin J, Cheng Y. Unusual liver MR findings of Wilson's disease in an asymptomatic 2-year-old girl. Abdom Imaging 1998; 23:56–59.

174. Vogl TJ, Hammerstingl R, Schwartz S, et al. MRI of the liver in Wilson disease. Rofo Fortschr Geb Rontgenstr 1994; 160:40–45.

175. Mortele KJ, Ros PR. Imaging of diffuse liver disease. Sem in Liv Dis 2001; 21:195–212.

176. Mortele KJ, McTavish J, Ros PR. Current techniques of computed tomography. Helical CT, multidetector CT, and 3D reconstruction. Clin Liv Dis 2002; 6:29–52.

177. Young ST, Paulson EK, Washington K, et al. CT of the liver in patients with metastatic breast carcinoma treated by chemotherapy: Findings simulating cirrhosis. AJR 1994; 163:1385.

178. Ryan J, Straus DJ, Lange C, et al. Primary lymphoma of the liver. Cancer 1988; 61:370.

179. Weissleder R, Stark DD, Elizondo G, et al. MRI of hepatic lymphoma. Magn Reson Imaging 1988; 6:675.

180. Mitchell DG, Nazarian LN. Hepatic vascular diseases: CT and MRI. Sem Ultrasound CT MRI 1995:49–68.

181. Soyer P, Rabenandrasana A, Barge J, et al. MRI of the Budd-Chiari syndrome. Abdom Imaging 1994; 19:325.

182. Spritzer CE. Vascular diseases and MR angiography of the liver. MRI Clin North Am 1997; 5:377–396.
183. Stark DD, Hahn PF, Trey C. MRI of Budd-Chiari syndrome. AJR 1986; 146:1141.
184. Brown B, Abu-Yousel M, Farner R, et al. Doppler sonography: a noninvasive method for evaluation of hepatic venocclusive disease. AJR 1990; 154:721.
185. Mortele KJ, Van Vlierberghe H, Wiesner W, Ros PR. Hepatic veno-occlusive disease: MR imaging findings. Abdom Imaging 2002; 27: 523–526.

4

Applications of Microbubbles in Liver Ultrasound

Christopher J. Harvey, Adrian K. P. Lim, Martin J. K. Blomley, and David O. Cosgrove
Hammersmith Hospital, Imperial College Faculty of Medicine,
London, England

INTRODUCTION

Ultrasound microbubble contrast agents were originally developed to improve or rescue Doppler studies where there is low volume/slow flow or the signals are weak because of attenuation by overlying tissues. Microbubbles are composed of air or complex gas particles of less than 10 μm in diameter which are stable enough to cross capillary beds and provide safe, effective systemic acoustic enhancement when given intravenously. Recent technological advances have produced novel imaging modes which exploit the nonlinear behavior of microbubble contrast agents and have dramatically extended the clinical and research applications of ultrasound. Ultrasound (US) is commonly the first imaging modality used in the diagnosis and assessment of both focal and diffuse liver disease. However, US is less sensitive than computed tomography (CT) and magnetic resonance (MR) in the detection of metastatic liver disease, and all imaging modalities are inaccurate in the diagnosis of cirrhosis. The advent of US microbubbles imaged with contrast-specific modes promises to improve the sensitivity and specificity of ultrasound in the detection and characterization of focal liver lesions to rival that of other cross-sectional modalities. This chapter reviews the current and potential applications of ultrasound contrast agents in the diagnosis of focal and diffuse liver disease.

MICROBUBBLE CONTRAST AGENTS

Ultrasound, unlike all other imaging modalities, has lacked effective contrast agents until comparatively recently. This was rectified in the 1990s with the introduction of microbubbles that have revolutionized clinical and research applications in this field (1–3). Microbubbles are made less than 10 µm in diameter so they can cross capillary beds and are safe, effective echo enhancers. When administered intravenously, microbubbles remain within the vascular compartment, though some agents have been shown to exhibit a hepatosplenic-specific phase (Table 1). To be effective as clinical tools, microbubbles must survive passage through the cardiopulmonary circulation to produce useful systemic enhancement. Microbubbles consist of a gas (usually air or a perfluorocarbon), stabilized by an ingenious range of methods (Table 1). When given intravenously, microbubbles produce marked augmentation of the ultrasound signal for several minutes, in grey-scale and Doppler, of up to 25 dB (greater than 300-fold increase). Levovist (SH U 508A; Schering AG, Germany) is licensed in many countries worldwide and consists of galactose microaggregates whose surfaces provide nidation sites on which air bubbles form when it is suspended in water; stabilized by a trace of palmitic acid. SonoVue (Bracco, Italy) is a blood pool agent containing sulfur hexafluoride, which prolongs longevity due to its lower solubility and has recently been licensed for clinical use in Europe. Additionally some agents have a late liver-splenic tropic phase where the bubbles accumulate in normal liver and splenic parenchyma 2–5 minutes after injection when the vascular enhancement has faded.

Microbubbles known to exhibit liver-specific behavior are Levovist (4,5), Sonavist (both Schering AG, Germany)(6), and Sonazoid (NC100100; Amersham, UK) (7) (Table 1). In the late phase the bubbles are stationary or extremely slow moving, as shown by the absence of conventional Doppler signals. The mechanism of hepatic accumulation is not completely understood. Possible explanations are mediation by the reticuloendothelial system phagocytosis or pooling and endothelial adherence in the liver sinusoids. Late phase imaging is optimally achieved using microbubble specific nonlinear imaging techniques, described below, to produce maximal lesion to background contrast differentiation.

TABLE 1   Classification of Ultrasound Microbubbles

Microbubble	Gas	Stabilization	Company
Blood pool agents			
Levovist (SHU 508A)[a]	Air	Palmitic acid	Schering
Echovist[a]	Air	None	Schering
Albunex[b]	Air	Sonicated albumin	Tyco
Quantison	Air	Dried albumin	Andaris Ltd
Imavist (Imagent, AFO150)	Perfluorohexane	Surfactant	Schering
Optison[a] (FS069)	Perfluoropropane	Sonicated albumin	Tyco/ Amersham
Echogen (QW3600)	Dodecafluoropentane	Liquid droplet, surfactant	Sonus
SonoVue (BR1)[a]	Sulfur hexafluoride	Phospholipids	Bracco
Definity, (DMP115)	Perfluoropropane	Phospholipids	Bristol-Myers Squibb
BR14	Perfluorobutane	Phospholipids	Bracco
Liver-specific agents			
Levovist (SHU 508A)[a]	Air	Palmitic acid	Schering
Sonavist (SHU 563A)	Air	Cyanoacrylate	Schering
Sonazoid[TM] (NC100100)	Perfluorocarbon	Not public information	Amersham

[a]Licensed for clinical use.
[b]No longer commercially available

INTERACTIONS OF MICROBUBBLES WITH ULTRASOUND WAVES

The interactions of microbubbles with an ultrasound beam are complex (8). Since a microbubble is more compressible than soft tissue, alternating expansion and contraction occurs when it is exposed to an oscillating acoustic signal. At low acoustic power these oscillations are equal and symmetrical (linear behavior) and the frequency of the scattered signal is unaltered with the scattering intensity linearly related to that of the incident beam. As the acoustic power increases [mechanical index (MI) > 0.3], more complex nonlinear interactions occur as the expansion and contraction phases become unequal because the microbubbles resist compression more strongly than expansion. Microbubbles resonate (in the diagnostic ultrasound range 1–20 MHz) and behave like a musical instrument, emitting harmonic signals at multiples (and fractions) of the insonating frequency. These harmonic signals are microbubble specific and may be regarded as a signature or fingerprint unique to that agent. At still higher powers (MI > 1.0), although within accepted limits for diagnostic imaging, highly nonlinear behaviour occurs, resulting in bubble disruption/scintillation.

MICROBUBBLE IMAGING MODES AND STRATEGIES

Microbubbles were originally developed to improve or rescue Doppler ultrasound studies where there is low volume/slow flow or the signals are weak because of attenuation from surrounding tissues, e.g., in the assessment of portal venous patency in cirrhosis. With advances in the sensitivity of ultrasound Doppler equipment, this application has become less important.

Over the last few years microbubbles have been used in novel ways to derive functional and anatomical information in the liver. There are two main approaches to the imaging of microbubbles. First, by tracking their passage through a region of interest, time-intensity curves may be derived (analogous to dynamic radionuclide tests). Second, microbubbles may be imaged to map the distribution of normal or diseased liver. These approaches may be applied to ultrasound of the liver to improve the detection and characterisation of liver lesions using a combination of vascular and liver-specific imaging.

Harmonics may be used to image US contrast agents by tuning the receiver to listen to a band of frequencies centred on the microbubble harmonic signal, thus excluding the fundamental signals that arise from tissue. However, tissues also produce harmonics, especially when higher acoustic powers are used and separating these out is challenging. The goal of separating them can be achieved in two ways. In the first to be discovered, a high MI beam is used to deliberately disrupt the microbubbles. Using a color Doppler mode, the sudden disappearance of signal is seen as a large Doppler shift resulting in a characteristic mosaic of color signal. This method works well for fragile air-filled agents, although microbubble destruction has the disadvantage that the effect is very transient, lasting only a few frames. This approach is known as stimulated acoustic emission (SAE) or loss of correlation (LOC) (Fig. 1) (4,5) and is particularly successful with microbubbles that have a liver-specific phase. In the late phase of liver-specific agents malignancies appear as defects surrounded by the bright normal liver (Figs. 1,2). It has the advantage of displaying

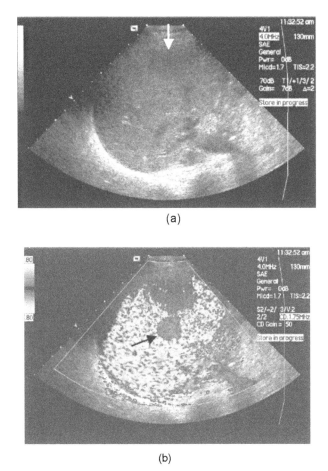

(a)

(b)

FIGURE 1   Section through the right lobe of liver in a 76-year-old man with pancreatic carcinoma. (a) The baseline B-mode image shows a subtle metastasis (arrow). (b) Imaging in stimulated acoustic emission (SAE) mode 3 minutes after Levovist not only improves the conspicuity of the metastasis but also reveals a further metastasis (arrow) which cannot be seen in B-mode. (From Ref. 33.) (See color insert)

the distribution of the microbubbles as a separate color overlay on the traditional B mode image and does not rely on the bubble movement so that the microcirculation can be detected. In a study of specificity a spectrum of benign and malignant focal liver lesions were assessed for SAE activity in the late phase of Levovist (9). Metastases and hepatocellular carcinoma

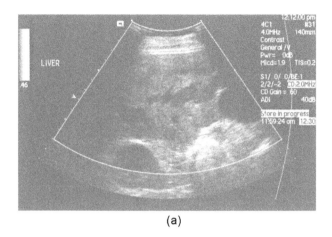

(a)

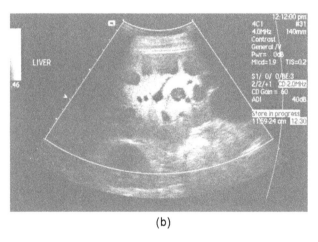

(b)

FIGURE 2 Section through the right lobe of liver in a 68-year-old man with metastatic melanoma. (a) B-mode shows multiple ill-defined echopoor lesions. (b) Three minutes after Levovist, using Agent Detection Imaging (ADI, Siemens, USA), a microbubble specific mode based on loss of correlation, the conspicuity of the metastases is improved with "extra" lesions revealed not seen on B-mode. (From Ref. 33.) (See color insert)

(HCC) showed no or very low SAE signals, while significantly higher uptake was observed in hemangiomas and focal nodular hyperplasia (FNH) (9).

While this method is very sensitive and specific to the presence of microbubbles, it is limited by the spatial resolution of color Doppler (several times worse than grey-scale) and by the focal zone dependence (site of maximal power deposition) of the LOC effect. Other novel modes such as cadence agent detection imaging (ADI; Siemens, USA) (Fig. 2) based on LOC retain the benefits of complete separation of tissue from bubble signal but also have high spatial resolution, have less focal zone dependence, and allow the removal of the color overlay so the co-registered B-mode can be inspected for abnormalities (10). However, SAE/LOC techniques rapidly destroy the contrast agent and preclude the use of real-time scanning, so a sweep-and-review approach has to be used.

The alternative approach relies on the fact that with newer microbubbles (particularly those with phospholipid shells) harmonics can be elicited at much lower acoustic powers than are necessary to generate tissue harmonics. Thus, if a very low acoustic power can be used without the image being lost in noise, the microbubble signals (harmonics) can be separated from the tissue signal (fundamental). An important step in the progress to this ideal was the development of pulse/phase inversion techniques that evolved from the desire to detect microbubble harmonics but to avoid frequency filtering because the narrow bandwidth that this method requires degrades spatial resolution. Phase/pulse inversion mode (PIM) is a grey-scale nonlinear mode, which combines the spatial resolution of grey-scale with a high microbubble sensitivity (11). In the PIM a pair of pulses is sent sequentially along each scan line, the second being 180 degrees out of phase with respect to the first. The returning echoes from the pair are summed so that the linear echoes cancel while the harmonics remain and are used for image formation. PIM gives excellent quality images in both vascular and late phases and, like the high MI SAE mode, detects the presence of microbubbles without relying on their motion. As initially implemented, PIM required a relatively high MI and therefore tissue harmonics contaminated the microbubble signal. Special approaches are required to operate PIM at the very low powers needed to avoid tissue harmonics without too much noise in the images. One ingenious approach to this is to send a continuous stream of alternating phase inverted pulses and use color Doppler circuitry to pick out the harmonics; essentially this method (known as power pulse inversion, PPI; Philips, USA) exploits the high sensitivity of Doppler to overcome the signal-to-noise limitation. Because the Doppler circuitry is used for the microbubble signature, PPI achieves the twin goals of complete separation of the contrast from the tissue information and of displaying each in a separate image layer (PPI in color, B-mode in grey) that can be viewed separately or as a mix. Another approach to solving the problem also uses a series of pulses, though usually only around three per line. Here, as well as inverting the phase, the amplitude of the pulses is also changed; this has the useful effect of shifting the harmonics that result from the subtraction into the fundamental frequency band of the transducer where it is at its most sensitive. Known as contrast pulse sequencing (CPS, Siemens, USA) the harmonics are displayed in a color tint over the B-mode picture and, as with PPI, either or both can be viewed as required. In a variant of the subtraction approaches, the direction of flow of the microbubbles (and therefore of blood) in larger vessels is depicted rather as with color Doppler, while slow moving and stationary microbubbles are shown in green. This mode, known as vascular recognition imaging (VRI, Toshiba, Japan) (Fig. 3), also allows the microbubble signature to be displayed separately from or combined with the B-mode and has the advantage of providing additional information on the flow direction in larger vessels. All of these modes operate at very low powers (MI < 0.2 and sometimes as low as 0.02), and, as well as suppressing the tissue harmonics, this has the major advantage that bubble destruction is minimized.

These technological advances combined with the availability of more stable microbubbles (e.g., SonoVue) have facilitated the development of real-time nondestructive (low MI) imaging modes that can demonstrate the capillary bed as well as larger vessels. Contrast enhanced imaging of focal liver lesions may be divided into arterial (20–25 s) and portal (45–90 s) phases, and real-time imaging allows these phases to be followed successively so that the dynamic enhancement pattern and vascular

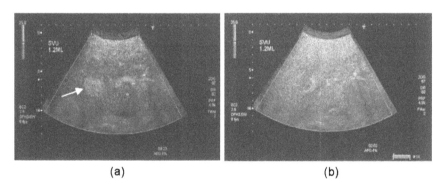

(a)   (b)

FIGURE 3 Section through the right lobe of liver. (a) Arterial phase (23 s postinjection of 1.2 mL SonoVue) image of a hypervascular metastasis in segment 7 (arrow) using vascular recognition imaging (VRI, Aplio, Toshiba, Japan). The green pixels depict stationary microbubbles in liver tissue, and the red and blue depict directional flow of microbubbles in vessels. (b) Late phase (2 minutes postinjection of 1.2 mL SonoVue) imaging shows that the metastasis now contains fewer green pixels in relation to the surrounding liver parenchyma and is clearly outlined with a "halo." (See color insert)

morphology may be assessed. The low MI means that continuous imaging can be performed for as long as the agent persists (5–10 minutes after a full dose of SonoVue). This technique has replaced the laborious intermittent imaging necessary with the destructive high MI approaches.

An additional opportunity offered by the latest contrast specific modes is the use of a destructive (high MI) pulse to destroy the bubbles in the particular scan plane and to observe reperfusion of the lesion using a low MI mode. The rate of replenishment in the field allows calculation of indices such as microcirculatory flow rate, a measure of tissue perfusion as well as fractional vascular volume. Three-dimensional displays can be constructed demonstrating anatomical vascular structure, which may prove important in defining tumor grade and response to therapy. These methods have great potential especially with the recent interest in monitoring response to angiogenesis inhibitors (12).

CHARACTERISTICS OF FOCAL LIVER LESIONS

The enhancement pattern characteristics of focal liver lesions following microbubble administration are summarized in Table 2 .

HEMANGIOMA

This common benign tumor often presents a clinical problem in the differentiation from malignancy. Although they are vascular, because the blood flow is very slow, they appear hypovascular on unenhanced Doppler. Imaging using low MI modes after IV administration of microbubbles shows a characteristic peripheral nodular pattern with progressive centripetal filling over several minutes (Fig. 4) analogous to that seen on CT and MRI (13–15). Interval delay imaging (30, 60, 120 s, etc) and real-time low MI modes are particularly useful in demonstrating this feature. A variable amount of uptake is seen in the late phase of liver-specific agents according to the time of imaging.

FOCAL NODULAR HYPERPLASIA

Focal nodular hyperplasia (FNH) is a highly vascular lesion even on unenhanced Doppler. Using low MI real-time contrast-enhanced modes, a stellate or spoke-wheel pattern can be seen in the arterial phase (16) (Fig. 5). A central scar may be seen as a hypoechoic area. FNH exhibits marked contrast uptake in the late parenchymal phase of liver-specific agents (9,17) (Fig. 5).

TABLE 2 Enhancement Pattern Characteristics of Focal Liver Lesions Following Microbubble Administration

Lesion	Characteristic features	Arterial phase (low MI imaging)	Portal phase (low MI imaging)	Late liver-specific phase (parenchymal uptake)[a]
Hypervascular metastases	Iso- or hypoechoic defect in portal and liver-specific phases	Hyperechoic (hypervascular)	Iso- or hypoechoic	No contrast uptake (appears as a defect)
Hypovascular metastases	Hypoechoic defect in portal and liver-specific phases	Little change in echopattern with variable rim enhancement	Hypoechoic	No contrast uptake (appears as a defect)
Hepatocellular carcinomas	Vascular lakes and tortuous vessels	Hyperechoic (typically basket pattern hypervascularity)	Hyper-, iso-, or hypoechoic	Variable but mostly little or no uptake with high grade tumors
Hemangiomas	Progressive globular, centripetal enhancement	Hypoechoic with peripheral globular enhancement	Centripetal filling in	Variable contrast uptake, but often less than adjacent liver
Focal nodular hyperplasia	Stellate central scar, which remains echopoor	Hyperechoic (hypervascular) spoke-wheel enhancement pattern emanating from a central artery	Hyper- or isoechoic	Marked contrast uptake, comparable or greater than adjacent liver

[a]Only applicable for microbubbles with a liver-specific phase.
Source: Ref. 32.

FOCAL FATTY CHANGE/SPARING

Focal fatty change/sparing may present as a diagnostic problem especially in patients on chemotherapy. Imaging with contrast agents shows that the vascularity is equal to the rest of the liver as is the signal in the late phase of liver-specific agents, thus distinguishing it from metastases (Fig. 6).

HEPATOCELLULAR CARCINOMA

Hepatocellular carcinomas (HCCs) are hypervascular, and continuous low MI scanning demonstrates tortuous corkscrew vessels in the arterial phase (13–15,17). The presence of cirrhosis may diminish the effects of contrast enhancement because of beam attenuation, especially if the HCC is deep seated. Typically HCCs appear as signal defects in the late parenchymal phase surrounded by a bright liver (13–15,17–19). However, liver-specific phase contrast uptake has been reported in well-differentiated HCCs. Allowing for this observation, the technique may be a promising way of distinguishing HCC from regenerating nodules which show contrast uptake in the late phase as they contain normal liver constituents.

Another useful application of contrast agents is in the assessment of residual viable HCC following ablative therapy (Fig. 7). In a study by Choi et al. (20) 6 of 40 patients with HCCs treated with radio-frequency ablation showed residual tumour on microbubble-enhanced Doppler US, all confirmed by CT. Thus this technique allows accurate assessment of the success of tumor ablation during the procedure.

METASTASES

The vascular appearances of metastases are variable on contrast-enhanced imaging depending on vessel density, size, and whether they have been treated. Metastases from the same cell type may exhibit a range of appearances, and different primary cell types may show identical features. Typically hypovascular metastases (e.g., from colon, stomach, lung) show some peritumoral vessels in the arterial phase and appear as filling defects during the portal phase on continuous low MI imaging. In contrast, hypervascular metastases (carcinoid, neurendocrine tumors, melanoma) show marked enhancement in the arterial phase (Fig. 8). In late phase imaging with liver-specific agents both types of metastases appear as signal defects surrounded by bright normal liver (13–15,17–19,21–25) (Fig. 9). A bright halo may be seen around some metastases, and this has been shown to be specific to malignancy; the cause is unknown, but it may represent compressed normal liver tissue (Fig. 10) (26).

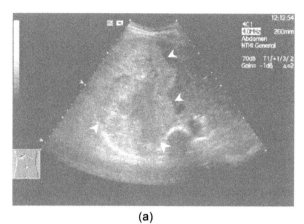

(a)

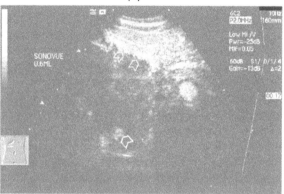

(b)

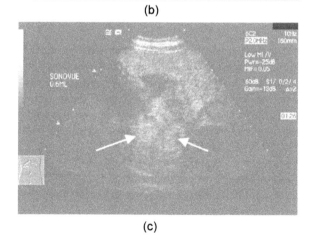

(c)

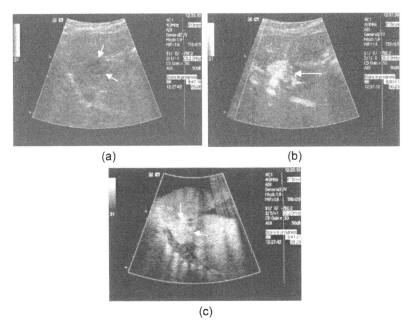

(a)   (b)

(c)

FIGURE 5   This 34-year-old man presented with abdominal pain. (a) The B-mode image shows an echo-poor lesion in the left lobe of liver (arrows). (b) Twenty-five seconds after a bolus injection of Levovist, the vascular phase was imaged in agent detection imaging mode (ADI; Siemens, USA) and shows the lesion to be hypervascular (arrow), suggesting focal nodular hyperplasia (FNH). (c) Imaging in the liver-specific phase of Levovist (5 minutes after injection) in ADI mode shows signals within the lesion (arrows), equal to adjacent liver parenchyma, which supports the diagnosis of FNH, which was subsequently confirmed. (From Ref. 33.) (See color insert)

FIGURE 4   Hemangioma in a 47-year-old woman. (a) The baseline US shows a large heterogeneous liver lesion (arrowheads). (b) Following a bolus injection of SonoVue (Bracco, Italy), the vascular phase was imaged using the novel real-time low MI nondestructive contrast pulse sequencing mode (CPS; Siemens, USA). Characteristic peripheral globular enhancement (arrows) is present. (c) After several minutes of continuous imaging, centripetal lesion filling-in (arrows) is seen strongly suggestive of a hemangioma. (From Ref. 33.) (See color insert)

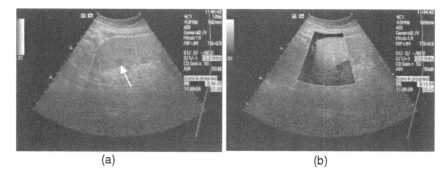

(a)   (b)

FIGURE 6   Longitudinal section through the left lobe of liver in a 76-year-old man receiving aduvant chemotherapy for colorectal carcinoma. (a) The baseline US shows an echopoor lesion (arrow). The surrounding liver parenchyma is echogenic, consistent with fatty change. The differential for the focal lesion was between a metastasis and focal fatty sparing. (b) Imaging in the late liver-specific phase of Levovist using agent detection imaging mode (ADI, Siemens, USA) demonstrates that the lesion takes up the microbubbles as the signal in it is equal to the adjacent liver allowing a confident diagnosis of focal fatty sparing. (See color insert)

Imaging in the late phase of liver-specific microbubbles using PIM has been shown to increase sensitivity in the detection of focal liver malignancies improving both subjective and objective conspicuity (21,22,25). Also, the detection of subcentimeter metastases was significantly improved, with the smallest lesions detected decreasing to a mean of 3 mm in PIM after Levovist (22) (Fig. 9). Real-time imaging has also been used in the detection of residual viable tumor in metastases treated by radio-frequency ablation with good correlation demonstrated with CT (27).

DIFFUSE LIVER DISEASE

There is no accurate noninvasive test to assess diffuse liver disease. At present biopsy is the gold standard, but even this may be limited by sampling error. However, following a bolus injection of microbubbles, their passage through a tissue of interest such as a tumor or organ can be quantified to generate time intensity curves from which functional information can be derived. The development of micro arterio-venous shunting in the liver cirrhosis and arterialization of the vascular supply in malignancy is well known. Thus, the study of hepatic vascular transit times after a peripheral bolus injection of Levovist, while performing

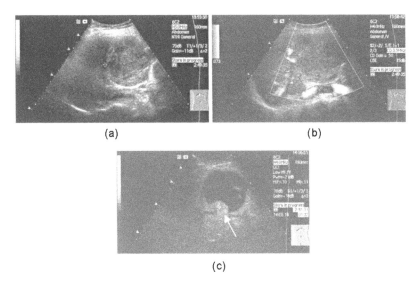

(a)   (b)

(c)

FIGURE 7 Follow-up US in a 46-year-old woman who had undergone chemo-embolization of an hepatocellular carcinoma (HCC). (a) The baseline US shows an HCC with areas of necrosis (indicated by callipers). (b) Power Doppler interrogation shows no evidence of tumour recurrence. (c) Following a bolus injection of the microbubble SonoVue (Bracco, Italy), the vascular phase was imaged using coherent contrast imaging low mechanical index (MI) mode (CCI; Siemens, USA) and shows an avidly enhancing peripheral lesion (arrow) which was confirmed to be a recurrent HCC. (From Ref. 33.) (See color insert)

spectral Doppler of a hepatic vein, has proved a useful application. The audio output from the ultrasound system is fed to a computer, which records the mean spectral intensity over each second, allowing a time intensity curve to be derived. An exponential smoothing algorithm is applied to the curve, and the arrival time of the contrast bolus (defined as a 10% rise in intensity above baseline) can be calculated.

In normal subjects the arrival time usually occurs after 40 seconds. However, in cirrhosis and malignancy an early arrival time (< 24 s) and a "left shift" of the time intensity curve is found because of an increased hepatic arterial supply and arterio-venous shunting. This technique has been shown to be a highly sensitive indicator of cirrhosis and metastases (28,29). A study comparing 15 patients with biopsy-proven cirrhosis, 12 with biopsy-proven noncirrhotic diffuse liver disease, and 11 normal controls showed that an arrival time of 24 s or less in a hepatic vein was extremely sensitive in separating cirrhotics from the other two groups (28).

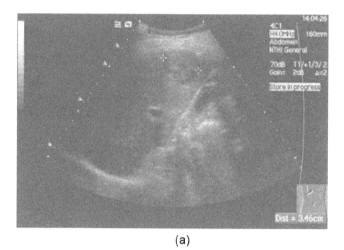

(a)

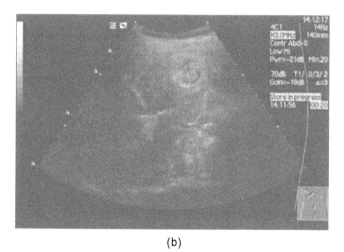

(b)

FIGURE 8   Longitudinal section of the right lobe of liver in a patient with a gastro-intestinal stromal tumor (GIST). (a) Baseline B-mode image shows a predomi-nantly echo-poor lesion (indicated by callipers). (b) Arterial phase imaging using a low mechanical index (MI 0.2) mode 20 seconds after IV SonoVue shows a hypervascular enhancement pattern. (c) In the portal phase (54 s postinjection) the lesion echogenecity has faded while the surrounding parenchyma has enhanced. (d) In the late phase (3 min postinjection) the lesion is seen as a defect with normal enhancement of the surrounding liver. The vascular and late phase enhancement characteristics are consistent with a hypervascular metastasis.

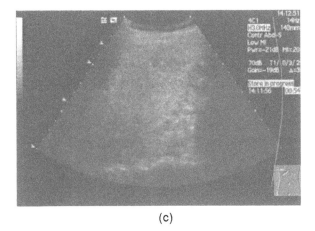

(c)

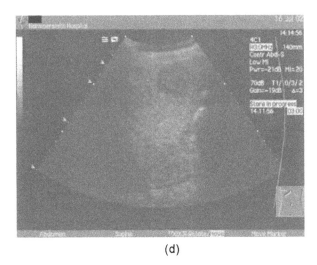

(d)

FIGURE 8   (continued)

Large prospective trials are presently underway to assess the predictive value of this technique in the development of metastases in cancer patients (30) and as a noninvasive method of grading diffuse liver disease (31).

SUMMARY

Microbubble contrast agents have markedly extended the clinical and research applications of ultrasound in hepatology. Using a combination of

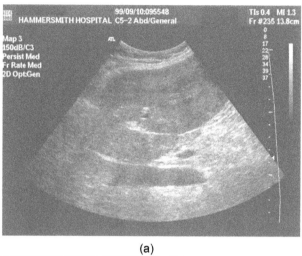

(a)

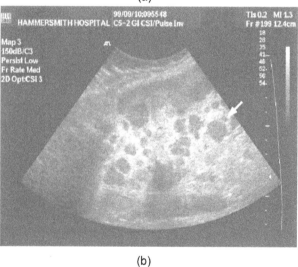

(b)

FIGURE 9 Longitudinal section of the left lobe of liver in a 74-year-old man with carcinoma of the colon. (a) Conventional B-mode shows a heterogeneous liver echotexture but no definite focal lesions. (c) Examination of the same area in pulse inversion mode (PIM) (ATL, Philips, USA) following Levovist reveals multiple metastases, some as small as 3 mm (arrow). Note the characteristic bright halo around the metastases. (From Ref. 21.)

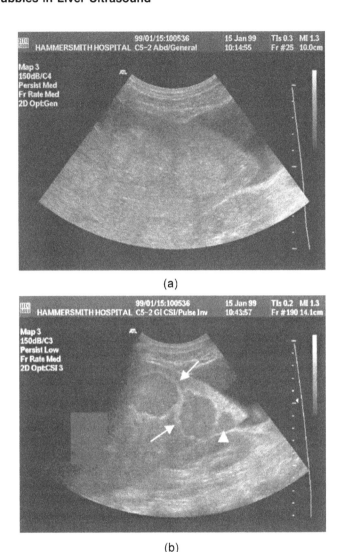

(a)

(b)

FIGURE 10 Section through the right lobe of liver in a 58-year-old male with metastatic insulinoma. (a) Conventional B-mode longitudinal image showing two echogenic metastases. (b) Three minutes postinjection of Levovist scanning in pulse inversion mode (ATL, Philips, USA), the metastases show relative reversal of echogenecity, with respect to the adjacent liver, because of the elevated parenchymal intensity. An intensely echogenic "halo" effect (arrows) around the metastases is present. A subtle metastasis, not seen on the B-mode image, is made conspicuous (arrowhead). (From Ref. 22.)

real-time and liver-specific imaging, microbubbles improve the sensitivity and specificity of ultrasound for the detection and characterization of focal liver lesions which rivals that of both CT and MR. Functional studies are promising for assessment of diffuse liver disease and for prediction of occult metastatic disease.

REFERENCES

1. Cosgrove DO. Ultrasound contrast agents. In: Dawson P, Cosgrove DO, Grainger RG, eds. Textbook of Contrast Media. Oxford, UK: ISIS Medical Media, 1999:451–587.
2. Goldberg BB, Raichlen JS, Forsberg F, eds. Ultrasound contrast agents. 2nd ed. London: Martin Dunitz, 2001.
3. Harvey CJ, Blomley MJK, Eckersley RJ, Cosgrove DO. Developments in ultrasound contrast media. Eur Radiol 2001; 11:675–689.
4. Blomley MJK, Albrecht T, Cosgrove DO, Jayaram V, Butler-Barnes J, Eckersley R. Stimulated acoustic emission in the liver parenchyma with the US contrast agent Levovist. Lancet 1998; 351:568.
5. Blomley MJK, Albrecht T, Cosgrove DO, Eckersley R, Jayaram V, Butler-Barnes J, Bauer A, Schlief R. Stimulated acoustic emission to image a late liver and spleen-specific phase of Levovist in normal volunteers and patients with and without liver disease. US Med Biol 1999; 25:1341–1352.
6. Forsberg F, Goldberg BB, Liu JB, et al. Tissue-specific US contrast agent for evaluation of hepatic and splenic parenchyma. Radiology 1999; 210:125–132.
7. Leen E, Ramnarine K, Kyriakopoulou, K, et al. Improved characterization of focal liver tumors: dynamic doppler imaging using NC100100: a new liver specific echo-enhancer. Eur J Ultrasound 2000; 11:95–104.
8. Forsberg F, Shi WT. Physics of contrast microbubbles. In: Goldberg BB, Raichen JS, Forsberg F, eds. Ultrasound Contrast Agents. 2nd ed. London: Martin Dunitz, 2001:15–24.
9. Blomley MJK, Sidhu PS, Cosgrove DO, Albrecht T, Harvey CJ, Heckemann R, Butler-Barnes J, Eckersley RJ, Basilico R. Do different types of liver lesions differ in their uptake of the microbubble contrast agent SH U 508A in the late liver phase? Early experience. Radiology 2001; 220:661–667.
10. Bryant TH, Basilico R, Pilcher J, Albrecht, T, Sidhu P, Blomley M. Characterisation of liver lesions as benign or malignant is aided by analysis of their uptake of a liver-specific microbubble imaged using a new non-linear technique (ADI): a multicenter trial. Radiology 2002; 225(P):245.
11. Hope Simpson D, Chin CT, Burns PN. Pulse inversion doppler: a new method for detecting non-linear echoes from microbubble contrast agents. IEEE Trans Ultrason Ferroelectr Frequency Control 1999; 46:372–382.
12. Folkman J. What is the evidence that tumours are angiogenesis dependent? J Natl Cancer Inst 1990; 82:4–6.

13. Wilson SR, Burns PN, Muradali D, Wilson JA, Lai X. Harmonic hepatic US with microbubble contrast agent: Initial experience showing improved characterization of hemangioma, hepatocellular carcinoma and metastasis. Radiology 2000; 215:153–161.

14. Bertolotto M, Dalla Palma L, Quaia E, Locatelli M. Characterization of unifocal liver lesions with pulse inversion harmonic imaging after Levovist injection: preliminary results. Eur Radiol 2000; 10:1369–1376.

15. Kim TK, Choi BI, Han JK, Hong HS, Park SH, Moon SG. Hepatic tumors: contrast agent-enhancement patterns with pulse inversion harmonic US. Radiology 2000; 216:411–417.

16. Uggowitzer M, Kugler C, Groll R, Mischinger H, et al. Sonographic evaluation of focal nodular hyperplasias (FNH) of the liver with a trans-pulmonary galactose-based contrast agent (Levovist). Br J Radiol 1998; 71: 1026–1032.

17. Dill-Macky MJ, Burns PN, Khalili K, Wilson SR. Focal hepatic masses: Enhancement patterns with SH U 508A and pulse-inversion US. Radiology 2002; 222:95–102.

18. Burns PN, Wilson SR, Hope Simpson D. Pulse inversion imaging of liver blood flow. Improved method for characterizing focal masses with microbubble contrast. Invest Radiol 2000; 35:58–71.

19. Choi B, Kim T, Han J, et al. Vascularity of hepatocellular carcinoma: assessment with contrast-enhanced second harmonic versus conventional power Doppler US. Radiology 2000; 214:167–172.

20. Choi D, Lim HK, Kim SH, Lee WJ, Jang HJ, Lee JY, Paik SW, Koh KC, Lee JH. Hepatocellular carcinoma treated with percutaneous radio-frequency ablation: usefulness of power Doppler US with a microbubble contrast agent in evaluating therapeutic response-preliminary results. Radiology 2000; 217:558–563.

21. Harvey CJ, Blomley MJK, Eckersley RJ, Heckemann R, Butler-Barnes J, Cosgrove DO. Pulse inversion mode imaging of liver specific microbubbles: improved detection of subcentimetre metastases. Lancet 2000; 355:807–808.

22. Harvey CJ, Blomley MJK, Eckersley RJ, Cosgrove DO, Patel N, Heckemann R, Butler-Barnes J. Hepatic malignancies: improved detection with pulse inversion US in late phase of enhancement with SH U 508A—early experience. Radiology 2000; 216:903–908.

23. Albrecht T, Hoffmann CW, Schmitz SA, et al. Phase inversion sonography during the liver-specific late phase of contrast enhancement with Levovist: improved detection of liver metastases. AJR 2001; 176:1191–1198.

24. Blomley MJK, Albrecht T, Cosgrove DO, Patel N, Jayaram V, Butler-Barnes J, Eckersley R, Bauer A, Schlief R. Improved imaging of liver metastases with stimulated acoustic emission in the late phase of enhancement with the US contrast agent SH U 508A: early experience. Radiology 1999; 210: 409–416.

25. Albrecht T, Blomley MJK, Burns PN, Wilson S, Harvey CJ, Leen E, Claudon M, Calliada F, Correas JM, LaFortune M, Campani R, Hoffmann CW, Cosgrove DO, LeFevre F. Improved detection of hepatic metastases with

pulse inversion ultrasonography during the liver-specific phase of SHU 508A (Levovist)—a multicenter study. Radiology 2003; 227:361–370.

26. Harvey CJ, Blomley MJK, Cosgrove DO, Eckersley R, Heckemann R, Butler-Barnes J. Is the presence of an echogenic rim around focal liver lesions imaged in the late phase of liver-specific ultrasound microbubbles in phase inversion mode specific to malignancy?. Radiology 2000; 217(P):304.

27. Solbiati L, Goldberg SN, Ierace T, et al. Radio-frequency ablation of hepatic metastases: postprocedural assessment with a US microbubble contrast agent—early experience. Radiology 1999; 211:643–649.

28. Albrecht T, Blomley MJK, Cosgrove DO, Taylor-Robinson S, Jayaram V, Eckersley R, Bauer A, Schlief R. Non-invasive diagnosis of hepatic cirrhosis by transit-time analysis of an ultrasound contrast agent. Lancet 1999; 353:1579–1583.

29. Blomley MJK, Albrecht T, Cosgrove DO, Jayaram V, Eckersley R, Patel N, Taylor-Robinson S, Bauer A, Schlief R. Liver vascular transit time analyzed with dynamic hepatic venography with bolus injections of an US contrast agent: early experience in 7 patients with metastases. Radiology 1998; 209:862–866.

30. Harvey CJ, Blomley MJK, Lynch M, Eckersley R, Pilcher J, Cosgrove DO. Liver vascular transit time measured using carotid delay time with bolus injections of the microbubble Levovist can predict the presence of occult metastases in colorectal cancer. Radiology 2001; 221(P):269.

31. Blomley MJK, Lim ALP, Harvey CJ, Patel N, Eckersley RJ, Basilico R, Heckemann R, Butler-Barnes J, Urbank A, Cosgrove DO, Taylor-Robinson SD. Liver microbubble transit time compared with histology in diffuse liver disease: A cross sectional study. Gut 2003; 52:1188–1193.

32. Leen E. The role of contrast-enchanced ultrasound in the characterization of focal liver lesions. Eur Radiol 2001; 11(suppl 3):E27–E34.

33. Harvey CJ, Pilcher JM, Eckersley RJ, Blomley MJ, Cosgrove DO. Advances in ultrasound. Clin Radiol 2002; 57(3):157–177.

5

Liver Imaging: Multislice CT

Christiane Kulinna and
Wolfgang Schima
University of Vienna, Vienna, Austria

INTRODUCTION

Computed tomography (CT) has proved to be a versatile tool for assessment of focal liver lesions and diffuse liver disease. Although less expensive imaging methods, such as sonography, are widely available, patients with equivocal findings at sonography often need helical CT for definitive diagnosis. Indications for liver CT imaging include differentiation of benign liver lesions [e.g., simple cysts, hemangiomas, adenomas, focal nodular hyperplasia (FNH)] from those that are malignant [e.g., metastasis, hepatocellular carcinoma (HCC), cholangiocarcinoma]. In the acutely ill patient, a suspected liver abscess or blunt abdominal trauma may well warrant CT examination. In transplant surgery, preoperative assessment of vascular anomalies and follow-up after surgery frequently requires CT.

Compared with MR imaging, CT has had historical advantages of increased availability, shorter imaging times, and lower cost. On the other hand, MRI offers superior soft tissue contrast, lack of ionizing radiation, and imaging in virtually any plane of view desired. With the increasing availability of liver-specific MR contrast agents, MR imaging is superior to single-slice helical CT imaging for detection of liver metastases and HCC (1,2). However, with the advent of multislice CT (MSCT), body imaging

121

has become much faster. Furthermore, the possibility of thinner slices has remarkably improved detection of small focal liver lesions (3) when using 3D image reconstruction from MSCT data sets. Multiplanar reconstructions and sophisticated three-dimensional reconstruction tools have substantial added value for abdominal CT angiography, and, in general, increasing experience with MSCT has created new opportunities in the diagnostic imaging of liver disorders (4,5).

In this chapter, current MSCT imaging protocols will be presented, including advanced techniques for multiplanar reconstructions of the liver. The clinical utility of various contrast phases will be discussed with particular regard to the detection and characterization of benign and malignant tumors. The use of multidetector CT for assessment of the hepatic vasculature and the added value of MSCT in trauma imaging will be highlighted.

TECHNICAL CONSIDERATIONS

Since Hounsfield presented the first clinical CT image in 1972, the improvements in CT image quality and scan performance have been enormous. The most significant development came with the development of helical CT in 1989 (6), which broadened the diagnostic applications of CT and established CT as a true volume imaging modality. More recently, the introduction of multislice CT in 1998 has opened up a whole range of new applications, including thin collimation scanning of the liver within one breathhold. Current MSCT scanners feature up to 16 parallel rows of x-ray detectors that operate simultaneously at individual collimations of about 0.5–0.75 mm (7). Tube cooling has been improved and tube rotation time has decreased to 0.5 seconds or, with the newest generation of 16-row detector machines, to 0.4–0.43 seconds. The upper abdomen from the diaphragm to the pelvis can be covered with submillimeter collimation during a single breathhold. The pelvis can additionally be imaged with very thin collimation while the patient slowly breathes out. MSCT allows the examination of the liver with practically isotropic data sets, such that image reformatting in planes other than the axial is possible without loss of diagnostic quality. This is a prerequisite for optimal assessment of very small liver lesions in all planes. The advantages of multislice CT can be employed either to reduce the time to cover a given volume or to use narrower beam collimation to increase the z-axis resolution and reduce volume averaging.

Nevertheless, true isotropic resolution has not been reached with 4-slice MSCT: for a typical abdomen examination, the in-plane resolution is about 0.5 mm using a standard body kernel (8). The new generation of MSCT scanners that offer simultaneous acquisition of up to 16 submillimeter slices represent an important step on the path towards true isotropic scanning. The reduced gantry rotation time (under 500 ms, up to 0.4 s) has an important impact on temporal resolution and dose utilization. The relative dose utilization of a representative 4-slice CT scanner is 70% for 4×1 mm collimation and 85% for 4×2.5 mm collimation. The evaluated 16-slice CT system has an improved dose utilization of 76% resp. 82% for 16×0.75 mm collimation and 85% resp. 89% for 16×1.5 mm collimation, depending on the size of the focal spot (large resp. small) (8). Thus, MSCT with 16-slice scanners are no longer restricted to special applications but are ready for routine applications. The simultaneous acquisition of 16×0.75 mm slices with 16-slice MSCT rather than 4×1 mm slices reduces both scan time and motion artifacts facilitates the examination of uncooperative patients, reduces the amount of contrast medium needed, and improves axial resolution. Abdominal CTA using 16-slice MSCT showed equivalent morphological information to selective catheter angiography for assessment of hepatic and mesenteric vasculature up to the fourth-generation of vessels (9). Improved spatial resolution enables high-quality three-dimensional (3D) visualization.

INTRAVENOUS CONTRAST—WHAT HAS CHANGED WITH MSCT?

Hepatic enhancement depends on injected iodine load relative to body weight (10). For single slice CT, injection of either 2 mL/kg b.w. of contrast material or a fixed volume of 120–150 mL of contrast material (at 300 mg/mL iodine), corresponding to a total iodine load of 36–45 g per patient, is necessary to achieve adequate liver enhancement (11–13). For the same iodine load, faster contrast injection rates result in earlier maximum liver enhancement. Slower injection rates provide delayed, but otherwise equivalent, hepatic enhancement (10). When MSCT was first introduced, the total iodine load or the contrast volume could not be reduced (14,15) because maximum enhancement of the liver parenchyma is dependent on the total iodine load and largely independent of examination time (12). However, recent studies have found that higher iodine concentrations with a constant iodine load have a positive impact on abdominal enhancement during the arterial phase. For example, MSCT detection of hypervascular HCC in the arterial phase is improved at higher contrast material concentrations (16). However, concentration has no influence on enhancement during the portal venous phase of abdominal MSCT (15).

Due to the shortened scan times of MSCT, it has become even more important to time image acquisition appropriately with regard to contrast material injection (17). A major challenge of MSCT is not to miss the arterial phase before maximum arterial liver enhancement is reached. Thus, standard scanning delays do not reliably provide optimal timing for the arterial-dominant phase of CT scanning (18). Individual circulation time can be assessed by administering a small bolus (15 mL at 5 mL/s) of contrast material and a 40 mL saline flush, followed by a series of single-level low-dose (10 mA) scans at the level of the celiac trunk. A cursor is placed over the abdominal aorta, and the interval to peak aortic enhancement is measured to determine the vascular transit time. Currently, automatic bolus-tracking systems are in use: after the start of contrast material injection, dynamic low-dose scans are acquired at the level of the celiac trunk with measurements of aortic enhancement: the scan is automatically started when aortic enhancement exceeds a preset threshold level, usually 100–150 HU. With 4-row MSCT and rapid scanning of the liver in a minimum of 6 seconds, injection rates can be increased at earlier peak enhancement with a narrow acquisition interval. The injection rate influences greatly the bolus venous flow velocity and determines the shape of the contrast bolus (19). In order to obtain optimal liver enhancement during the arterial phase, the amount of contrast that enters the liver during this phase must be as great as possible. Because of the very short duration of imaging this phase when using MSCT (6–8 s), this can be best achieved only by using a concentrated contrast bolus with a steep upslope; i.e., a high injection rate must be used (19). In recent years, experienced authors recommended at least 3.0–6.0 mL/s injection rates to achieve a sufficient conspituity for hypervascular tumors enhanced in the arterial-dominant phase (5,20,21). At the authors' institution, an injection rate of 5–8 mL/s is employed in order to optimize liver tumor imaging (Fig. 1) and depiction of the hepatic vasculature.

HOW MANY SCANS ARE NEEDED?

The faster z-axis speed and improved longitudinal resolution of MSCT enables faster hepatic scan acquisitions. It has been shown that the true arterial-dominant phase in liver helical CT scanning may be shorter than 9 seconds (19), which is too short to cover the entire liver with a single-slice scanner. Thus, MSCT provides a significant advantage over single-slice helical CT, because it allows liver scanning in defined organic perfusion phases, e.g., early and late arterial phases, portal-venous phase, and equilibrium phase, all with very thin collimation in a single breath-hold. Alternatively, the ease of performing multiple scans in different perfusion phases would result in a dramatic increase in radiation exposure for the patient and a flood of imaging data for the radiologist (22).

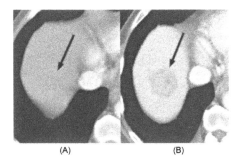

(A)   (B)

FIGURE 1   Effect of flow rate on lesion detection: 50-year-old woman with large metastasis from colon cancer in segment 6. (A) The first scan was done on single-row helical CT with a flow of 2 mL/s. Portal venous phase scan (enhancement of the inferior cava vein) shows insufficient delineation of the lesion. (B) The second scan 2 weeks later was done on a 4-row multidetector scanner with a flow rate of 8 mL/s, which shows an excellent enhancement of the parenchyma with delineation of the metastasis.

There is still debate about whether an unenhanced scan should be performed routinely. Increased radiation exposure may be outweighed by additional information provided by an unenhanced scan, at least initially, i.e., better delineation of calcifications, hemorrhage, and embolization material, increased detection of HCC (23), better differentiation between cysts and small hypovascular metastases, and demonstration of extrahepatic abnormalities (such as adrenal masses or renal stones). For follow-up studies, unenhanced scans may be omitted or acquired, depending on the diagnostic question. An additional native phase is also needed for an enhanced diagnostic MSCT tool, which is hepatic perfusion imaging for indirect detection of hepatic lesions and for differentiation of preexisting cirrhosis (24).

The first contrast-enhanced scan should be during the hepatic arterial phase. It has been shown that two "arterial phase" scans can be performed with MSCT (Fig. 2). The first or early arterial phase, with no or only a minimal admixture of enhanced portal venous blood, provides a suitable imaging template for CT arteriography. Preoperative visualization is important in patients who are candidates for hepatic resection, cryoablation, or arterial chemoembolization. The second phase or late arterial phase, with portal venous inflow, maximizes hypervascular tumor detection. These two scans last for not more than 7–10 seconds each if a high-speed scan mode is instituted. Including an interscan delay of approximately 5 seconds for table movement, these two scans can be performed within one breath-hold. Murakami et al. (18) reported that a double arterial

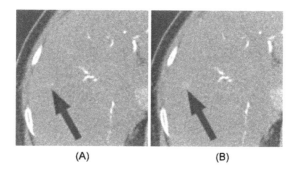

(A)   (B)

FIGURE 2 Double-arterial phase scan: 66-year-old man with hypervascular HCC in segment 8 of the liver. (A) Early arterial phase MSCT gives a CT-angiographic picture with excellent enhancement of the arteries, but there is only faint enhancement of the mass (arrow) in segment 8 of the liver. Note that portal vessels do not show contrast enhancement yet. (B) In the late arterial phase MSCT portal venous inflow has already begun. The mass shows significant enhancement. Degree of contrast enhancement of mass is greater on this late arterial than on early arterial phase scan.

phase scan is much better than single arterial phase scans for the detection of hypervascular HCC (sensitivity 86% for the double arterial phase versus 54% and 78%, respectively, for the single arterial phase scans). The third pass of the acquisition begins 60 seconds after the beginning of the contrast injection. This corresponds in timing to the portal venous phase of a biphasic helical scan using a single-slice system. During the third pass, hepatic veins that were unenhanced during the arterial phase, or the portal venous inflow phase, are now enhanced.

Regarding the value of delayed phase scanning, several authors report significant benefits for diagnosis of hypovascular tumors. Hwang et al. (25) explained that peak enhancement of the hepatic parenchyma on delayed phase imaging because of portal hypertension in cirrhotic patients maximizes the contrast between the relatively hypovascular hepatocellular carcinomas and the surrounding hepatic parenchyma. In addition, the delayed phase has further value in the characterization of hepatic masses because of the better visualization of the capsule or mosaic pattern of hepatocellular carcinoma. Delayed peripheral enhancement of cholangiocarcinoma and "filling-in" patterns of hemangioma are well-established signs sought for the differential diagnosis of hepatic masses (26). Other authors reported that the portal venous phase is equal to the delayed phase in the detection and characterization of liver lesions (27). Most authors prefer two or, at maximum, three different contrast-enhanced phases, depending on the indication, e.g., evaluation of suspected of HCC or metastases or follow-up (14,22).

Radiologists should recognize that acquisition of multiple scans as standard practice in every patient, regardless of the indication, poses a serious problem. Increased radiation exposure for patients has become an issue for public discussion and, furthermore, huge amounts of imaging data flood both workstations and reporting radiologists. Great consideration should be taken to establish the indication for each patient's referral before applying multiple phase imaging.

SLICE THICKNESS

For dynamic hepatic CT with a single-detector helical scanner, a reconstructed slice thickness of 7–10 mm has been commonly used (28–33). Multidetector technology facilitates thinner slices for the same breathhold and retrospective reconstruction with different slice thickness, obtained from the original data. Thinner slices are useful for reconstructing multiplanar images and 3D CT angiography (34–37). Weg et al.(3) used a dual-detector CT scanner to study the benefits of thin collimation when evaluating small (diameter < 10 mm) liver lesions, primarily hypovascular metastases. In this study, more lesions were found on images obtained with a 2.5 mm collimation than on those obtained with a 5, 7.5, or 10 mm collimation. Using multidetector CT for detection of focal liver lesions, other investigators have described conflicting findings regarding optimal slice thickness. Kopka and Grabbe (38) were able to demonstrate that thin sections of 2–4 mm from 4×2 mm collimation were superior to thicker sections via increased detection rates and confidence for small liver lesions. Similar results were found by Basilico et al. (39), where 3 mm thick sections was found superior to 5 mm sections for detection of small hypervascular liver lesions. Conversely, Haider et al. found no improvement in the detection or characterization of focal liver lesions when using 2.5 and 3.75 mm collimation compared with 5 mm collimation (40). However, some study limitations may account for this discrepancy; only portal-venous phase scanning with a fixed scan delay was used, which does not account for each individual patient's circulation time. In addition, image noise was much higher than in other studies (3), and interobserver agreement was suboptimal for the detection of small lesions, which might have minimized the differentiation between benign and malignant lesions with thin collimation. The present authors' experience with different slice thickness suggests improved detection and characterization of small liver lesions when using a 1, 3, or 5 mm slice thickness compared to a 7 mm slice thickness. However, the use of very thin sections (i.e., images reconstructed at 1 mm slice

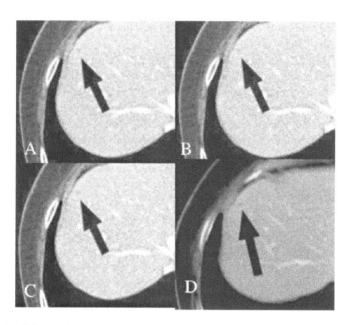

FIGURE 3 Effect of slice thickness on lesion detection: liver metastasis in 72-year-old woman with breast cancer. Images reconstructed from the same 16 × 1.5 collimation scan in portal-venous phase with 2 (A), 3 (B), 4 (C), and 8 mm (D) sections show 4 mm metastasis in segment 5, which can be well visualized on 2, 3, and 4 mm thick sections, whereas the lesion is difficult to see on the 8 mm reconstruction due to partial volume effect. Please note the increased image noise on 2 mm thick sections compared to 3 or 4 mm thick images.

thickness) decreased signal-to-noise ratio and did not result in any improvement compared to 3 mm sections (Fig. 3). In addition, the radiation exposure is considerably increased. Images from 3–5 mm thickness seem to provide the optimal combination of adequate signal-to-noise ratio and spatial and contrast resolution.

SCAN PROTOCOLS/EXAMINATION PROTOCOLS

Most examination protocols can be performed with only two different detector collimations when MSCT is used in for routine clinical work versus research studies. In day-to-day practice, MSCT data with a 4-row scanner can be acquired with 4 × 1–1.25 mm, 4 × 2.5 mm, or 4 × 3.75–5 mm collimation; or, with a 16-row scanner, with 16 × 0.5–0.75 mm or 16 × 1–1.5 mm collimation, depending on the scanner type and vendor.

If any postprocessing, such as multiplanar reconstructions, (MPR), maximum intensity projection (MIP) or a virtual rendering technique (VRT) is planned, a high-resolution protocol (in the z-axis) with a 4×1–1.25 mm (16×0.5–0.75 mm) mode for abdominal, and particularly liver examination, is appropriate in 95% of cases. The 4×2.5–5 mm (16×1.5 mm) mode is useful when the entire abdomen must be examined with one acquisition for patients referred for oncology follow-up, or for studies that do not require postprocessing. The 4×5 mm scan is used only for trauma patients, where the head, chest, abdomen, spine, and parts of legs must be scanned quickly. The 2×0.5 mm mode employed by 4-row scanners offers great possibilities for postprocessing, but has two big disadvantages. Compared to the 4×1 mm mode, the 2×0.5 mm scan has a four times higher scan time and tube load (41) and markedly decreased z-axis coverage. The result is that this mode can only be used for small structures like the skull base or wrist, but it has no role in liver imaging.

Sixteen-row detector scanners have the potential to cover large scan volumes with submillimeter collimation in combination with reasonable scan times. CT angiography, in particular, will benefit from this potential because of improved spatial resolution. CT angiography in the pure arterial phase will become feasible. For example, an abdominal CTA with a collimation of 16×0.5–0.75 mm, and a table feed of 12 mm/rotation requires only 19 seconds (9). When true isotropic resolution is not a prerequisite, a 16×1–1.5 mm collimation provides even shorter examination times or wider scan range for abdominal or liver examination. Standard examination protocols for different MSCT scanners are shown in Tables 1 and 2.

IMAGE REFORMATTING

MSCT allows the reconstruction of images in additional planes of view, obtained from thin-slice source images, either at the time of scanning or later if data can be retrieved from electronic storage devices and post-processed on a PACS workstation. Particularly for liver lesions near the diaphragm, assessment of extent may be easier on coronal or sagittal views than on axial images. With the breakthrough toward isotropic resolution of MSCT, image reformatting with multiplanar reconstructions (MPR) will result in high-quality MSCT images in almost any plane with 1 mm collimation. Generally, images of the liver should be reconstructed in two different planes, as is standard in MSCT. Axial reconstructions should always be performed, because they represent the plane of view convention-ally provided by both CT and MRI, permitting correlation if required. The

TABLE 1 MSCT Protocols for Liver Tumor Imaging: 4-Row Scanners

	GE light speed[a]				Toshiba Aquilion[b]				Siemens VolumeZoom[c]				Siemens VolumeZoom[d]			
	Pre	ADP	PVP	Delayed	Pre	Early ADP	Late ADP	PVP	Pre	ADP	PVP	Delayed	Pre	ADP	PVP	Delayed
Collimation(mm)	4×3.75	4×1.25	4×2.5	4×2.5	4×2	4×2	4×2	4×2	4×2,5	4×2,5	4×2,5	4×2,5	4×2,5	4×2,5	4×2,5	4×2,5
Feed/rotation	22.5	7.5	15	15	11	11	11	11	15	15	15	15	20	20	20	20
Rotation time (s)		0.8				0.5				0.5				0.5		
kV		120				120				120				120		
mAs	120	160	160	160		150				165				180		
Matrix size		512 × 512				512 × 512				512 × 512				512 × 512		
Scan direction		Cranio-caudal				Cranio-caudal				Cranio-caudal				Cranio-caudal		
Slice thickness (mm)	5	2.5	5	5	2	2	2	2	5	5	5	5		3	3	3
Reconstruction interval (mm)	5	2.5	5	5	5	2	2	5	5	5	5	5		2	2	2
Contrast material		120 mL				120 mL				120 mL				90	40	
Flow rate		3–4 mL/s				4 mL/s				5 mL/s				3–4	1	
Scan delay		Bolus tracking	Interscan delay 30 s	200 s		Bolus tracking	Total delay 40 s	Total delay 60 s	[e]	Bolus tracking	Interscan delay 40 s	200 s[f]		Care bolus	50–60 s	600 s[f]

ADP: arterial-dominant phase; PVP: portal-venous phase.
[a] Courtesy of: Reto Bale, M.D., Department of Radiology, University of Innsbruck.
[b] Courtesy of: Martin Uggowitzer, M.D., Department of Radiology, University of Graz.
[c] Courtesy of: Thomas Helmberger, M.D., Department of Radiology, University of Munich.
[d] Protocol used at the Department of Radiology, University of Vienna.
[e] Unenhanced scan only used in case of HCC.
[f] Delayed scan only used in case of CCC.

TABLE 2 MSCT Protocols for Liver Tumor Imaging: 16-Row Scanners

	Siemens Sensation 16[a]				Siemens Sensation 16[b]			
	Pre	ADP	PVP	Delayed	Pre	ADP	PVP	Delayed
Collimation (mm)	16 × 1.5	16 × 1.5	16 × 1.5		16 × 1.5	16 × 1.5	16 × 1.5	16 × 1.5
Feed/rotation	24	24	24		30	30	30	30
Rotation time (s)			0.5				0.5	
kV			120				120	
mAs			165		120	160	160	160
Matrix size			512 × 512				512 × 512	
Scan direction			Cranio-caudal				Cranio-caudal	
Slice thickness (mm)	5	5	5		3	3	3	3
Reconstruction interval (mm)	5	5	5		2	2	2	2
Contrast material			120 mL				120 mL	
Flow rate			3–4 mL/s				5 mL/s	
Scan delay	c	Bolus tracking	Interscan delay 30 s	200 s[d]		Bolus tracking	Interscan delay 40 s	200 s[d]

ADP: arterial-dominant phase; PVP: portal-venous phase.
[a]Courtesy of: Thomas Helmberger, M.D., Department of Radiology, University of Munich.
[b]Protocol used at the Department of Radiology, University of Vienna.
[c]Unenhanced scan only used in case of HCC.
[d]Delayed scan only used in case of CCC.

second "standard" plane of view for liver MSCT should be coronal, an orientation that facilities comparative evaluation of both right and left liver lobes and which well represents vessels. Most liver surgery is performed via the subcostal access route, with the patient supine, and the coronal view most closely resembles the intraoperative situation from the surgeon's point of view. Additional planes of view, such as the sagittal view, may be useful in some instances. For diagnosis, image reconstruction with contiguous 3–5 mm slices is sufficient. Secondary image reformatting is possible when either the raw data set or axial 1 mm source images have been archived on a picture archiving and communicating system (PACS), which allows a secondary reformatting. In view of the increased number of images gathered by MSCT, a combination with a PACS unit appears very beneficial.

The MIP postprocessing technique is well known from MR angiography. After application of a threshold, the contiguous images of the volume data set are superimposed. For example, this technique is used to enhance detectability of pulmonary nodules for lung cancer screening. Many authors have also used this 3D reconstruction tool for visualization of hepatic vessels in different planes (42). Others prefer volume rendering (VR) for generating three-dimensional images, because MIPs and shaded surface displays also have significant limitations. Unlike MIP and shaded surface display techniques, both of which use less than 10% of the image data, VR can display nearly all of the volume data (43). This allows VR 3D CTA to display multiple overlapping vessels by providing vessel depth similar to DSA. However, creation of adequate "pseudo-anatomical" visualization of vessels is relatively time-consuming. Various colors or grey levels are mapped to precise ranges of Hounsfield units with the additional option of thresholding out or editing any unnecessary anatomical sytructures.

MCST scanners produce a large data load for clinical networks: there are approximately 300–500 slices per patient for an abdominal study using 4×1 mm collimation and additional multiplanar reconstructions, and there can be up to 1000 images when using 3D CT angiography. This requires considerable storage capability. Since it is not feasible to both print and read hundreds of images for every patient, innovative display methodologies for the acquired data are required. Until such methods are developed, reading in cine mode on a PACS system is a viable alternative. Quick visualization of complex anatomical structures and vessels is possible using this approach. Not all received images should be archived, and any archiving should be report-oriented. In the future we will need increasingly highpower workstations and automatic archiving systems to handle these volumes of data.

FOCAL LIVER LESIONS

Metastases

The most frequent reason for performing imaging studies of the liver is to assess focal liver lesions. The most frequent indication (approximately 90%) is to exclude or assess liver metastases, which are approximately 10 times more common than primary malignant tumors of the liver (44). In one third of all malignant tumors, liver metastases are found at the time of diagnosis of the primary tumor or occur during follow-up. Complicating this, autopsy studies suggest benign focal liver lesions are present in 20–50% of the general population (45,46). Even in patients with malignant disease, the majority of of small liver lesions are benign (47,48). Thus, the preferred liver imaging technique should combine both high sensitivity for lesion depiction and good characterization. In addition, any imaging technique should provide information as to number, size, and topographic assessment relating lesions to segments and the vascular environment so that appropriate management can be planned. Currently, sonography is the mainstay of routine radiological staging for patients at low risk for liver metastases. CT or MRI should be employed in equivocal cases and in those at high risk of developing liver metastases. Contrast-enhanced MRI has been found to be more sensitive than contrast-enhanced helical CT and almost equivalent to CT arterial portography for detection of liver metastases (1,49,50). Indeed, contrast-enhanced MRI has been found to be the most sensitive diagnostic tool for detecting liver metastases, with sensitivities of 78–97% and specificities of 71–87% (1,2,51). With the introduction of helical CT in 1989, the sensitivity of CT was improved to 62–87% (52,53). To adequately differentiate malignant from benign lesions and to characterize these lesions with CT, high spatial resolution, dynamic contrast enhancement imaging, and multiplanar 2D and 3D are all required to varying degrees.

The introduction of MSCT has provided significant competition for MRI in oncological imaging. Using MSCT, the regular combination of a chest, abdomen, and pelvis study is feasible, while remaining both less expensive and faster than MRI, thereby increasing patient through-put. Early experience suggests indicates that contrast-enhanced MSCT might match MRI for lesion detection. Given this, the use of thin sections, viewed at a workstation, is mandatory to facilitate detection of small liver lesions. However, detection of more small lesions alone, without increased confidence in characterization, would not be of great clinical value. It has been shown that significant improvement in diagnostic accuracy for detection and characterization of focal liver lesions is possible when scan protocols are optimized (3,18,38). Best results were obtained with slice thickness of 3.75 and 5 mm. Correct differentiation between benign and malignant lesions was achieved in 93% with 3.75 mm thickness and in 91% using a 5 mm thickness, whereas only 84% of lesions could be correctly characterized at 7 mm (38).

Hepatocellular Carcinoma

Hepatocellular carcinoma has a poor prognosis. Five-year survival is less than 30%, the resectability rate is 17%, and the mean survival time after diagnosis is 6 months (54). Treatment consists of surgical resection, percutaneous ablation, if possible, and/or chemotherapy, with remission of up to 3 years achieved in more than 40% of these patients. Thus, early tumor detection and accurate radiological assessment of tumor extent is crucial for optimal management.

HCC is usually hypervascular and helical CT has improved detection by allowing acquisition of both arterial-dominant and portal venous phases during separate breath-holds (31–33). Using single detector helical CT, Baron et al. (32) established the addition of a hepatic arterial-dominant phase acquisition, which significantly increases HCC detection compared to portal venous phase imaging alone. Multidetector CT scanners acquire multiple CT data sets with each rotation of the x-ray tube; the ability to scan through the liver in less than 10 seconds allows acquisition of two separate sets of CT images of the liver within the time generally regarded as the hepatic arterial-dominant phase (double arterial phase) (55). Murakami et al. (18) emphasized the usefulness of double arterial phase imaging for detecting hypervascular HCC with multidetector CT. However, Kim et al. reported that three-phase MSCT (single arterial phase, portal-venous and delayed phase) is, overall, as good as four-phase MSCT (double arterial phase, portal-venous and delayed phase) for detection of HCC (33).

Multislice technology also enables us to work with thinner slices during the same breath-hold and to retrospectively reconstruct images with a different slice thickness via the original CT data. MSCT allows the reconstruction of images in additional planes of view with nearly isotropic voxels. For the assessment of vascular infiltration, reconstructions perpendicular to, and along the axis of, the vessels are very useful (Fig. 4). As already stated, axial reconstructions should be the norm, but the second "standard" plane of view for MSCT of the liver should be coronal in order to better visualize vascular anatomy and best simulate the surgeon's intraoperative perspective. Sagittal reconstructions are mandatory for the depiction of infiltration of the portal vein or diaphragm.

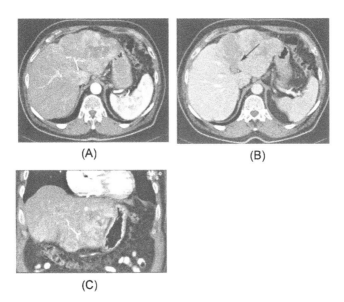

(A)   (B)

(C)

FIGURE 4   49-year-old man with large, multifocal HCC with portal vein thrombus. (A) Transverse scan in the arterial phase shows the hyperattenuating nodules of the HCC. (B) Portal venous phase scan shows extension of the tumor into the left portal vein (arrow). (C) The coronal MPR better shows the multifocal extension of the HCC.

Biliary Disease

The search for noninvasive diagnostic tools in patients with suspected obstructive biliary disease is an emerging medical need. Interventional procedures such as endoscopic retrograde cholangiopancreatography (ERCP) or percutaneous transhepatic cholangiography (PTC) are costly, physician-intensive procedures, are not feasible in all patients, and carry a high complication rate. The role of MRI is well established as the most reliable noninvasive technique. However, certain contraindications, for example, long examination times and limited scanner availability, still restrict use of MRI. The role of CT has been extensively discussed in the literature, and the long acquisition time required by conventional or single-slice helical CT scanners is known to adversely influence both image quality and patient compliance (57). MSCT raises the possibility of thinner collimation and shorter scan times, resulting in better compliance and reduced motion artifact. Due to the improved z-axis resolution, high-quality multiplanar and 3D reconstructions can be performed (Fig. 5). Axial and MPR images allow determination of the site and cause of obstruction, but the use of

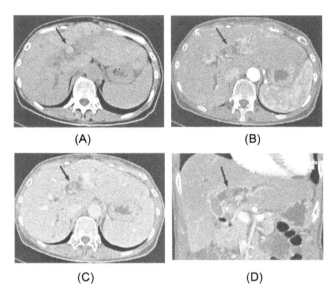

(A)   (B)

(C)   (D)

FIGURE 5   59-year-old woman with stenosis of biliodigestive anastomosis and intrahepatic stones. Stone (arrow) in projection on the left hepatic duct in unenhanced (A), arterial (B) and portal-venous (C) scan with dilatation of intrahepatic bile ducts. (D) Severe stenosis (white arrow) of the biliodigestive anastomosis is better revealed by the coronal MPR. Multiple bile duct stones pile up proximal to the stenosis.

high-quality MPR with MSCT can be considered a real improvement when assessing the biliary tract and the exact relationship between biliary and extrabiliary structures (57). Maximum intensity projection (MIP) images provide a panoramic, cholangiographic-like view of the bile ducts and are particularly useful in complex situations, such as those encountered in the detection of anatomical variations or when assessing the biliary extension of cholangiocarcinoma.

Cholangiocellular carcinoma (CCC) arises from the intra- or extrahepatic bile ducts. Intrahepatic or peripheral CCCs arise from the small bile ducts. It is the second most common primary hepatic neoplasm, but only 8–13% of all CCCs occur in the liver alone. More often, CCCs occur at the bifurcation of the hepatic duct, often referred to as a Klatskin tumor (58). Less than 20% of CCCs are resectable at presentation, and 5-year survival is only 30%. On gross pathology specimens, CCCs appear as firm, hypovascular masses with a significant amount of fibrous stroma. CCCs tend to encase the portal vein and the hepatic artery. In contrast to HCC, CCCs rarely show intravascular growth by tumor thrombus. Hilar CCCs

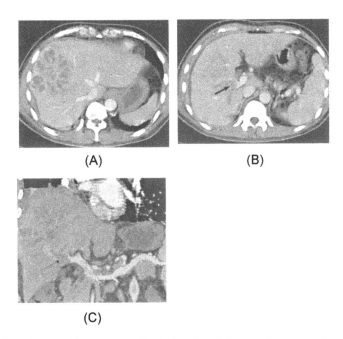

(A)   (B)

(C)

FIGURE 6   52-year-old woman with cholangiocellular carcinoma and portal vein invasion. (A) Portal venous scan shows the large hypodense cholangiocarcinoma. (B) Axial image (caudad of the previous) shows extension of the CCC into the right portal vein. (C) Curved planar reconstruction along the portal vein better delineates intravascular tumor growth (arrow).

tend to produce biliary dilatation more often than does HCC, which is often the first diagnostic hint of a CCC (Fig. 6). The high temporal resolution offered by MDCT can be used for thin collimation scanning in multiple planes for a better understanding of the individual pathology. Curved planar reconstructions along the right and left bile ducts and along the portal vein bifurcation may demonstrate the presence or absence of tumor infiltration much better than axial images alone. However, the additional diagnostic value of CPR has not been quantified in large series of CCC patients.

Benign Lesions

Small hemangiomas may rapidly achieve homogeneous enhancement during the arterial phase on CT scans, potentially simulating a vascular neoplasm. While hypervascular neoplasms demonstrate a washout of contrast material and become isoattenuating or hypoattenuating with liver parenchyma, hemangiomas retain contrast material and demonstrate enhancement matching that of vessels during the portal venous phase and on any additional equilibrial phase. Other benign lesions can also appear as enhancing foci during the arterial-dominant phase.

The most common lesions are FNH, which are very vascular and may not be seen on conventional CT scans. Now that MSCT allows the entire liver to be scanned during the arterial phase, detection of FNH has become more common. These lesions can be seen as homogeneously enhancing lesions with a characteristic central, branching, hypodense scar (Fig. 7). Small lesions, however, may not demonstrate a central scar and may appear homogeneously, simulating a hypervascular metastasis. The shorter acquisition times of MSCT allow imaging during periods of more intense enhancement, as well as more precise imaging during specific phases of

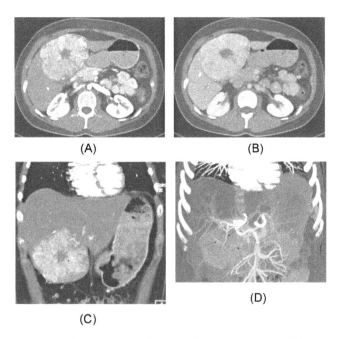

(A)   (B)

(D)

(C)

FIGURE 7   46-year-old woman with focal nodular hyperplasia. (A) Axial image in arterial phase shows marked FNH enhancement and the typical central scar. (B) There is rapid contrast material wash-out of the lesion in the portal-venous phase. Lesion is nearly isodense to background hepatic parenchyma. (C) Coronal MPR from arterial phase data set. Please note that image quality of coronal MRP is comparable to axial view. (D) Coronal maximum intensity projection demonstrates the arterial feeding vessels of the FNH (arrows).

enhancement. In addition, 3D reconstructions may provide valuable information about lesion extension and vascular supply in cases needing surgery.

LIVER TRANSPLANTATION

Preoperative Evaluation

Living donor-related liver transplantation is a relatively new development in liver transplantation, a response to the critical shortage of cadaveric organs. For pediatric recipients, usually the left lobe is donated. For adult-to-adult living donor transplantation, a right lobe donor hepatectomy is required to obtain a graft of adequate size for the recipient (59). Careful donor selection and thorough preoperative evaluation is necessary to avoid any donor risk, minimize complications, and to assure graft function. The role is to define when graft donation is contraindicated and to identify anatomical variations that may alter the surgical approach (60). The following anatomical features must be assessed during imaging evalutation of the donor organ (4,61):

1. Volume of the liver and of the right lobe: either hand tracing or automated tracing of the liver outline is performed on axial portal-venous phase images. The right lobe is usually of adequate size for the recipient, but it is also critical to assess the volume of the remaining left lobe (segments I–IV) to support the donor postoperatively.
2. Hepatic arterial anatomy: identification of the replaced or accessory right hepatic arteries may alter the surgical approach. Identification of the arterial supply to segment IV is of the utmost importance (62) (Fig. 8A-B.). Predominant arterial supply via the right hepatic artery may leave the donor without vascularization of segment IV postoperatively, which may lead to segmental atrophy of the donor liver, already markedly reduced in size by the surgical procedure.
3. Portal venous anatomy: venous anatomy is best displayed on coronal reformations of the portal-venous phase images. Surgically relevant variations include a separate origin for the right posterior portal vein and portal vein trifurcation (37)
4. Hepatic venous anatomy: special attention should be given to the presence of an accessory inferior right hepatic vein, which must be separately dissected during surgery. The hepatic veins are best visualized either in the axial plane or on curved planar reformations along their course (Fig. 8C)

5. Biliary anatomy: detection of anatomical variations of biliary
    anatomy is essential for donor evaluation, in particular where
    right intrahepatic ducts drain directly into the left hepatic duct.
    Either CT cholangiography after slow infusion of a biliary con-
    trast agent, endoscopic retrograde cholangiography, or MR cho-
    langiography may be used for this purpose.

Postoperative Complications

Hepatic artery stenosis and thrombosis are important complications in
liver transplantation. The incidence of such complications varies between

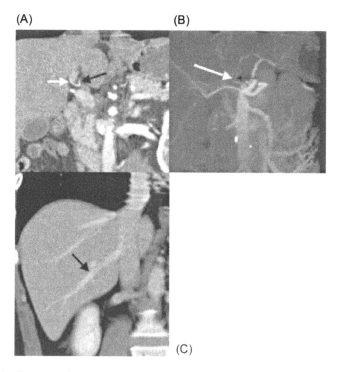

(A)   (B)

(C)

FIGURE 8   Preoperative evaluation of a living related right lobe liver donor: surgically relevant vascular variants. (A) Assessment of arterial supply to segment 4
is crucial: coronal MPR shows the left hepatic artery (black arrow) and a branch
supplying segment 4 (white arrow). (B) The maximum intensity projection better
demonstrates left hepatic artery to segment 2/3 (black arrow) and a branch to segment 4 (white arrow). (C) Curved coronal reconstruction along the right hepatic
vein shows right hepatic vein and an accessory inferior right hepatic vein (arrows),
which is large enough to be reanastomosed during right lobe transplantation

6% and 11% (63,64) and reduces 6-month survival to 70% (63). If diagnosed early in the postoperative period, surgical repair may be successful. Digital subtraction angiography (DSA) has served as the gold standard for diagnosis. However, the invasive nature of DSA makes it less attractive as a diagnostic tool in the early postoperative period. While color Doppler sonography has been proposed as an alternative means of detecting vascular complications, many authors have reported frequent false-negative sonographic exams, primarily due to flow-through collateral vessels after thrombosis of the hepatic artery. Hepatic arterial insufficiency may lead to biliary duct necrosis and stenosis since they have an exclusively arterial blood supply.

Multiphasic multislice CT allows, in a single examination, a comprehensive evaluation for both potential liver donors and graft recipients. 3D-CTA with maximum intensity projection, multiplanar reconstructions, shaded surface display, and volume rendering techniques has become a strong competitor for DSA. The development of MSCT allows scan times fast enough to image the liver during a pure arterial phase of contrast opacification, which offers the possibility of 3D CTA for a variety of clinical applications.

Some authors prefer an MIP technique, which projects the highest CT values of voxels encountered in a ray through the scan volume onto an image and provides excellent visualization of the relevant vessels (65). Volume-rendering and surface shaded displays are excellent tools for three-dimensional visualization of collaterals. With these tools, the spatial relationship of these vessels can be depicted (65). A problem with SSD and VR is that soft tissues surrounding the portal venous system and hypervas-cular organs, such as the pancreas and intestinal mucosa, are also markedly enhanced in this phase and may thus interfere with image interpretation and result in inferior image quality compared to MIP (65). Other authors prefer volume rendering because it utilizes the entire CT dataset to construct 3D images. In any event, whatever 3D visualization technique is chosen for demonstration purposes, thorough evaluation of the thin axial source images in cine mode remains the mainstay of diagnostic assessment. In addition, MSCT allows depiction of ischemia-related biliary compli-cations, such as bilomas and abscesses that would not be detectable with conventional angiography, and making MSCT a "one-stop-shop" for evaluation of these patients.

TRAUMA

Liver injury may occur in patients who sustain blunt abdominal trauma. Rapid deceleration, typically seen in motor vehicle accidents, may lead to

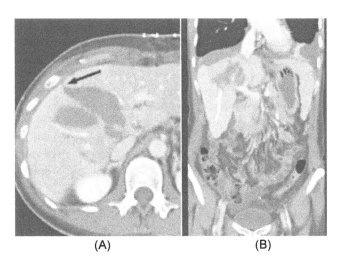

(A)   (B)

FIGURE 9   Liver laceration: 28-year-old woman after motorbike crash. (A). Post-contrast MSCT demonstrates a linear leaceration (arrow) of the capsule with a deep intraparenchymal hematoma. (B) On the coronal reconstruction the whole amount of laceration is better appreciated. Examination of the whole body reveals blood in the peritoneal cavity (white arrow).

parenchymal injury and even tears of the supporting ligaments. Acute laceration of the liver is considered a life-threatening condition, potentially resulting in severe blood loss and circulatory instability. Liver laceration is often part of the spectrum of injuries in polytrauma patients. Therefore, a rapid and reliable diagnostic procedure is mandatory to facilitate timely and appropriate therapy. The faster scanning and large volume coverage of MSCT help avoid motion-related artefacts while narrow collimation with improved spatial resolution enables a more detailed assessment of parenchymal organs and vessels than single-detector helical CT. In addition, MSCT allows three-dimensional visualization of liver laceration (Fig. 9) and permits quantification that is unattainable when only using axial slices. The important CT findings in liver injury are linear lacerations, which may follow the portal vein or hepatic vein branches, and subcapsular and intraparenchymal hematomas. The CT classification of liver injuries by Mirvis et al. (66) is based on the differentiation between superficial (less than 3 cm from the liver surface) and deep (more than 3 cm from the surface) lacerations.

Another major advantage of using MSCT for trauma cases is the ability to combine an arterial vascular phase of the thorax (when searching for traumatic aortic disruption) with a parenchymal phase examination of the abdomen. Even with a "high-speed" polytrauma protocol (e.g., 4×5 mm collimation, 6 mm slice thickness) from head to symphysis pubis, the high spatial resolution of MSCT enables improved detectabiliy of small lacerations in the hepatic parenchyma or vessel injury.

CONCLUSION

MSCT integrates the advantages of high scanning speed and high spatial resolution for liver imaging. The new generation of 16-row scanners represents a breakthrough toward isotropic resolution in routine clinical practice. This results in improved detection and characterization of focal liver lesions. Multiplanar display and advanced 3D reconstruction tools have a substantial value for liver CT. However, the dramatic increase in image data will require an innovative approach to image handling by the reporting radiologist and solutions to storage problems for selected data.

ACKNOWLEDGMENTS

The authors thank Dominique Sandner, RT, Silvia Kiss, RT, Gabriela Biechl, RT, Isabella Prohaska, RT, and Sylvia Unterhumer, RT, for their invaluable help in preparation of the 3D-image reconstructions.

REFERENCES

1. Oudkerk M, Torres CG, Song B, Konig M, Grimm J, Fernandez-Cuadro J, Op de Beeck B, Marquardt M, van Dijk P, de Groot JC. Characterization of liver lesions with mangafodipir trisodium-enhanced MR imaging: multicenter study comparing MR and dual-phase spiral CT. Radiology 2002; 223: 517–524.
2. Hori M, Murakami T, Kim T, Tsuda K, Takahashi S, Okada A, Takamura M, Nakamura H. Detection of hypervascular hepatocellular carcinoma: comparison of SPIO-enhanced MRI with dynamic helical CT. J Comput Assist Tomogr 2002; 26:701–710.
3. Weg N, Scheer MR, Gabor MP. Liver lesions: improved detection with dual-detector-array CT and routine 2.5-mm thin collimation. Radiology 1998; 209:417–426.
4. Schroeder T, Nadalin S, Stattaus J, Debatin JF, Malago M, Ruehm SG. Potential living liver donors: evaluation with an all-in-one protocol with multi-detector row CT. Radiology 2002; 224:586–591.
5. Ichikawa T, Kitamura T, Nakajima H, Sou H, Tsukamoto T, Ikenaga S, Araki T. Hypervascular hepatocellular carcinoma: can double arterial phase imaging

with multidetector CT improve tumor depiction in the cirrhotic liver? Am J Roentgenol 2002; 179:751–758.

6. Kalender W, Seissler W, Klotz E et al. Spiral volumetric CT with single-breath-hold technique, continuous transport and continuous scanner rotation Radiology 1989; 173(P):456.

7. Ohnesorge B, Flohr T, Schaller S, Klingenbeck-Regn K, Becker C, Schopf UJ, Bruning R, Reiser MF. The technical bases and uses of multi-slice CT. Radiologe 1999; 39:923–931.

8. Flohr T, Stierstorfer K, Bruder H, Simon J, Schaller S. New technical developments in multislice CT-Part 1: approaching isotropic resolution with sub-millimeter 16-slice scanning. Rofo Fortschr Geb Rontgenstr Neuen Bildgeb Verfahr, 2002; 174:839–845.

9. Wintersperger BJ, Helmberger TK, Herzog P, Jakobs TF, Waggershauser T, Becker CR, Reiser MF. New abdominal CT angiography protocol on a 16 detector-row CT scanner—first results. Radiologe 2002; 42:722–727.

10. Chambers TP, Baron RL, Lush RM. Hepatic CT enhancement. Part I. Alterations in the volume of contrast material within the same patients. Radiology 1994; 193:513–517.

11. Kopka L, Rodenwaldt J, Fischer U, Mueller DW, Oestmann JW, Grabbe E. Dual-phase helical CT of the liver: effects of bolus tracking and different volumes of contrast material. Radiology 1996; 201:321–326.

12. Silverman PM, Brown B, Wray H, Fox SH, Cooper C, Roberts S, Zeman RK. Optimal contrast enhancement of the liver using helical (spiral) CT: value of SmartPrep. Am J Roentgenol 1995; 164:1169–1171.

13. Kopka L, Funke M, Fischer U, Vosshenrich R, Oestmann JW, Grabbe E. Parenchymal liver enhancement with bolus-triggered helical CT: preliminary clinical results. Radiology 1995; 195:282–284.

14. Foley WD, Mallisee TA, Hohenwalter MD, Wilson CR, Quiroz FA, Taylor AJ. Multiphase hepatic CT with a multirow detector CT scanner. Am J Roentgenol 2000; 175:679–685.

15. Engeroff B, Kopka L, Harz C, Grabbe E. Impact of different iodine concentrations on abdominal enhancement in biphasic multislice helical CT. Rofo Fortschr Geb Rontgenstr Neuen Bildgeb Verfahr 2001; 173:938–941.

16. Awai K, Takada K, Onishi H, Hori S. Aortic and hepatic enhancement and tumor-to-liver contrast: analysis of the effect of different concentrations of contrast material at multi-detector row helical CT. Radiology 2002; 224:757–763.

17. Kulinna C, Helmberger T, Kessler M, Reiser M. Improvement in diagnosis of liver metastases with the multi-detector CT. Radiologe 2001; 41:16–23.

18. Murakami T, Kim T, Takahashi S, Nakamura H. Hepatocellular carcinoma: multidetector row helical CT. Abdom Imaging 2002; 27:139–146.

19. Bader TR, Grabenwoger F, Prokesch RW, Krause W. Measurement of hepatic perfusion with dynamic computed tomography: assessment of normal values and comparison of two methods to compensate for motion artifacts. Invest Radiol 2000; 35:539–547.

20. Kim T, Murakami T, Takahashi S, Tsuda K, Tomoda K, Narumi Y, Oi H, Nakamura H. Effects of injection rates of contrast material on arterial phase hepatic CT. Am J Roentgenol 1998; 171:429–432.

21. Tublin ME, Tessler FN, Cheng SL, Peters TL, McGovern PC. Effect of injection rate of contrast medium on pancreatic and hepatic helical CT. Radiology 1999; 210:97–101.

22. Kopka L, Rogalla P, Hamm B. Multislice CT of the abdomen—current indications and future trends. Rofo Fortschr Geb Rontgenstr Neuen Bildgeb Verfahr 2002; 174:273–282.

23. Oliver JH 3rd, Baron RL, Federle MP, Jones BC, Sheng R. Hypervascular liver metastases: do unenhanced and hepatic arterial phase CT images affect tumor detection? Radiology 1997; 205:709–715.

24. Kopka L, Rodenwaldt J, Hamm BK. Value of hepatic perfusion imaging for indirect detction of different liver lesions: feasibility study with multi-slice helical CT. Radiology 2000; 217(P):457.

25. Hwang GJ, Kim MJ, Yoo HS, Lee JT. Nodular hepatocellular carcinomas: detection with arterial-, portal-, and delayed-phase images at spiral CT. Radiology 1997; 202:383–388.

26. Lim JH, Choi D, Kim SH, Lee SJ, Lee WJ, Lim HK, Kim S. Detection of hepatocellular carcinoma: value of adding delayed phase imaging to dual-phase helical CT. Am J Roentgenol 2002; 179:67–73.

27. Choi BI, Lee HJ, Han JK, Choi DS, Seo JB, Han MC. Detection of hypervascular nodular hepatocellular carcinomas: value of triphasic helical CT compared with iodized-oil CT. Am J Roentgenol 1997; 168:219–224.

28. Merine D, Takayasu K, Wakao F. Detection of hepatocellular carcinoma: comparison of CT during arterial portography with CT after intraarterial injection of iodized oil. Radiology 1990; 175:707–710.

29. Yoshimatsu S, Inoue Y, Ibukuro K, Suzuki S. Hypovascular hepatocellular carcinoma undetected at angiography and CT with iodized oil. Radiology 1989; 171:343–347.

30. Ohashi I, Hanafusa K, Yoshida T. Small hepatocellular carcinomas: two-phase dynamic incremental CT in detection and evaluation. Radiology 1993; 18:851–855.

31. Hollett MD, Jeffrey RB Jr, Nino-Murcia M, Jorgensen MJ, Harris DP. Dual-phase helical CT of the liver: value of arterial phase scans in the detection of small (< or = 1.5 cm) malignant hepatic neoplasms. Am J Roentgenol 1995; 164:879–884.

32. Baron RL, Oliver JH 3rd, Dodd GD 3rd, Nalesnik M, Holbert BL, Carr B. Hepatocellular carcinoma: evaluation with biphasic, contrast-enhanced, helical CT. Radiology 1996; 199:505–511.

33. Kim T, Murakami T, Oi H, Matsushita M, Kishimoto H, Igarashi H, Nakamura H, Okamura J. Detection of hypervascular hepatocellular carcinoma by dynamic MRI and dynamic spiral CT. J Comput Assist Tomogr 1995; 19:948–954.

34. Rubin GD, Dake MD, Napel SA, McDonnell CH, Jeffrey RB Jr. Three-dimensional spiral CT angiography of the abdomen: initial clinical experience. Radiology 1993; 186:147–152.

35. Winter TC 3rd, Freeny PC, Nghiem HV, Hommeyer SC, Barr D, Croghan AM, Coldwell DM, Althaus SJ, Mack LA. Hepatic arterial anatomy in transplantation candidates: evaluation with three-dimensional CT arteriography. Radiology 1995; 195:363–370.

36. Raptopoulos V, Steer ML, Sheiman RG, Vrachliotis TG, Gougoutas CA, Movson JS. The use of helical CT and CT angiography to predict vascular involvement from pancreatic cancer: correlation with findings at surgery. Am J Roentgenol 1997; 168:971–977.

37. Kamel IR, Kruskal JB, Pomfret EA, Keogan MT, Warmbrand G, Raptopoulos V. Impact of multidetector CT on donor selection and surgical planning before living adult right lobe liver transplantation. Am J Roentgenol 2001; 176: 193–200.

38. Kopka L, Grabbe E. Biphasic liver diagnosis with multiplanar-detector spiral CT. Radiologe 1999; 39:971–978.

39. Basilico R, Filipone A, Ricciardi M, Iezzi A, Bonomo. Impact of slice thickness on the detction of liver lesions with multislice CT. Radiology 2000; 217(P):368.

40. Haider MA, Amitai MM, Rappaport DC, O'Malley ME, Hanbidge AE, Redston M, Lockwood GA, Gallinger S. Redston M, Lockwood GA, Gallinger S. Multi-detector row helical CT in preoperative assessment of small (< or = 1.5 cm) liver metastases: is thinner collimation better? Radiology 2002; 222:137–142.

41. Loos R, Oldendorf M, Deichen JT, Wucherer M. Multidetector CT: What to do with all the data?. Reiser MF, Takahashi M, Modic M, Bruening R, ed. Multislice CT. New York: Springer-Verlag, 2001:3–8.

42. Kamel IR, Raptopoulos V, Pomfret EA, Kruskal JB, Kane RA, Yam CS, Jenkins RL. Living adult right lobe liver transplantation: imaging before surgery with multidetector multiphase CT. Am J Roentgenol 2000; 175: 1141–1143.

43. Calhoun PS, Kuszyk BS, Heath DG, Carley JC, Fishman EK. Three-dimensional volume rendering of spiral CT data: theory and method. Radiographics 1999; 19:745–764.

44. Winkeltau G, Kraas E. Liver, malignancies. Schumpelick V, Bleese NM, Mommsen USurgery. Stuttgart: Enke, MVS, 1994:667–669.

45. Karhunen PJ. Benign hepatic tumours and tumour like conditions in men. J Clin Pathol 1986; 39:183–188.

46. Ishak KG. Benign tumors and pseudotumors of the liver. Appl Pathol 1988; 6:82–104.

47. Jones EC, Chezmar JL, Nelson RC, Bernardino ME. The frequency and significance of small (less than or equal to 15 mm) hepatic lesions detected by CT. Am J Roentgenol 1992; 158:535–539.

48. Schwartz LH, Gandras EJ, Colangelo SM, Ercolani MC, Panicek DM. Prevalence and importance of small hepatic lesions found at CT in patients with cancer. Radiology 1999; 210:71–74.
49. Seneterre E, Taourel P, Bouvier Y, Pradel J, Van Beers B, Daures JP, Pringot J, Mathieu D, Bruel JM. Detection of hepatic metastases: ferumoxides-enhanced MR imaging versus unenhanced MR imaging and CT during arterial portography. Radiology 1996; 200:785–792.
50. Ba-Ssalamah A, Heinz-Peer G, Schima W, Schibany N, Schick S, Prokesch RW, Kaider A, Teleky B, Wrba F, Lechner G. Detection of focal hepatic lesions: comparison of unenhanced and SHU 555 A-enhanced MR imaging versus biphasic helical CTAP. J Magn Reson Imaging 2000; 11:665–672.
51. Helmberger T, Gregor M, Holzknecht N, Rau H, Scheidler J, Reiser M. Effects of biphasic spiral CT, conventional and iron oxide enhanced MRI on therapy and therapy costs in patients with focal liver lesions. Rofo Fortschr Geb Rontgenstr Neuen Bildgeb Verfahr 2000; 172:251–259.
52. Kopka L, Rodenwaldt J, Kunz P, Grabbe E. Impact of different contrast material iodine concentrations on hepatic parenchymal enhancement in helical CT of the portal venous phase. Radiology 1998; 209(P):216.
53. Leuwert MS van, Nordzij J, Feldberg M, Hennipman AH, Doornewaard H. Focal liver lesions: characterisation with triphasic spiral CT. Radiology 1996; 201:327–336.
54. Oliver JH 3rd, Baron RL. Helical biphasic contrast-enhanced CT of the liver: technique, indications, interpretation, and pitfalls. Radiology 1996; 201:1–14.
55. Thoeni RF. Malignant focal liver lesions. In: Heuck A, ed. Abdominal and Pelvic MRI. New York: Springer-Verlag, 1998:34–49.
56. Kawata S, Murakami T, Kim T, Hori M, Federle MP, Kumano S, Sugihara E, Makino S, Nakamura H, Kudo M. Multidetector CT: diagnostic impact of slice thickness on detection of hypervascular hepatocellular carcinoma. Am J Roentgenol 2002; 179:61–66.
57. Zandrino F, Benzi L, Ferretti ML, Ferrando R, Reggiani G, Musante F. Multislice CT cholangiography without biliary contrast agent: technique and initial clinical results in the assessment of patients with biliary obstruction. Eur Radiol 2002; 12:1155–1161.
58. Soyer P, Bluemke DA, Reichle R, Calhoun PS, Bliss DF, Scherrer A, Fishman EK. Imaging of intrahepatic cholangiocarcinoma: 2. Hilar cholangiocarcinoma. Am J Roentgenol 1995; 165:1433–1436.
59. Marcos A, Olzinski AT, Ham JM, Fisher RA, Posner MP. The interrelationship between portal and arterial blood flow after adult to adult living donor liver transplantation. Transplantation 2000 27; 70:1697–1703.
60. Cheng YF, Huang TL, Lee TY, Chen TY, Chen CL. Overview of imaging in living related donor hepatic transplantation. Transplant Proc 1996; 28:2412–2414.
61. Ishifuro M, Horiguchi J, Nakashige A, Tamura A, Marukawa K, Fukuda H, Ono C, Akiyama Y, Kushima T, Ito K. Use of multidetector row CT with

volume renderings in right lobe living liver transplantation. Eur Radiol 2002; 12:2477–2483.

62. Krupski G, Rogiers X, Nicolas V, Berdien E, Maas R, Malago M, Broelsch CE, Bucheler E. The significance of the arterial vascular supply of segment IV in living liver donation. Rofo Fortschr Geb Rontgenstr Neuen Bildgeb Verfahr 1997; 167:32–36.

63. Langnas AN, Marujo W, Stratta RJ, Wood RP, Shaw BW Jr. Vascular complications after orthotopic liver transplantation. Am J Surg 1991; 161:76–82.

64. Wozney P, Zajko AB, Bron KM, Point S, Starzl TE. Vascular complications after liver transplantation: a 5-year experience. Am J Roentgenol 1986; 147:657–663.

65. Nakayama Y, Yamashita Y, Takahahi M. CT portography by multidetector row CT. Reiser MF, Takahashi M, Modic M, Bruening R, eds. Multislice CT. New York: Springer-Verlag, 2001:187–196.

66. Mirvis SE, Whitley NO, Vainwright JR, Gens DR. Blunt hepatic trauma in adults: CT-based classification and correlation with prognosis and treatment. Radiology 1989; 171:27–32.

6

Multislice CT Angiography of the Hepatic and Mesenteric Vasculature

Andrea Laghi, Riccardo Ferrari,
Franco Iafrate, Pasquale Paolantonio,
Michela Celestre, and
Roberto Passariello
University of Rome—"La Sapienza", Rome, Italy

INTRODUCTION

Computed tomographic angiography (CTA) is a valuable diagnostic modality for imaging the vascular system. CTA is a minimally invasive, safe, relatively comfortable and low-cost technique (1). Using dedicated scanning protocols, low-dose acquisitions can be obtained, minimizing the impact of radiation exposure (2). As a result, CTA provides a potential alternative to diagnostic conventional angiography.

The development of multislice spiral CT technology represents a significant advancement for CTA studies (3), particularly in the evaluation of splanchnic vessels (4–6). Multislice spiral CT involves acquisition times that are considerably faster than conventional single-slice spiral CT scanners enabling greater anatomical coverage and fewer misregistration and respiratory motion artifacts. Implementation of thin-slice collimation protocols increases spatial resolution along the longitudinal axis, providing virtually isotropic three-dimensional voxels. Consequently, image quality is improved with better diagnostic evaluation of small peripheral vascular

149

branches (7,8). Finally, use of intravenous contrast is more efficient due to more accurate timing and optimal separation between the arterial and portal venous phases.

In order to optimally exploit the benefits of using multislice CT, it is of paramount importance not only to optimize study protocols, but also to improve image display (9). This requires that three-dimensional datasets are reconstructed and interactively evaluated on dedicated workstations using axial and two-dimensional multiplanar images as well as more complex rendering techniques, such as maximum intensity projections (MIP), surface shaded displays (SSD), and volume rendering (10–12).

MULTISLICE CTA TECHNIQUE

Optimizing technique in order to acquire a three-dimensional dataset of high quality is critically important when attempting to evaluate the hepatic and mesenteric vasculature. The components of the examination include patient preparation, image acquisition, image reconstruction, three-dimensional reconstruction, and data analysis.

Patient Preparation

No specific patient preparation is required except for the standard pre-cautions (i.e., fasting) necessary for intravenous injection of an iodinated contrast medium. Before the study, patients receive 800 mL of water as an oral contrast agent in order to produce negative contrast in the stomach and small bowel. The use of a positive oral contrast agent creates difficulties when generating three-dimensional reconstructions and requires additional operator time for data segmentation to remove overlying high-density small bowel content.

Image Acquisition

Image acquisition parameters to be considered are longitudinal spatial resolution (depending on slice collimation, effective slice thickness, and pitch) and optimal timing of contrast medium injection (in order to acquire pure arterial and portal venous phases).

Contrast medium injection is generally performed using an automatic power injector. Adequate venous access is required since a fast flow rate is necessary to obtain adequate separation between the arterial and portal venous phases as well as optimal peak arterial enhancement. Slower flow rates impair optimal opacification of smaller arterial vessels due to inadequate intravascular concentration of contrast material. Usually 120–140 mL of nonionic iodinated contrast medium are infused intravenously at a flow rate of 4–5 mL/s into a peripheral (typically antecubital) vein. Following a test bolus injection of 20 mL of contrast medium, sequential dynamic slices are acquired at the level of the celiac trunk origin in order to assess the optimal delay. Two spiral CT scans of the abdomen and pelvis are obtained at the arterial phase (delay calculated based on bolus test injection) and portal venous phase (delay of 60–70 s). Depending on the type of scanner, optimal imaging parameters may differ. In our experience (5), using a four-slice multislice spiral CT scanner (Somatom Plus 4 Volume Zoom; Siemens, Erlangen, Germany) equipped with a flying focal spot, an adaptive array matrix, and a gantry rotation time of 0.5 s, images should be acquired using 1 mm slice collimation, 1–1.25 mm slice thickness, 6 mm/s table feed, 120 mAs, and 120 kVp. Breath-hold times range from 30 to 35 seconds, depending on the size of the patient. Patients are instructed to hyperventilate before scanning and to exhale slowly if they cannot suspend respiration for the entire examination time.

Image Reconstruction

Image reconstruction interval is another important factor that affects the quality of three-dimensional images. In principle, in order to obtain optimal image quality, a 20–40% overlap should be employed. This requires a reconstruction index of 0.6–0.8 mm. However, since the use of a sub-millimeter reconstruction thickness produces a considerable number of images (800–1000 images per scan per patient), it is sometimes beneficial to limit the image reconstruction interval to 1 mm with no image overlap in order to reduce the workload on the workstation. This will only minimally affect the quality of three-dimensional reconstructions.

Three-Dimensional Reconstructions and Data Analysis

Once acquired, images are downloaded to an off-line dedicated workstation in order to generate three-dimensional reconstructions. Three-dimensional data sets can be examined using different reconstruction techniques, starting with multiplanar reformations in three orthogonal axes and in oblique planes. Three-dimensional reconstructions can be obtained by using either maximum intensity projection (MIP) or surface-rendering or volume-rendering algorithms (Fig. 1). For better anatomical representation and evaluation of spatial relationships as well as faster and easier interaction with three-dimensional datasets, volume rendering is the preferred reconstruction algorithm, although the final diagnosis is derived using combined evaluation of source and reconstructed images. With volume rendering, selective vessel representation is obtained using different rendering curves. A panoramic overview of the entire major

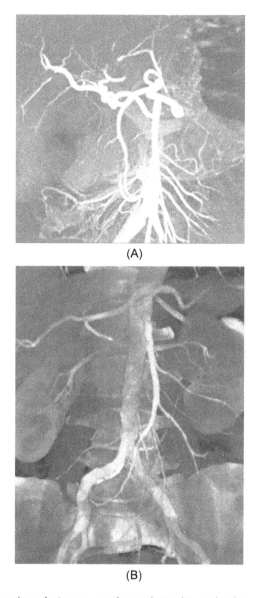

(A)

(B)

FIGURE 1   Comparison between maximum intensity projection (A) and volume-rendered (B) reconstructions of splanchnic vessels. On maximum intensity projection, detailed evaluation of thin peripheral branches is obtained, but with overlapping of vascular structures. Three-dimensional relationships among vessels are evident on volume-rendered reconstructed image.

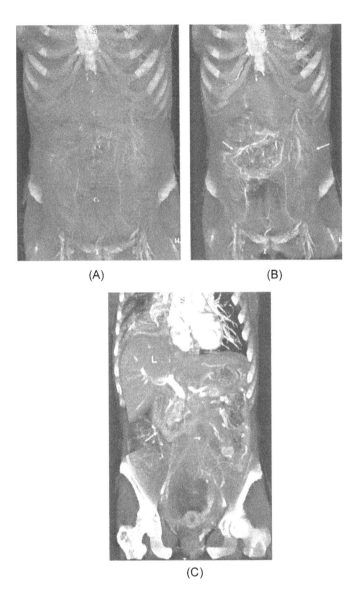

(A)   (B)

(C)

FIGURE 2 The use of interactive "cut planes" permits a virtual dissection of the body volume. On the surface view of the abdomen, (A) cutaneous plane is depicted with some superficial vessels observed in transparency. Coronal cut planes progressively open the body volume showing omental vessels (B) (arrows) and liver parenchyma (L) and duodenal lumen (C) (arrow).

abdominal branches can be obtained using a preset opacity curve showing only the vascular surface. Evaluation of minor vessels (i.e., second, third, and more distal orders of collateral branches) requires analysis of three-dimensional data sets using interactive multiplanar cut planes ("oblique

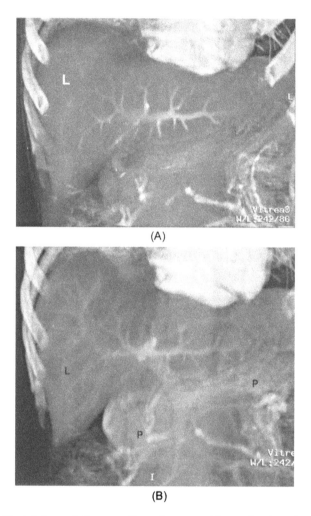

(A)

(B)

FIGURE 3   Modulation of the opacity values provides selective visualization of different anatomical structures. (A) Opacity curve showing liver parenchyma together with left branch of portal vein. (B) Increasing the transparency, the portal venous system, together with the liver and pancreas, are observed. L, liver; P, pancreas.

trim") (Fig. 2) as well as modulation of the opacity of anatomical structures under evaluation and alterations in window width and level parameters in order to see vessels "through" abdominal organs (Fig. 3). Image analysis, therefore, requires direct operator interpretation at the workstation where two-dimensional axial, multiplanar reconstructions, and three-dimensional images are simultaneously available. In this manner a complete analysis of arterial and venous vessels can be obtained within a mean interpretation time of 20 minutes.

HEPATIC AND MESENTERIC VESSELS:
ANATOMY AND VARIANTS

Arterial Vascular System

The celiac trunk and main arterial branches (common hepatic, left gastric, and splenic arteries) are routinely identified at CTA (Fig. 4) as well as intrahepatic vessels up to tertiary order branches as small as 1 mm in diameter. In particular, the artery to segment IV, an important anatomical landmark before liver transplantation from a living liver donor, is clearly depicted (Fig. 5). In a recent study, major arterial trunks (celiac, hepatic, superior mesenteric, and left gastric) were depicted in all cases. Visualization of small arteries was as follows: right and left hepatic, 62 (100%) of 62; middle hepatic, 52 (87%) of 60; cystic, 47 (90%) of 52; right gastric, 50 (89%) of 56; and right and left inferior phrenic, 57 (92%) and 55 (89%) of 62, respectively (13).

Arterial anomalies (the right hepatic artery arising from either the superior mesenteric artery or the abdominal aorta; the left hepatic artery arising from the left gastric artery; the left gastric artery arising as a separate branch of the abdominal aorta; a common origin of the celiac and superior mesenteric arteries) are easily evaluated on high-resolution CT angiography images (Figs. 6,7).

The superior mesenteric artery (SMA) is usually identified in its entirety, including its origin and major branches (Fig. 8). The SMA usually arises less than 1.5 cm below the origin of the celiac trunk. Major collateral branches are represented by (a) the inferior pancreatico-duodenal artery (Fig. 9), which may arise either from the right or left side of the SMA, and has an oblique course anastomosing superiorly with the superior pancreatico-duodenal artery, a branch of the gastro-duodenal artery; (b) the right and middle colic arteries, with the latter absent in up to 80% of normal individuals, supplying blood to the ascending colon; (c) the jejunal branches (Fig. 10), arising from the left side of the SMA; and (d) the

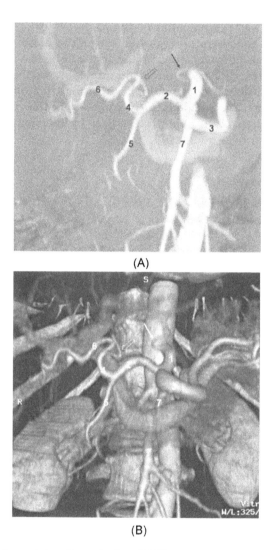

(A)

(B)

FIGURE 4 Maximum intensity projection (MIP) and volume-rendering reconstruction of the celiac trunk. (A) On MIP image, a panoramic overview of the arterial vessels is provided, but three-dimensional spatial relationships are missing. (B) On volume-rendered three-dimensional image, using high opacity values with surface representation of vessels, the use of virtual lighting and shading provides a better three-dimensional evaluation of the spatial relationships among different arteries. Celiac trunk (1); common hepatic artery (2); splenic artery (3); hepatic artery (4); gastroduodenal artery (5); right hepatic artery (6); superior mesenteric artery (7). Left hepatic artery (open arrow); left gastric artery (black arrow).

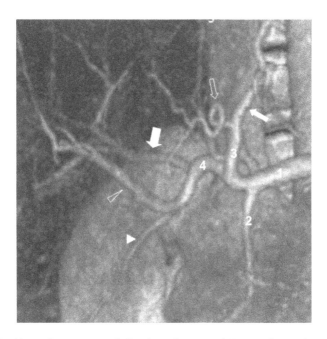

FIGURE 5 Normal anatomy of the hepatic vasculature using volume-rendered three-dimensional surface reconstruction. Three-dimensional image shows common hepatic artery (1), gastroduodenal artery (2), left (3) hepatic artery with branch to segments II and III (arrow), as well as intrahepatic segmentary branch to segment IV (open arrow). Right hepatic artery (4) with intrahepatic branches to segments VI (arrowhead), VII (open arrowhead), and VIII (large white arrow) are also depicted.

ileo-colic artery and ileal branches, arising from the right side of the SMA, supplying blood to the ileum and cecum.

The high resolution of multislice CT angiography also allows for the identification of the marginal arteries of Dwight and Drummond, which supply the vasa recta to the small intestine and colon and provide a continuous channel of potential collateral blood supply to the entire gut (14,15). The marginal artery is defined as the artery closest to and parallel with the wall of the intestine supplying the vasa recta. The vasa recta are fine branches that arise from the marginal artery and supply the bowel wall (Fig. 11).

The inferior mesenteric artery (IMA), which arises from the left side of the aorta around 7 cm below the origin of the SMA, can be visualized together with its major branches: (a) the left colic artery, which has a straight superior course, supplying the transverse and descending colon; by anastomosing with the middle colic artery, it provides a communication

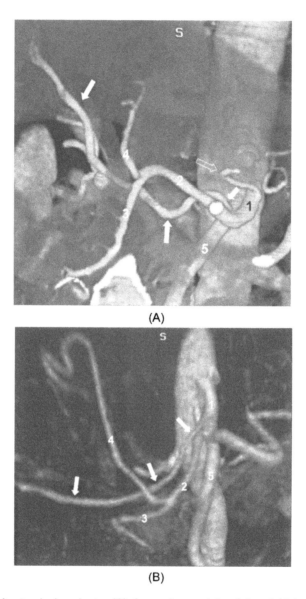

(A)

(B)

FIGURE 6 Anatomical variants. (A) Anomalous origin of the right hepatic artery
(white arrows) from the superior mesenteric artery. (B) Right hepatic artery (white
arrows) originating from the celiac trunk. Celiac trunk (1); common hepatic artery
(2); gastroduodenal artery (3); left hepatic artery (4); superior mesenteric artery
(5); left gastric artery (open arrow).

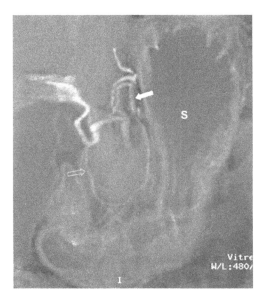

FIGURE 7   Gastric arcade as a result of the anastomosis between the left (arrow) and right (open arrow) gastric arteries. Volume rendering allows the visualization of soft tissue density structures, like the stomach (S), together with arterial vessels.

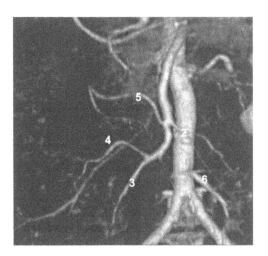

FIGURE 8   Volume-rendered surface reconstruction of the superior mesenteric artery (1) with major collaterals: jejunal branches (2); terminal ileal branch (3); ileocolic artery (4); and right colic artery (5). The origin of the inferior mesenteric artery (6) is also noted.

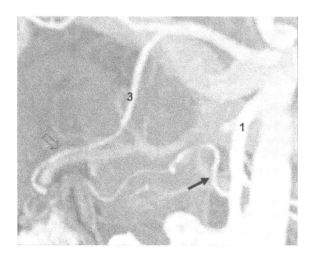

FIGURE 9   Maximum intensity projection reconstruction of the inferior pancreatico-duodenal artery (arrow), the first branch of the superior mesenteric artery (1). The inferior pancreatico-duodenal artery has an oblique course, anastomosing superiorly with the superior pancreatico-duodenal artery (open arrow), a branch of the gastro-duodenal artery (3).

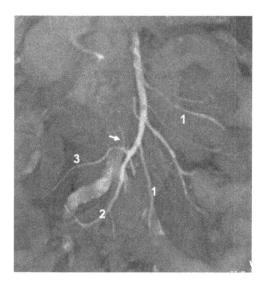

FIGURE 10   Detailed view of jejunal and ileal arteries (1), with terminal ileal branch (2) and ileocolic artery (3). The origin of the right colic artery from the ileocolic artery is also noted (arrow).

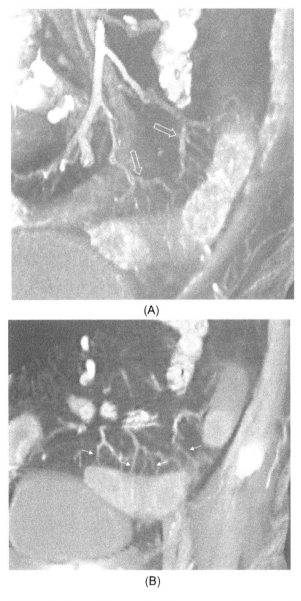

(A)

(B)

FIGURE 11 (A) Arterial vascular arcade (open arrows) of the sigmoid colon with vasa recta (small arrows) feeding the bowel wall. (B) On coronal oblique thick multiplanar image reconstruction, the vasa recta (small arrows) are better appreciated.

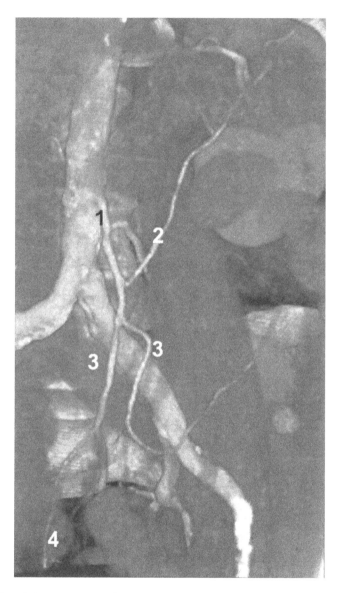

FIGURE 12   Inferior mesenteric artery (1) with major collateral branches: the left colic artery (2), which has a straight superior course, supplying the transverse and descending colon; the sigmoid arteries (3); two to four vessels supplying the sigmoid colon; and the superior hemorrhoidal artery (4), the terminal branch for the upper rectum.

between the SMA and IMA vascular systems and when absent its function is performed by the sigmoid arteries; (b) the sigmoid arteries, two to four vessels supplying the sigmoid colon; and (c) the superior hemorrhoidal (rectal) artery, the terminal branch supplying the upper rectum (Fig. 12).

Venous Vascular System

All major venous vessels (portal vein, splenic vein, superior mesenteric vein, and inferior mesenteric vein) and collateral branches can be accurately depicted using CTA. The major technical problem when evaluating the venous system is in discerning small arteries from veins, both of which are opacified on delayed images. Correct image analysis requires additional interpretation time on the workstation.

The portal vein is usually visualized along its entire course with demonstration down to the level of intrahepatic segmentary branches

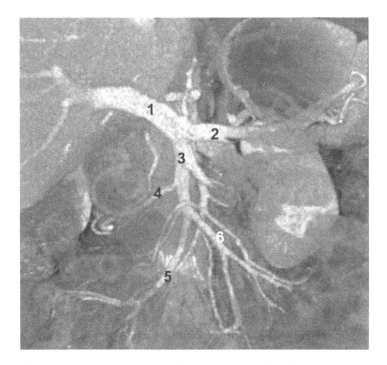

FIGURE 13 Portal venous system. The portal vein (1) with its oblique course is entirely depicted, together with the splenic vein (2) and the superior mesenteric vein (3). Major collaterals of the superior mesenteric vein are shown: right colic (4); ileocolic (5); and intestinal (6) veins.

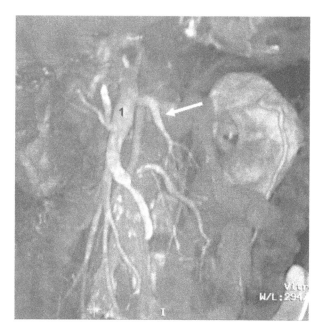

Figure 14   Inferior mesenteric vein (arrow) joining the superior mesenteric vein (1).

(Fig. 13). A clear depiction of the portal venous bifurcation is usually obtained allowing evaluation of the presence of vascular anomalies (i.e., portal trifurcation).

The SMV is usually a single trunk, receiving blood from the middle and right colic veins, the ileocolic vein, the gastrocolic vein, and from the jejunal and ileal branches. The IMV receives blood from the left colic vein, the sigmoid veins and the superior hemorrhoidal vein; it can terminate at the splenic vein or at the splenoportal angle or may drain into the SMV (Fig. 14) (16).

IMAGING FINDINGS IN PATHOLOGICAL CONDITIONS

Hepatic Vessels

Assessment of the hepatic vasculature is extremely useful in order to plan both interventional vascular procedures and surgical operations. For instance a vascular "road-map" showing major arterial vessels to hypervascular hepatic lesions may guide the interventional radiologist in planning chemoembolization therapy (Fig. 15) while demonstration of hepatic and portal venous segmentary branches may help the surgeon prior to a hepatic

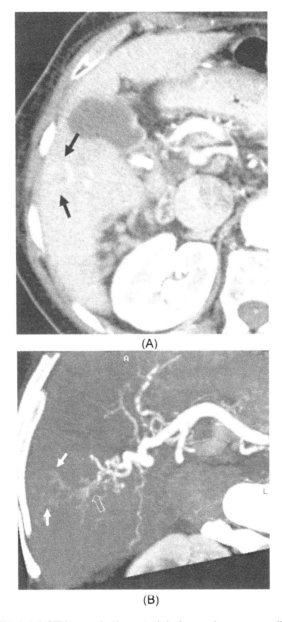

(A)

(B)

FIGURE 15   (A) Axial CT image in the arterial phase shows a small hypervascular hepatocarcinoma (arrows). (B) Axial maximum intensity projection demonstrates tumoral arterial vessels with typical "basket pattern" (arrows), supplied by a branch of the artery of segment V (open arrow).

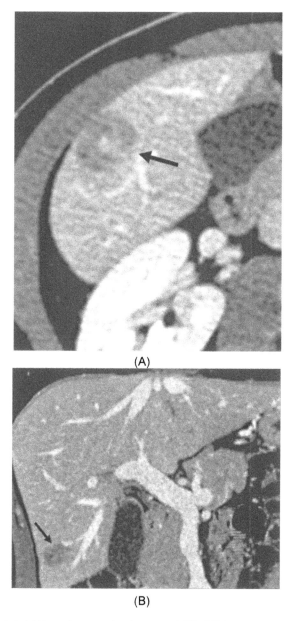

(A)

(B)

FIGURE 16 Axial (A) and coronal reformatted (B) CT images showing a hepatic metastasis (arrow) located in segment VI. MIP-reconstructed (C) vascular image of the portal vein and hepatic vessels demonstrates vascular relationship, which helps to plan the surgical approach (1, right hepatic vein).

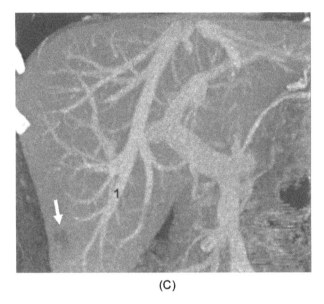

(C)

FIGURE 16   (continued)

resection (Fig. 16). Portal cavernomatous transformation (Fig. 17) following occlusion of the main portal trunk may be demonstrated in cirrhotic patients as well as esophago-gastric, omental, and spleno-renal collateral vessels.

Mesenteric Vessels

Pathological conditions where evaluation of mesenteric vessel involvement is required include pancreatic cancer, mesenteric ischemia, and inflammatory diseases affecting the small and large bowel.

In the case of pancreatic cancer, infiltration of the SMA is a known contraindication to surgery (17). It has been demonstrated that simultaneous evaluation of axial and multiplanar reformatted planes is useful for assessing vascular invasion and that sagittal planes in particular provide excellent evaluation of the posterior fat plane between the SMA and the abdominal aorta, which is especially useful in excluding vascular encasement (18,19) (Fig. 18). Precise evaluation of the SMV and the portal vein is also extremely important as venous infiltration of less than 2 cm is one criterion for performing pancreatic surgery in combination with a vascular graft. Again, multiplanar reformatted images, in this case along

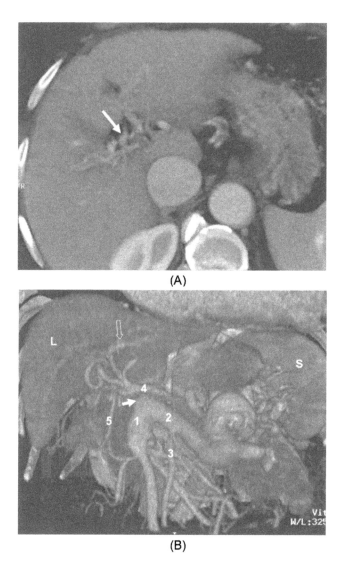

(A)

(B)

FIGURE 17   Portal occlusion with cavernous transformation. (A) The axial thick slab shows dilatation of vasa vasorum (arrow), typical of cavernous portal transformation. (B) Volume-rendered reconstruction shows portal occlusion at the spleno-mesenteric confluence (arrow) as well as partial patency of the left branch (open arrow). Superior mesenteric vein (1), splenic vein (2), inferior mesenteric vein (3), hepatic artery (4), gastroduodenal artery (5), liver (L) and spleen (S).

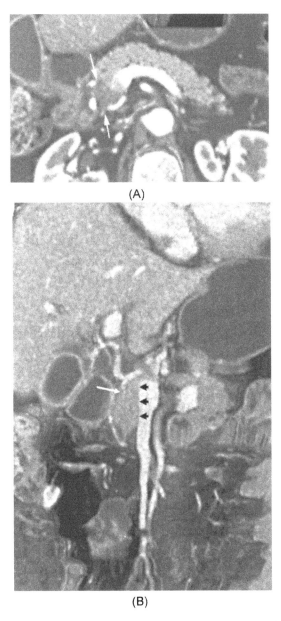

(A)

(B)

FIGURE 18 (A) Axial CT image in the pancreatic phase demonstrates a hypodense mass lesion, referred to as a pancreatic head carcinoma (arrows). (B) On the coronal reformatted image, the mass lesion is shown infiltrating the gastroduodenal artery (arrow) as well as the aortal vein (arrowheads).

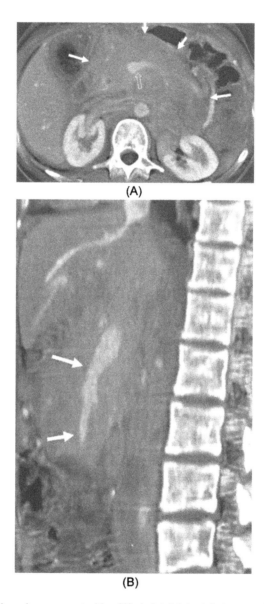

(A)

(B)

FIGURE 19   Sclerosing mesenteritis. (A) Axial thick-slab image demonstrates an infiltrating mass (arrows) encasing the mesenteric vein (open arrow) and its branches. Significant small bowel thickening is also noted. (B) Encasement of the vessels by the mass (arrows) is better demonstrated on sagittal reformatted image. (C) Maximum intensity projection image provides a panoramic overview of omental collateral vessels.

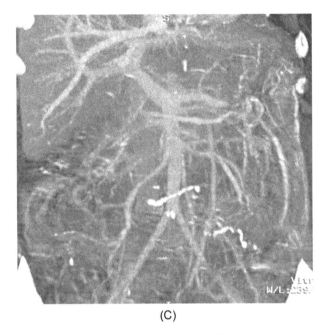

(C)

FIGURE 19   (continued)

the coronal or coronal oblique planes, provide excellent evaluation of possible vascular infiltration.

In the case of mesenteric ischemia, multislice spiral CT angiography may provide all the diagnostic information necessary for treatment planning. Multislice spiral CT angiography is useful in demonstrating the various causes of ischemia including narrowing or occlusion of the SMA due to either atherosclerotic plaque or thrombus or neoplastic vascular occlusion due to either thrombosis or neoplastic encasement of the SMV (17).

Finally, multislice spiral CTA may have a role in the assessment of vascular changes related to inflammatory bowel disease, small bowel tumors (i.e., carcinoid, lymphoma), and less common pathological conditions (i.e., metastases, sclerosing mesenteritis, etc.) (Fig. 19).

CONCLUSION

Because of its greatly enhanced image resolution, multislice CTA is capable of overcoming the technical challenges of depicting small mesenteric vessels, providing a detailed anatomical view similar to digital subtraction angiography, but with the added advantages provided by image postprocessing. Image postprocessing is an essential part of the technique and should be performed interactively by the operator at a dedicated workstation using several reconstruction algorithms (20). Because of its ability to display the 3D spatial relationships between vessels and surrounding organs, volume-rendering is the most appropriate algorithm for managing volumetric datasets. The clinical applications of volume-rendered three-dimensional vascular maps include cancer staging, surgical planning, and evaluating patients with suspected mesenteric ischemia (14). More widespread use of this technique can be expected in the near future with the greater availability of multislice CT technology, improvements in workstation design and performance, and specific education of radiologists in the use of dedicated computer software. A cost-benefit analysis is required in order to better understand the impact of this new imaging modality on patient management and outcomes.

REFERENCES

1. Rubin GD, Shiau MA, Schmidt AJ, et al. Computed tomographic angiography: historical perspective and new state-of-the-art using multi detector-row helical computed tomography. J Comput Assist Tomogr 1999; 23(S1): S83–S90.
2. van Gelder RE, Venema HW, Serlie IW, Nio CY, Determann RM, Tipker CA, Vos FM, Glas AS, Bartelsman JF, Bossuyt PM, Lameris JS, Stoker J. CT colonography at different radiation dose levels: feasibility of dose reduction. Radiology 2002; 224(1):25–33.
3. Rubin GD, Shiau MC, Kee ST, Logan LJ, Sofilos MC. Aorta and iliac arteries: single versus multiple detector-row helical CT angiography. Radiology 2000; 215:670–676.
4. Horton KM, Fishman EK. Volume-rendered 3D CT of the mesenteric vasculature: normal anatomy, anatomic variants and pathologic conditions. Radiographics 2002; 22:161–172.
5. Laghi A, Iannaccone R, Catalano C, Passariello R. Multislice spiral computed tomography angiography of mesenteric arteries. Lancet 2001; 358:638–639.
6. Johnson PT, Heath DG, Kuszyk BS, Fishman EK. CT angiography with volume rendering: advantages and applications in splanchnic vascular imaging. Radiology 1996; 200:564–568.
7. Hu H, He HD, Foley WD, Fox SH. Four multidetector-row helical CT: image quality and volume coverage speed. Radiology 2000; 215:55–62.
8. McCollough CH, Zink FE. Performance evaluation of a multi-slice CT system. Med Phys 1999; 26:2223–2230.
9. Rubin GD. Data explosion: the challenge of multi detector-row CT. Eur J Radiol 2000; 36:74–80.

10. Heath DG, Soyer PA, Kuszyk BS, et al. Three-dimensional spiral CT during arterial portography: comparison of 3D rendering techniques. Radiographics 1995; 15:1001–1011.

11. Kuszyk BS, Heath DG, Ney DR, et al. CT angiography with volume rendering: imaging findings. AJR 1995; 165:445–448.

12. Hong KC, Freeny PC. Pancreaticoduodenal arcades and dorsal pancreatic artery: comparison of CT angiography with three-dimensional volume rendering, maximum intensity projection, and shaded-surface display. AJR 1999; 172:925–931.

13. Takahashi S, Murakami T, Takamura M, Kim T, Hori M, Narumi Y, Nakamura H, Kudo M. Multidetector row helical CT angiography of hepatic vessels: depiction with dual-arterial phase acquisition during slicw breath hold. Radiology 2002; 222:81–88.

14. Horton KM, Fishman EK. Volume-rendered 3D CT of the mesenteric vasculature: normal anatomy, anatomic variants and pathologic conditions. Radiographics 2002; 22:161–172.

15. Lin PH, Chaikof EL. Embryology, anatomy and surgical exposure of the great abdominal vessels. Surg Clin North Am 2000; 80:417–433.

16. Graf O, Boland GW, Kaufman JA, Warshaw AL, Fernandez-del-Castillo C, Mueller PR. Anatomic variants of mesenteric veins: depiction with helical CT venography. AJR Am J Roentgenol 1997; 168:1209–1213.

17. Raptopoulos V, Steer ML, Sheiman RG, Vrachliotis TG, Gougoutas CA, Movson JS. The use of helical CT and CT angiography to predict vascular involvement from pancreatic cancer: correlation with findings at surgery. AJR 1997; 168:971–977.

18. Laghi A, Iannaccone R, Catalano C, Carbone I, Sansoni I, Mangiapane F, Passariello R. Multislice spiral computer tomography in diagnosis and staging of pancreatic carcinoma: preliminary experience. Digest Liver Dis 2002; 34:732–738.

19. Procacci C, Biasiutti C, Carbognin G, Bicego E, Graziani R, Franzoso F, Pesci A, Megibow AJ. Spiral computer tomography assesment of resectability of pancreatic ductal adenocarcinoma: analysis of result. Digest Liver Dis 2002; 34:739–747.

20. Fishman EK. CT Angiography: clinical applications in the abdomen. Radiographics 2001; (900001)S3–16.

7

Positron Emission Tomography of the Gastrointestinal Tract

Stephen J. Skehan

St Vincent's University Hospital, Dublin, Ireland

INTRODUCTION

Positron emission tomography (PET) has progressed over the last 15 years from a research tool to a routine clinical investigation. It is now available in many centers, and some knowledge of its technique and applications is important for physicians who deal with diseases of the gastrointestinal (GI) tract. Current clinical applications of PET relate mostly to the management of patients with malignant disease, and this chapter will discuss GI cancer applications of PET in detail. Although much evidence has been produced to support the use of PET in GI malignancies, important questions still remain regarding its exact role, and these will also be explored. In addition to its use in oncology, PET may also be used to assess bowel inflammation. The advantages and disadvantages of the technique for this application will be discussed. The chapter will begin with a brief description of the physical and biological principles that underlie the use of PET, and throughout the chapter the relative and complementary roles of PET and "traditional" anatomical imaging will be emphasized.

BASIC PHYSICS AND BIOLOGY OF PET

PET is similar to single photon radionuclide techniques such as bone scinti-graphy in that a radioactive tracer is injected into the patient and an image of tracer distribution within the patient is subsequently generated by detection of emitted radiation. However, the physics of tracer localization are significantly different from single photon radionuclide imaging. A positron-emitting isotope, such as fluorine-18, decays by emission of a positron, which is a tiny particle with the same mass as an electron but the opposite charge. When a positron is emitted, it travels a very short distance in tissue (approximately 1 mm) before it combines with an electron. The two particles annihilate each other and their mass is converted to energy in the form of two 511 KeV gamma rays that travel in diametrically opposed directions. Detection of each positron emission occurs by the simultaneous detection of these two gamma rays by detectors placed in a ring around the patient. The imaging computer draws an imaginary "line of response" between the two detectors that register a simultaneous event. Standard reconstruction techniques such as filtered back projection or iterative reconstruction are then used to transform many thousands of these lines of response into a three-dimensional image of the tracer distribution within the patient.

Unlike single photon imaging, localization of activity with PET relies on accurate temporal resolution of detected photons (a window of the order of 10 ns is used to determine "coincidence") rather than the use of a lead collimator to filter out scattered activity. Avoidance of the need for collimation results in greater sensitivity for photon detection and therefore an improved signal-to-noise ratio for PET compared with single photon imaging. The spatial resolution of PET is approximately 4 mm, which is also better than single photon scintigraphy. Evolution of detector crystals and associated electronics has resulted in greater temporal resolution and greater sensitivity, with shorter scan times.

Another advantage of PET over single photon emission computed tomography (SPECT) is the relative ease with which attenuation correction can be performed. This technique uses an external radiation source to obtain a transmission (rather than emission) image of the patient. These data are used to map the tissue attenuation of emitted photons arising from different depths and different organs within the patient, so that appropriate corrections can be made to the final image to give a true representation of tracer distribution in the patient.

The main positron emitting isotopes in clinical use are (half-life in brackets) ^{15}O (2 min), ^{13}N (10 min), ^{11}C (20 min), and ^{18}F (110 min). They are produced in a particle accelerator known as a cyclotron. The chemistry of ^{18}F is such that it frequently substitutes for hydrogen. Indeed one of the major advantages of these tracers over single photon tracers such as ^{99m}Tc is that they occur naturally in almost all biological molecules. Therefore, rapid radiochemistry techniques allow the synthesis of a wide range of naturally occurring tracers that are handled by the body in exactly the same way as the nonradioactive molecule. The short half-life of the tracers is advantageous in reducing the effective dose to the patient, but it creates practical problems for the synthesis and subsequent distribution of PET radiopharmaceuticals. For practical purposes, ^{18}F is the only tracer that can be used when the cyclotron is not in the same facility as the PET scanner. Fortunately ^{18}F is the isotope with the most widespread applications in clinical imaging.

^{18}F-Fluoro-deoxyglucose (FDG) is a glucose analogue that is readily synthesized from ^{18}F. It is the workhorse radiopharmaceutical of oncology imaging with PET. Malignant cells accumulate glucose and FDG more avidly than normal cells, predominantly because of increased expression of cell surface glucose transporters (1,2). Malignant cells also make more efficient use of this excess glucose in the glycolytic pathway by virtue of increased intracellular hexokinase production (1). Unlike glucose, however, FDG is not metabolized by hexokinase so it remains trapped in the malignant cell. This is the basis of oncology imaging with FDG—malignant cells accumulate more of the tracer than normal cells.

Assessment of oncology patients with anatomical imaging techniques such as computed tomography (CT) or magnetic resonance (MR) relies on distortion of normal anatomy, the presence of abnormal masses, and a change in structure over time. Any of these abnormalities may be seen in an oncology patient who has been successfully treated, making posttreatment evaluation difficult. Similarly, detection of disease in enlarged lymph nodes is based on the statistical probability of nodes that are greater than a certain size containing malignant rather than reactive cells. This is not a foolproof technique in that malignant cells can be found in nodes that are invisible or barely visible on CT, while reactive nodes measuring greater than 1 cm in diameter are a frequent finding. By detecting malignant disease because of its altered biology regardless of the presence or absence of anatomical alteration, PET provides an extremely useful alternative assessment of disease status.

SCAN TECHNIQUE

Patient preparation for PET is relatively straightforward. Patients fast for 4–6 hours prior to tracer injection in order to avoid high plasma glucose levels. This has been shown to increase tracer uptake in tumors, particularly pancreatic cancers, although the effect is not very marked for other tumors (3,4). A small dose of an anxiolytic, such as diazepam 5 mg administered orally 30 minutes prior to injection, is helpful to reduce artefact from skeletal muscle uptake. This can be particularly troublesome in the neck. FDG is administered intravenously with the patient sitting or lying in a quiet room. The typical dose is 370 MBq, which results in an effective dose of 5–10 mSv. Frusemide 20 mg administered intravenously just before the FDG injection results in useful clearance of activity from the kidneys and ureters in addition to dilution of bladder activity. With this protocol it is rarely necessary to insert a urinary catheter, except occasionally for subtle abnormalities located very close to the bladder (5). Bowel cleansing is not necessary. Image acquisition begins 45–60 minutes postinjection of FDG and takes approximately 30–60 minutes depending on the type of scanner and the area to be scanned. A typical "whole body" study includes images from skull base to upper thighs.

Images should be reviewed on a workstation and correlated with anatomical imaging. The latest PET scanners combine a full ring of detectors with multislice CT on the same platform. The CT study is acquired first in the usual way, followed by the PET study. The major advantage of this is automatic registration of functional (PET) images with anatomical (CT) images. The CT study can also be used to provide a map for attenuation correction, avoiding the need for additional transmission images. Care must be taken during the CT part of the study to acquire images during quiet free breathing in order to minimize misregistration (6).

Normal FDG uptake may be seen in stomach, colon, stomas (Fig. 1), kidneys, ureters, bladder, and recent laparotomy wounds (7). Case reports of abnormal pelvic activity due to the menstruating retroverted uterus and pelvic kidneys have also been published (8,9).

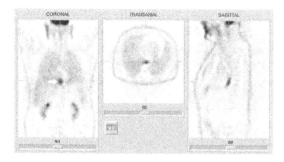

FIGURE 1   FDG PET image. Primary esophageal tumor (arrow) seen in all three orthogonal planes. Normal renal activity is visible bilaterally.

ESOPHAGEAL CANCER

Diagnosis of Primary Cancer

FOCAL, intense tracer accumulation is the hallmark of primary esophageal cancer with PET (Fig. 1). The sensitivity of FDG PET for diagnosis of esophageal cancer is between 94 and 100% (10–14). These figures are based on studies of patients with known esophageal malignancy, so no data are available for specificity. The ability of FDG PET to differentiate between benign and malignant lesions of the esophagus has not been evaluated. It is unlikely that this would be useful since histological diagnosis is essential and is also readily obtained with minimal risk to the patient (15,16). The normal stomach and esophagus may demonstrate mildly increased tracer uptake relative to background activity (Fig. 2). Inflammation in the stomach may be associated with a significant increase in tracer uptake, which can mimic malignancy (17). Moderately increased tracer uptake has been described with Barrett's esophagus, but this tends to be less prominent than any associated malignancy (18). The limited spatial resolution of FDG PET (approximately 5 mm) means that it cannot be used to assess the depth of invasion of the primary tumor unlike endoscopic ultrasound.

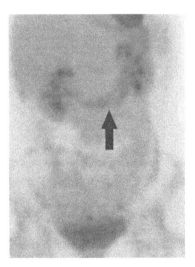

FIGURE 2 Anterior maximum intensity projection FDG PET image. Normal gastric activity in the body of the stomach (arrow). Bilateral renal activity is projected over the fundus and duodenum, and normal myocardial uptake is seen at the top of the image.

Local Nodal Staging

The accuracy of FDG PET for local nodal staging in esophageal cancer varies widely in the published literature. Accuracy figures range from 24 to 90% for PET compared with 40 to 78% for CT in the same patient groups (10–12,19–21). Three published studies were performed prospectively and used a uniform histological gold standard (14,20,21). Choi et al. prospectively evaluated 48 patients who underwent FDG PET and CT prior to esophagectomy and lymph node dissection (20). Endoscopic ultrasound was performed in 45 of the patients, but was unsuccessful in 12 due to esophageal stenosis, an important limitation of this technique. For assessing metastasis to individual nodal groups, FDG PET showed 57% sensitivity, 97% specificity, and 86% accuracy, whereas CT showed 18% sensitivity ($p < 0.0001$), 99% specificity ($p = 0.033$), and 78% accuracy ($p = 0.003$). However, for overall N staging, FDG PET was correct in 83% (40/48) of the patients, whereas CT and endoscopic ultrasound were correct in 60% (29/48; $p = 0.006$) and 58% (26/45; $p = 0.003$), respectively. Kim et al. prospectively studied 50 patients with esophageal cancer using PET and CT (14). Sensitivity and specificity of PET for detecting involved nodal groups were 51.9% and 94.2%, respectively, compared with 14.8% and 96.7% for CT. In Lerut's study FDG PET had a lower accuracy (48%) than combined CT and endoscopic ultrasound (69%) due to a significant lack of sensitivity (21). The limited sensitivity of PET is likely explained by the spatial resolution of the technique, which makes identification of small malignant nodes adjacent to the primary tumor difficult if not impossible in some cases (Fig. 3). In a retrospective study of 29 patients who underwent curative esophagectomy, PET and CT accurately revealed the extent

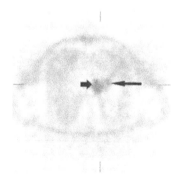

FIGURE 3 Axial FDG PET image. Esophageal primary tumor (short arrow) is not clearly distinguishable from adjacent involved lymph node (long arrow) due to limited spatial resolution.

of nodal disease in 76% (22/29) and 45% (13/29) of patients, respectively (10). In another recent retrospective study of 24 patients with esophageal cancer, there was no significant difference between CT and PET for local nodal staging, although a histological gold standard was not applied uniformly in this study (22).

The best available evidence therefore offers conflicting information on the diagnostic accuracy of FDG PET for local nodal staging in esophageal cancer. Even results from the more favorable studies demonstrate an important lack of sensitivity. However, it is important to note that the presence or absence of local nodes is not always critical in the surgical decision-making process, as a radical resection will generally include extensive nodal resection.

Distant Metastases

Identification of distant metastases is essential for appropriate management of patients with esophageal cancer as their presence is considered a contraindication to radical surgery. Lymph node metastases to supraclavicular, cervical, and celiac nodes are considered distant metastases (M1) rather than nodal metastases (N1) in the staging of esophageal cancer as their presence indicates stage IV (unresectable) disease (Fig. 4). PET offers a significant advantage over anatomical imaging modalities for the detection of metastatic disease. Figures for sensitivity and specificity are

FIGURE 4   Sagittal FDG PET image. Supraclavicular nodal metastasis (arrow) from esophageal carcinoma.

likely to be less accurate than for nodal staging because of the lack of a rigorous histological gold standard, but meaningful data about additional disease detection with PET are available. In three studies encompassing 97 patients with esophageal cancer, PET demonstrated additional metastatic disease in 21 patients (21.6%) (10,12,19). The greater sensitivity of PET was confirmed in a later study that evaluated the role of PET and CT in detecting distant metastases in 100 consecutive patients with esophageal cancer (23). PET detected 51 distant metastases in 27 of 39 cases (69% sensitivity, 93.4% specificity, 84% accuracy) in which metastases were confirmed by clinical follow-up or minimally invasive thoracoscopic/laparoscopic staging, compared with CT, which detected 26 metastases in 18 of 39 cases (46.1% sensitivity, 73.8% specificity, 63% accuracy) ($p < 0.01$). In another study of 52 patients with esophageal cancer who were assessed for resectablity, 17 were found to have metastatic disease (13). PET identified all 17 of these patients, while CT only identified 5.

A cautionary note was sounded by one more recent retrospective study of 24 patients staged with both PET and CT (22). For detection of metastatic disease, CT and PET showed no significant difference in sensitivity (83% and 67%, respectively) and specificity (75% and 92%, respectively). The relatively small number of patients in this study and the associated wide confidence intervals make it difficult to draw any definite conclusions. On balance, the ability of PET to detect distant metastases is very useful, as inappropriate major surgery can be avoided in a significant proportion of patients. Wallace et al. conducted a cost-effectiveness study of different staging strategies for esophageal cancer, including PET, CT, endoscopic ultrasound, and thoracoscopy/laparoscopy (24). They concluded that the combination of PET and endoscopic ultrasound with fine needle biopsy was the most cost-effective approach. In practice, locally available facilities and expertise will obviously determine the approach in any given institution and correlation of PET and anatomical imaging findings is essential. One of the problems with whole body staging with FDG PET is the relatively frequent finding of abnormal tracer uptake without any obvious corresponding abnormality on CT. In most cases it is essential to pursue these abnormalities with laparoscopy/thoracoscopy, particularly if they represent the only apparent site of metastasis.

Diagnosis of Recurrence

FDG PET is ideally suited to the diagnosis of tumor recurrence, as anatomical abnormalities that persist after treatment do not significantly affect its interpretation (Fig. 5). Some care is needed with this approach in

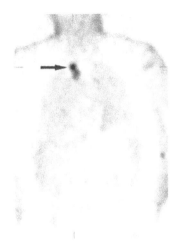

FIGURE 5 Coronal FDG PET image. Recurrence of disease in azygos nodes (arrow) 15 months post–total thoracic esophagectomy.

that recent surgery (within 4 weeks) may cause false-positive uptake of FDG so the examination should be delayed until after this interval if possible. The same caveat applies to radiotherapy, although the duration of this effect is not well established in the literature. Some authorities suggest that persistent increased tracer uptake more than 6 months after radiotherapy is very likely due to recurrent or residual disease rather than a treatment effect (25). In a study of 41 patients with clinical or radiological suspicion of recurrence of esophageal cancer, PET provided additional information in 11 of 41 (27%) patients (26). A major impact on diagnosis was found in 5 patients with equivocal or negative findings on complete diagnostic work-up in whom PET provided a true-positive diagnosis. In 5 other patients the diagnosis was staged upward from localized to extensive recurrent disease, and in 1 patient with an equivocal complete diagnostic work-up, PET correctly excluded malignancy.

Evaluation of Response to Therapy

Neo-adjuvant chemoradiotherapy has been used with some success prior to surgery for both adenocarcinoma and squamous cell carcinoma of the esophagus (27,28). Several authors have shown that PET can help predict the patients who benefit most from the neo-adjuvant therapy. In a recent prospective study of 39 patients with esophageal cancer, a reduction in the standardized uptake value (SUV) of FDG after neo-adjuvant therapy of greater than 60% was associated with 2-year disease-free and overall survival rates of 67% and 89%, respectively, compared with corresponding rates of 38% and 63% for patients with less than 60% reduction in SUV (29). Similar results were found in another study of 36 patients with locally advanced esophageal cancer in whom the PET response was strongly correlated with pathological response at the time of resection and survival (30).

These results are certainly promising, but the exact role of PET in this setting has yet to be defined. Studies to date are too small and the confidence intervals too wide to allow decisions about withholding surgery in poor responders to be made. PET has also been proposed as an early marker of response to chemotherapy in certain tumors such as lung cancer and lymphoma (31). The rationale is that early detection of a lack of response (after one cycle of therapy instead of the usual three or four) would allow an early change to more effective therapy. Unfortunately, the lack of any really effective chemotherapy for esophageal cancer means that this approach is not likely to be of any practical assistance in patient management at the time of writing.

COLORECTAL CANCER

Staging Prior to Hepatic Resection

The 5-year survival rate for patients with resectable hepatic metastases from colorectal cancer is between 35 and 55%, compared with negligible 5-year survival when surgery is not possible (32–37). Approximately 10–20% of patients with colorectal metastases to the liver are candidates for surgery, and the results of surgery have improved over recent years (33,38). Patient selection is based on the number and location of hepatic metastases and the presence or absence of extrahepatic metastases. Therefore the radiologist has a central role in patient selection, so that major surgery is avoided in patients who will not derive any long-term benefit from it and surgical resources are focused on patients who are likely to do well. Portal phase contrast enhanced helical or multidetector CT of the liver is the standard investigation in many institutions for evaluation of the liver. MRI and ultrasound may also be used. CT of the thorax and the remainder of the abdomen is also routinely performed to exclude extrahepatic disease. In spite of this extensive anatomical imaging, one of the main causes of treatment failure is undetetected disease at the time of surgery, with recurrences occurring in the liver and in extrahepatic locations in approximately equal proportions of patients (39).

PET detects additional disease in a significant number of patients who appear to have resectable liver metastases after assessment with anatomical

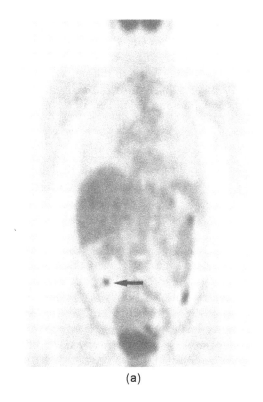

(a)

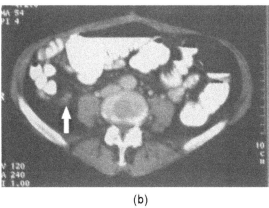

(b)

FIGURE 6 (a) Coronal FDG PET image. Focal extrahepatic abnormality (arrow) in a patient with colorectal metastases to the liver who was being considered for curative resection several months after right hemicolectomy. (b) Axial CT image confirms retroperitoneal recurrence (arrow).

imaging techniques (Fig. 6). In a prospective study Fong et al. found additional disease with PET in 9 of 40 patients considered resectable after anatomical imaging (40). Subcentimeter peritoneal implants were not detected with PET in 3 patients (7.5%) in the same study. In another study the sensitivity of PET for detecting extrahepatic disease was 94% compared with 64% for anatomical imaging (41). Ten of 91 patients with hepatic metastases in another study were found to have additional disease that precluded resection when imaged with PET (42). A false-negative rate of 7.7% was noted in the same study for small intra-abdominal lesions. Valk et al. studied 78 patients pre-operatively with PET and found that PET showed additional sites of disease in 23 patients in whom CT had identified only a single site of disease (43). Therefore PET is useful in detecting extrahepatic disease, but a small false-negative rate of less than 10% exists in the abdomen.

PET is also useful for detecting the presence of hepatic metastases (Fig. 7). Ultrasound, CT, PET, and MRI were compared in a recent meta-nalysis of techniques for the detection of hepatic metastases from gastro-intestinal primary tumors (44). In reviewing studies for inclusion, the authors set a threshold of 85% to represent the lowest clinically useful specificity of a diagnostic test in this setting. Having excluded studies with lower specificity, the mean weighted sensitivity was 55% [95% confidence intervals (CI): 41, 68] for ultrasound, 72% (95% CI: 63, 80) for CT, 76% (95% CI: 57, 91) for MRI, and 90% (95% CI: 80, 97) for FDG PET. Smaller lesions are more difficult to detect with PET, as with other imaging modalities. Fong et al. detected 85% of hepatic metastases larger than 1 cm in diameter with PET, but only 25% of metastases smaller than 1 cm (40). In practice it is essential to have CT images to hand at the time of reporting the PET examination. This is particularly helpful for segmental localization of lesions within the liver.

In addition to false-negative findings, false-positive findings of PET can also be a problem in clinical practice. The first step in evaluating an area of abnormal uptake is to correlate the PET with CT. This will sometimes reveal a previously undetected abnormality that in retrospect clearly represents a metastasis. Other imaging such as MRI or investigations such as laparoscopy, colonoscopy, or mediastinoscopy may be necessary to further investigate a PET abnormality, particularly if a true-positive finding would exclude the patient from potentially curative surgery.

The additional diagnostic accuracy of PET results in a change in diagnostic thinking and management for many patients with hepatic metastases. When compared with the original treatment plan based on anatomical imaging, management was changed in 11–29% of patients after PET in a variety of preoperative studies (40,42,43,45–47). In most cases

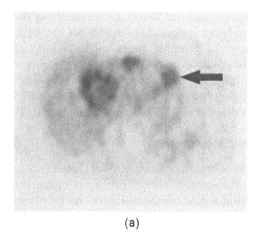

(a)

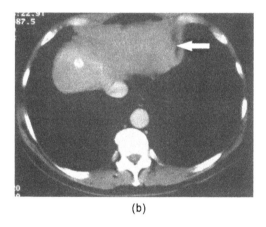

(b)

FIGURE 7   (a) Axial FDG PET image in a patient with hepatic metastases from colorectal carcinoma. An obvious lesion was present in the lateral segment of the left lobe of the liver (arrow). (b) Axial CT in the same patient. The small metastasis (arrow) was not identified prospectively on the preceding CT.

the planned change in management was from surgical to non-surgical treatment due to the detection of additional disease.

The success of PET in terms of diagnostic efficacy, diagnostic thinking, and management planning is proven, but at the time of writing there are few data about the impact of PET on postoperative survival after partial hepatectomy for colorectal metastases. A single prospective paper has addressed this issue in 43 patients deemed resectable after anatomical imaging (48). PET detected additional disease in 10 of the 43 patients, of whom 6 were considered inoperable because of the PET findings. After median follow-up of 24 months, the Kaplan-Meier estimate of 3-year survival in operated patients was 77%, with a lower 95% confidence interval of 60% for this estimate of survival. This is similar to actual 3-year survival rates in cohorts of patients not selected with PET, so more data are needed to see if this use of PET will improve outcome (49,50).

Diagnosis of Pelvic Recurrence

Patients with previous resection for rectal carcinoma are nearly always left with a soft tissue abnormality in the presacral space. The abnormality, which can range from a mass to streaking of the fat planes, is often more prominent and irregular when radiotherapy has also been used. Evaluation of the presacral region for tumor recurrence is therefore particularly difficult with anatomical imaging techniques. The options include a biopsy or follow-up imaging after an interval of several weeks to months. Biopsy may not be technically feasible and a negative result may give false reassurance. Follow-up is never a particularly palatable option for an anxious patient and may result in a significant delay in therapy.

As with other malignancies, PET is extremely useful in this setting as active malignant cells will show an increase in tracer uptake while fibrotic tissue will not (Fig. 8). Several studies have confirmed the role of PET in this setting. Sensitivity and specificity of 100% were reported in an early study of 15 patients (51). Keogan et al. prospectively investigated 18 patients with presacral masses or fat streaking and found that PET had sensitivity of 92.3% and specificity of 80% for detection of recurrent disease (52). In a different retrospective study the sensitivity and specificity of PET were 91% and 100%, respectively (53).

As noted previously, bladder catheterization is not generally necessary when investigating the pelvis with PET, particularly if frusemide is administered to promote urinary dilution. It is also advisable to wait at least 6 months after radiotherapy before performing PET, if possible, to avoid false-positive tracer uptake (25).

Rising CEA

Carcino-embryonic antigen (CEA) is a serum marker of disease activity in colorectal cancer that is routinely measured during follow-up of patients with previously treated colorectal cancer. It is reported to have a sensitivity of 59% and a specificity of 84% for detection of recurrence (54). In theory, early detection of recurrence can lead to further curative therapy. This benefit has also been demonstrated in practice, with 9–13% reduction in

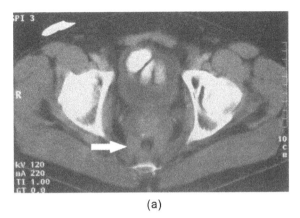

(a)

(b)

FIGURE 8 (a) Axial CT image in a patient with previous resection of rectal carcinoma. A large presacral mass is present (arrow). (b) Axial FDG PET image in the same patient shows normal urinary activity in the bladder, but no abnormal uptake in the mass, confirming a benign post-operative soft tissue mass.

cancer-related mortality in a cohort of patients who underwent intensive follow-up including frequent measurement of CEA (55).

When a rise in CEA occurs, the site of recurrence must be sought. However, even with CT and colonoscopy, it may not be possible to identify recurrence in many patients. The potential benefit of early diagnosis is therefore lost. PET has been used successfully in this situation to identify the site of recurrence (Fig. 9). Flanagan et al. studied 22 patients with rising CEA in whom anatomical imaging had failed to identify any recurrence (56). Seventeen had positive PET examinations (15 true positive), and 4 of these went on to surgery with curative intent. In another study of 15 similar patients, PET identified abnormalities in 14 and surgical procedures were performed in 9 with curative intent (57). Two of the nine were found to have

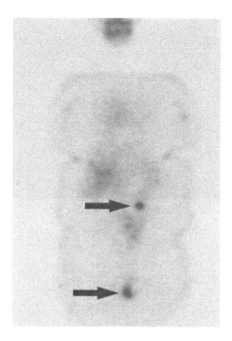

FIGURE 9   Coronal FDG PET image in a patient 2 years postresection for colorectal cancer with a rising CEA level demonstrates pelvic recurrence (arrow) and metastatic retroperitoneal lymphyadenopathy (arrow).

more extensive disease at surgery than PET had predicted and one of the PET studies proved falsely positive at operation. In a larger study of 50 patients with rising CEA levels and normal anatomical imaging, PET identified recurrence in 43 (58). Surgery was subsequently performed in 14 of these with curative intent. Therefore, PET can be used to direct surgery in cases of isolated recurrence and to avoid surgery when widespread recurrence is identified.

Diagnosis of Primary Colorectal Cancers

As with esophageal cancer, PET has a high sensitivity for the detection of primary colorectal cancer (96–100%), but its use is not currently recommended for this indication as histological diagnosis is necessary (59,60). Nevertheless, it is important to realize that synchronous or metachronous colonic tumors will demonstrate focal intense tracer uptake when a patient is being scanned for staging purposes or to detect recurrence (61). Colonic adenomas may also be detected with PET, although the sensitivity is poor, particularly for smaller lesions. PET identified only 14 of 59 adenomas visualized at colonoscopy in 110 asymptomatic patients who underwent both PET and colonoscopy as part of a health screening program (62).

Monitoring Therapy

Uptake of FDG decreases after neo-adjuvant chemoradiotherapy in patients with rectal cancer who demonstrate a pathological response to treatment (63). In a small study of 10 patients with unresectable hepatic metastases, a decrease in FDG uptake 72 hours after a single infusion of 5-fluorouracil and folinic acid was associated with a sustained response to therapy at 6 months (64). As yet, however, there is no clinically accepted role for PET in monitoring therapy for colorectal cancer.

PANCREATIC CARCINOMA

Differentiation of benign and malignant pancreatic masses with FDG PET has been studied extensively. Focal accumulation of FDG is considered evidence of a malignant lesion, while diffuse or less intense uptake is considered evidence of a chronic inflammatory mass (Fig. 10). Initial papers reported uniformly high diagnostic accuracy and recommended the technique for diagnosis of pancreatic masses. It is interesting to note the trend towards poorer results in more recent studies (Table 1). Most pancreatic cancers can be readily diagnosed with CT. Diagnostic difficulty arises in relatively few patients with pancreatic masses. Many of the earlier studies included patients with pancreatic cancers that were obvious on CT or ultrasound, which may have skewed their results. In Kasperk, et al.'s prospective study the authors concluded that PET did not reliably diagnose or exclude malignancy where anatomical imaging techniques were indeterminate, which is precisely the clinical setting where PET might be useful (65). Sendler et al. also concluded that PET did not allow exclusion of malignant tumors (66). This is really the critical question that imaging must answer—is it safe to observe the lesion rather than operate?

One of the recognized limitations of PET in pancreatic cancer is the reduction in sensitivity in patients with high levels of serum glucose (67–69). Diederichs et al. found that the detection rates for pancreatic malignancy were 86% and 42% if fasting plasma glucose levels were below and above 130 mg/dL, respectively (68). The same author has found that exclusion of patients with high plasma glucose or high C-reactive protein improves the diagnostic accuracy of the test, but in practice these are frequently the patients in whom diagnostic doubt exists (70). Shreve, however, found a high false-positive rate for malignancy even when clinical,

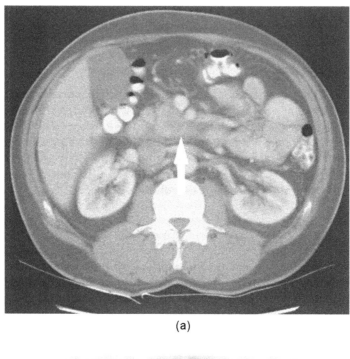

(a)

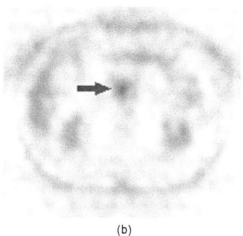

(b)

FIGURE 10   (a) Axial CT image in a 35-year-old patient with a history of chronic alcohol abuse and recurrent acute pancreatitis shows a poorly defined low attenuation mass in the pancreatic head (arrow). (b) Axial FDG PET image shows focal FDG uptake in the mass. Carcinoma of the pancreas was confirmed at laparotomy.

TABLE 1 Diagnostic Accuracy of FDG PET for Diagnosis of Malignancy in Pancreatic Masses

Year	n	Sensitivity (%)	Specificity (%)	Ref.
1994	40	92.6	84.6	67
1995	80	93.8	87.5	85
1995	41	94.3	81.8	86
1995	75	95.3	90	87
1997	106	85.1	84.4	69
1998	37	88.0	83.3	88
2000	42	71	64	66
2001	103	84	61	65

laboratory, or CT findings suggestive of inflammation were equivocal or absent (71).

Therefore, PET does not offer a simple solution to differential diagnosis of "difficult" pancreatic masses. It may give some additional information when viewed in conjunction with anatomical imaging and the clinical setting, but it is probably not warranted routinely. Similarly, diagnosis of lack of resectability due to local disease extension in pancreatic cancer is reliably performed with CT, and there is no evidence to suggest that PET has a role to play in this regard. In most cases of pancreatic cancer, local spread is the deciding factor in excluding resectability. Detection of metastatic disease is also important for determining resectability in a limited number of patients. Limited data indicate that, as with other tumors, PET can improve the detection of distant metastases (7 of 65 patients in one study), but further research is required to clarify its role in this setting (72).

HEPATOCELLULAR CARCINOMA AND CHOLANGIOCARCINOMA

PET cannot be used to exclude hepatocellular carcinoma (HCC) as the sensitivity of PET for HCC varies from 0 to 64% (73–78). Furthermore, few data exist about its specificity, so it also cannot be used to reliably confirm suspected hepatocellular carcinoma.

Very few published data exist for the diagnosis of cholangiocarcinoma with PET. Kluge et al. evaluated 54 patients, 26 with cholangiocarcinoma, 8 with benign biliary lesions, and 20 controls (79). They reported sensitivity of 92.3% and specificity of 92.9% for diagnosis of malignancy. Keiding et al. used a quantitative PET technique to diagnose cholangiocarcinoma in 15 patients with primary sclerosing cholangitis and 9 controls (80).

This approach allowed all 6 cholangiocarcinomas to be distinguished from benign lesions. In a small study of 11 patients with biliary strictures, the author found that PET had sensitivity of 40% (2/5) and specificity of 100% (6/6) for diagnosis of malignancy (81). Further studies are required to determine if PET has a significant role in the diagnosis of cholangio-carcinoma, particularly in patients with primary sclerosing cholangitis, in whom differentiation of benign and malignant strictures is diagnostically challenging.

INFLAMMATORY BOWEL DISEASE

Many early oncology studies with FDG PET noted that FDG was taken up at sites of inflammation, presumably representing increased glycolysis in the cellular infiltrate. Current evaluation of patients with suspected inflammatory bowel disease relies on endoscopy, barium studies, and cross-sectional imaging techniques. Some of these procedures are invasive and unpleasant for the patient. Leukocyte scintigraphy is a noninvasive method of evaluating bowel inflammation, but cell labeling is technically demanding and time-consuming. PET could potentially retain the advantages of leukocyte scintigraphy, including its accuracy, noninvasiveness and ability to evaluate the entire intestine in one examination, while also eliminating the need for labor-intensive cell labeling.

Using receiver operating characteristic curve analysis, it has been shown that activity greater than that in bone should be considered indicative of inflammation, while any activity less that is best interpreted as physiological (82). As with leukocyte scintigraphy or barium studies, the distribution of abnormalities often suggests the underlying disease process (Fig. 11). Few data exist about the accuracy of FDG PET for the detection

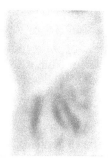

FIGURE 11 Coronal FDG PET image demonstrates discontinuous increased uptake in small bowel loops in a patient with Crohn's disease.

FIGURE 12   Coronal FDG PET image in 13-year-old girl with Crohn's colitis shows increased uptake in the ascending and descending colon. Colonoscopy had only reached the descending colon, so that more proximal disease extent could not be assessed.

of inflammatory bowel disease. A sensitivity of 81% and specificity of 85% (on a patient by patient basis) was reported in 25 pediatric patients with suspected inflammatory bowel disease, when compared with histological gold standards for the colon and histological or radiological (therefore less than perfect) gold standards for the small bowel (82). Importantly, in 8 of the 10 patients in whom colonoscopy could not be completed, FDG PET demonstrated inflammation proximal to the point reached endoscopically (Fig. 12). Similar results were reported for a prospective study of 59 patients with Crohn's disease (83). For endoscopically verified areas of inflammation, the sensitivity and specificity of PET were 85% and 89%, respectively.

Although more studies are needed, FDG PET appears to be a promising technique in inflammatory bowel disease, with clinical indications likely mirroring those of leukocyte scintigraphy. We have also noted a good correlation between FDG activity in the bowel and clinical disease activity in patients who have been treated, suggesting that this may be a useful technique for monitoring the success of therapy (84).

REFERENCES

1.   Brown RS, Goodman TM, Zasadny KR, Greenson JK, Wahl RL. Expression of hexokinase II and Glut-1 in untreated human breast cancer. Nucl Med Biol 2002; 29:443–453.
2.   Higashi T, Tamaki N, Torizuka T, Nakamoto Y, Sakahara H, Kimura T, Honda T, Inokuma T, Katsushima S, Ohshio G, Imamura M, Konishi J.

FDG uptake, GLUT-1 glucose transporter and cellularity in human pancreatic tumors. J Nucl Med 1998; 39:1727–1735.

3. Diederichs C, Staib L, Glatting G, Beger H, Reske S. FDG PET: elevated plasma glucose reduces both uptake and detection rate of pancreatic malignancies. J Nucl Med 1998; 39:1030–1033.

4. Neto CA, Zhuang H, Ghesani N, Alavi A. Detection of Barrett's esophagus superimposed by esophageal cancer by FDG positron emission tomography. Clin Nucl Med 2001; 26:1060.

5. Miraldi F, Vesselle H, Faulhaber PF, Adler LP, Leisure GP. Elimination of artifactual accumulation of FDG in PET imaging of colorectal cancer. Clin Nucl Med 1998; 23:3–7.

6. Goerres GW, Burger C, Schwitter MW, Heidelberg TN, Seifert B, Von Schulthess GW. PET/CT of the abdomen: optimizing the patient breathing pattern. Eur Radiol 2003; 13:734–739.

7. Zealley IA, Skehan SJ, Rawlinson J, Coates G, Nahmias C, Somers S. Selection of patients for resection of hepatic metastases: improved detection of extrahepatic disease with FDG pet. Radiographics 2001; 21(Spec No):S55–S69.

8. Bhargava P, Zhuang H, Hickeson M, Alavi A. Pelvic kidney mimicking recurrent colon cancer on FDG positron emission tomographic imaging. Clin Nucl Med 2002; 27:602–603.

9. Chander S, Meltzer CC, McCook BM. Physiologic uterine uptake of FDG during menstruation demonstrated with serial combined positron emission tomography and computed tomography. Clin Nucl Med 2002; 27:22–24.

10. Flanagan FL, Dehdashti F, Siegel BA, Trask DD, Sundaresan SR, Patterson GA, Cooper JD. Staging of esophageal cancer with 18F-fluorodeoxyglucose positron emission tomography. AJR Am J Roentgenol 1997; 168:417–424.

11. Kole AC, Plukker JT, Nieweg OE, Vaalburg W. Positron emission tomography for staging of oesophageal and gastroesophageal malignancy. Br J Cancer 1998; 78:521–527.

12. Rankin SC, Taylor H, Cook GJ, Mason R. Computed tomography and positron emission tomography in the pre-operative staging of oesophageal carcinoma. Clin Radiol 1998; 53:659–665.

13. Block MI, Patterson GA, Sundaresan RS, Bailey MS, Flanagan FL, Dehdashti F, Siegel BA, Cooper JD. Improvement in staging of esophageal cancer with the addition of positron emission tomography. Ann Thorac Surg 1997; 64:770–777.

14. Kim K, Park SJ, Kim BT, Lee KS, Shim YM. Evaluation of lymph node metastases in squamous cell carcinoma of the esophagus with positron emission tomography. Ann Thorac Surg 2001; 71:290–294.

15. Allum WH, Griffin SM, Watson A, Colin-Jones D. Guidelines for the management of oesophageal and gastric cancer. Gut 2002; 50(suppl 5): v1–v23.

16. Lightdale CJ. Esophageal cancer. American College of Gastroenterology. Am J Gastroenterol 1999; 94:20–29.

17. Shreve PD, Anzai Y, Wahl RL. Pitfalls in oncologic diagnosis with FDG PET imaging: physiologic and benign variants. Radiographics 1999; 19:61–77, 150–151.

18. Skehan SJ, Brown AL, Thompson M, Young JE, Coates G, Nahmias C. Imaging features of primary and recurrent esophageal cancer at FDG PET. Radiographics 2000; 20:713–723.

19. Luketich JD, Schauer PR, Meltzer CC, Landreneau RJ, Urso GK, Townsend DW, Ferson PF, Keenan RJ, Belani CP. Role of positron emission tomography in staging esophageal cancer. Ann Thorac Surg 1997; 64:765–769.

20. Choi JY, Lee KH, Shim YM, Lee KS, Kim JJ, Kim SE, Kim BT. Improved detection of individual nodal involvement in squamous cell carcinoma of the esophagus by FDG PET. J Nucl Med 2000; 41:808–815.

21. Lerut T, Flamen P, Ectors N, Van Cutsem E, Peeters M, Hiele M, De Wever W, Coosemans W, Decker G, De Leyn P, Deneffe G, Van Raemdonck D, Mortelmans L. Histopathologic validation of lymph node staging with FDG-PET scan in cancer of the esophagus and gastroesophageal junction: a prospective study based on primary surgery with extensive lymphadenectomy. Ann Surg 2000; 232:743–752.

22. Wren SM, Stijns P, Srinivas S. Positron emission tomography in the initial staging of esophageal cancer. Arch Surg 2002; 137:1001–1007.

23. Luketich JD, Friedman DM, Weigel TL, Meehan MA, Keenan RJ, Townsend DW, Meltzer CC. Evaluation of distant metastases in esophageal cancer: 100 consecutive positron emission tomography scans. Ann Thorac Surg 1999; 68:1133–1137.

24. Wallace MB, Nietert PJ, Earle C, Krasna MJ, Hawes RH, Hoffman BJ, Reed CE. An analysis of multiple staging management strategies for carcinoma of the esophagus: computed tomography, endoscopic ultrasound, positron emission tomography, and thoracoscopy/laparoscopy. Ann Thorac Surg 2002; 74:1026–1032.

25. Delbeke D. Oncological applications of FDG PET imaging: brain tumors, colorectal cancer, lymphoma and melanoma. J Nucl Med 1999; 40:591–603.

26. Flamen P, Lerut A, Van Cutsem E, Cambier JP, Maes A, De Wever W, Peeters M, De Leyn P, Van Raemdonck D, Mortelmans L. The utility of positron emission tomography for the diagnosis and staging of recurrent esophageal cancer. J Thorac Cardiovasc Surg 2000; 120:1085–1092.

27. Walsh TN, Noonan N, Hollywood D, Kelly A, Keeling N, Hennessy TP. A comparison of multimodal therapy and surgery for esophageal adeno-carcinoma. N Engl J Med 1996; 335:462–467.

28. Bosset JF, Gignoux M, Triboulet JP, Tiret E, Mantion G, Elias D, Lozach P, Ollier JC, Pavy JJ, Mercier M, Sahmoud T. Chemoradiotherapy followed by surgery compared with surgery alone in squamous-cell cancer of the esophagus. N Engl J Med 1997; 337:161–167.

29. Downey RJ, Akhurst T, Ilson D, Ginsberg R, Bains MS, Gonen M, Koong H, Gollub M, Minsky BD, Zakowski M, Turnbull A, Larson SM, Rusch V.

Whole body 18FDG-PET and the response of esophageal cancer to induction therapy: results of a prospective trial. J Clin Oncol 2003; 21:428–432.

30. Flamen P, Van Cutsem E, Lerut A, Cambier JP, Haustermans K, Bormans G, De Leyn P, Van Raemdonck D, De Wever W, Ectors N, Maes A, Mortelmans L. Positron emission tomography for assessment of the response to induction radiochemotherapy in locally advanced oesophageal cancer. Ann Oncol 2002; 13:361–368.

31. Shields AF, Mankoff DA, Link JM, Graham MM, Eary JF, Kozawa SM, Zheng M, Lewellen B, Lewellen TK, Grierson JR, Krohn KA. Carbon-11-thymidine and FDG to measure therapy response. J Nucl Med 1998; 39:1757–1762.

32. Belli G, D'Agostino A, Ciciliano F, Fantini C, Russolillo N, Belli A. Liver resection for hepatic metastases: 15 years of experience. J Hepatobiliary Pancreat Surg 2002; 9:607–613.

33. Choti MA, Sitzmann JV, Tiburi MF, Sumetchotimetha W, Rangsin R, Schulick RD, Lillemoe KD, Yeo CJ, Cameron JL. Trends in long-term survival following liver resection for hepatic colorectal metastases. Ann Surg 2002; 235:759–766.

34. Fong Y, Fortner J, Sun RL, Brennan MF, Blumgart LH. Clinical score for predicting recurrence after hepatic resection for metastatic colorectal cancer: analysis of 1001 consecutive cases. Ann Surg 1999; 230:309–321.

35. Hardy KJ, Fletcher DR, Jones RM. One hundred liver resections including comparison to non-resected liver-mobilized patients. Aust NZ J Surg 1998; 68:716–721.

36. Nakamura S, Suzuki S, Konno H. Resection of hepatic metastases of colorectal carcinoma: 20 years' experience. J Hepatobiliary Pancreat Surg 1999; 6:16–22.

37. Ohlsson B, Stenram U, Tranberg KG. Resection of colorectal liver metastases: 25-year experience. World J Surg 1998; 22:268–277.

38. Rees M, John TG. Current status of surgery in colorectal metastases to the liver. Hepatogastroenterology 2001; 48:341–344.

39. Yamada H, Kondo S, Okushiba S, Morikawa T, Katoh H. Analysis of predictive factors for recurrence after hepatectomy for colorectal liver metastases. World J Surg 2001; 25:1129–1133.

40. Fong Y, Saldinger PF, Akhurst T, Macapinlac H, Yeung H, Finn RD, Cohen A, Kemeny N, Blumgart LH, Larson SM. Utility of 18F-FDG positron emission tomography scanning on selection of patients for resection of hepatic colorectal metastases. Am J Surg 1999; 178:282–287.

41. Whiteford MH, Whiteford HM, Yee LF, Ogunbiyi OA, Dehdashti F, Siegel BA, Birnbaum EH, Fleshman JW, Kodner IJ, Read TE. Usefulness of FDG-PET scan in the assessment of suspected metastatic or recurrent adenocarcinoma of the colon and rectum. Dis Colon Rectum 2000; 43:759–770.

42. Topal B, Flamen P, Aerts R, D'Hoore A, Filez L, Van Cutsem E, Mortelmans L, Penninckx F. Clinical value of whole-body emission tomography in potentially curable colorectal liver metastases. Eur J Surg Oncol 2001; 27:175–179.

43. Valk PE, Abella-Columna E, Haseman MK, Pounds TR, Tesar RD, Myers RW, Greiss HB, Hofer GA. Whole-body PET imaging with [18F] fluorodeoxyglucose in management of recurrent colorectal cancer. Arch Surg 1999; 134:503–511.
44. Kinkel K, Lu Y, Both M, Warren RS, Thoeni RF. Detection of hepatic metastases from cancers of the gastrointestinal tract by using noninvasive imaging methods (US, CT, MR imaging, PET): a meta-analysis. Radiology 2002; 224:748–756.
45. Lai DT, Fulham M, Stephen MS, Chu KM, Solomon M, Thompson JF, Sheldon DM, Storey DW. The role of whole-body positron emission tomography with [18F] fluorodeoxyglucose in identifying operable colorectal cancer metastases to the liver. Arch Surg 1996; 131:703–707.
46. Vitola JV, Delbeke D, Sandler MP, Campbell MG, Powers TA, Wright JK, Chapman WC, Pinson CW. Positron emission tomography to stage suspected metastatic colorectal carcinoma to the liver. Am J Surg 1996; 171:21–26.
47. Ruers TJ, Langenhoff BS, Neeleman N, Jager GJ, Strijk S, Wobbes T, Corstens FH, Oyen WJ. Value of positron emission tomography with [F-18] fluorodeoxyglucose in patients with colorectal liver metastases: a prospective study. J Clin Oncol 2002; 20:388–395.
48. Strasberg SM, Dehdashti F, Siegel BA, Drebin JA, Linehan D. Survival of patients evaluated by FDG-PET before hepatic resection for metastatic colorectal carcinoma: a prospective database study. Ann Surg 2001; 233:293–299.
49. Yamamoto J, Shimada K, Kosuge T, Yamasaki S, Sakamoto M, Fukuda H. Factors influencing survival of patients undergoing hepatectomy for colorectal metastases. Br J Surg 1999; 86:332–337.
50. Finch MD, Crosbie JL, Currie E, Garden OJ. An 8-year experience of hepatic resection: indications and outcome. Br J Surg 1998; 85:315–319.
51. Ito K, Kato T, Tadokoro M, Ishiguchi T, Oshima M, Ishigaki T, Sakuma S. Recurrent rectal cancer and scar: differentiation with PET and MR imaging. Radiology 1992; 182:549–552.
52. Keogan MT, Lowe VJ, Baker ME, McDermott VG, Lyerly HK, Coleman RE. Local recurrence of rectal cancer: evaluation with F-18 fluorodeoxyglucose PET imaging. Abdom Imaging 1997; 22:332–337.
53. Ogunbiyi OA, Flanagan FL, Dehdashti F, Siegel BA, Trask DD, Birnbaum EH, Fleshman JW, Read TE, Philpott GW, Kodner IJ. Detection of recurrent and metastatic colorectal cancer: comparison of positron emission tomography and computed tomography. Ann Surg Oncol 1997; 4:613–620.
54. Moertel CG, Fleming TR, Macdonald JS, Haller DG, Laurie JA, Tangen C. An evaluation of the carcinoembryonic antigen (CEA) test for monitoring patients with resected colon cancer. Jama 1993; 270:943–947.
55. Renehan AG, Egger M, Saunders MP, O'Dwyer ST. Impact on survival of intensive follow up after curative resection for colorectal cancer: systematic review and meta-analysis of randomised trials. BMJ 2002; 324:813.

56. Flanagan FL, Dehdashti F, Ogunbiyi OA, Kodner IJ, Siegel BA. Utility of FDG-PET for investigating unexplained plasma CEA elevation in patients with colorectal cancer. Ann Surg 1998; 227:319–323.

57. Zervos EE, Badgwell BD, Burak WE, Jr., Arnold MW, Martin EW. Fluorodeoxyglucose positron emission tomography as an adjunct to carcino-embryonic antigen in the management of patients with presumed recurrent colorectal cancer and nondiagnostic radiologic workup. Surgery 2001; 130:636–644.

58. Flamen P, Hoekstra OS, Homans F, Van Cutsem E, Maes A, Stroobants S, Peeters M, Penninckx F, Filez L, Bleichrodt RP, Mortelmans L. Unexplained rising carcinoembryonic antigen (CEA) in the postoperative surveillance of colorectal cancer: the utility of positron emission tomography (PET). Eur J Cancer 2001; 37:862–869.

59. Abdel-Nabi H, Doerr RJ, Lamonica DM, Cronin VR, Galantowicz PJ, Carbone GM, Spaulding MB. Staging of primary colorectal carcinomas with fluorine-18 fluorodeoxyglucose whole-body PET: correlation with histopathologic and CT findings. Radiology 1998; 206:755–760.

60. Mukai M, Sadahiro S, Yasuda S, Ishida H, Tokunaga N, Tajima T, Makuuchi H. Preoperative evaluation by whole-body 18F-fluoro-deoxyglucose positron emission tomography in patients with primary colorectal cancer. Oncol Rep 2000; 7:85–87.

61. Drenth JP, Nagengast FM, Oyen WJ. Evaluation of (pre-)malignant colonic abnormalities: endoscopic validation of FDG-PET findings. Eur J Nucl Med 2001; 28:1766–1769.

62. Yasuda S, Fujii H, Nakahara T, Nishiumi N, Takahashi W, Ide M, Shohtsu A. 18F-FDG PET detection of colonic adenomas. J Nucl Med 2001; 42:989–992.

63. Guillem JG, Puig-La Calle J, Jr., Akhurst T, Tickoo S, Ruo L, Minsky BD, Gollub MJ, Klimstra DS, Mazumdar M, Paty PB, Macapinlac H, Yeung H, Saltz L, Finn RD, Erdi Y, Humm J, Cohen AM, Larson S. Prospective assessment of primary rectal cancer response to preoperative radiation and chemotherapy using 18-fluorodeoxyglucose positron emission tomography. Dis Colon Rectum 2000; 43:18–24.

64. Bender H, Bangard N, Metten N, Bangard M, Mezger J, Schomburg A, Biersack HJ. Possible role of FDG-PET in the early prediction of therapy outcome in liver metastases of colorectal cancer. Hybridoma 1999; 18:87–91.

65. Kasperk RK, Riesener KP, Wilms K, Schumpelick V. Limited value of positron emission tomography in treatment of pancreatic cancer: surgeon's view. World J Surg 2001; 25:1134–1139.

66. Sendler A, Avril N, Helmberger H, Stollfuss J, Weber W, Bengel F, Schwaiger M, Roder JD, Siewert JR. Preoperative evaluation of pancreatic masses with positron emission tomography using 18F-fluorodeoxyglucose: diagnostic limitations. World J Surg 2000; 24:1121–1129.

67. Bares R, Klever P, Hauptmann S, Hellwig D, Fass J, Cremerius U, Schumpelick V, Mittermayer C, Bull U. F-18 fluorodeoxyglucose PET in vivo

evaluation of pancreatic glucose metabolism for detection of pancreatic cancer. Radiology 1994; 192:79–86.

68. Diederichs CG, Staib L, Glatting G, Beger HG, Reske SN. FDG PET: elevated plasma glucose reduces both uptake and detection rate of pancreatic malignancies. J Nucl Med 1998; 39:1030–1033.

69. Zimny M, Bares R, Fass J, Adam G, Cremerius U, Dohmen B, Klever P, Sabri O, Schumpelick V, Buell U. Fluorine-18 fluorodeoxyglucose positron emission tomography in the differential diagnosis of pancreatic carcinoma: a report of 106 cases. Eur J Nucl Med 1997; 24:678–682.

70. Diederichs CG, Staib L, Vogel J, Glasbrenner B, Glatting G, Brambs HJ, Beger HG, Reske SN. Values and limitations of 18F-fluorodeoxyglucose-positron-emission tomography with preoperative evaluation of patients with pancreatic masses. Pancreas 2000; 20:109–116.

71. Shreve PD. Focal fluorine-18 fluorodeoxyglucose accumulation in inflammatory pancreatic disease. Eur J Nucl Med 1998; 25:259–264.

72. Rose DM, Delbeke D, Beauchamp RD, Chapman WC, Sandler MP, Sharp KW, Richards WO, Wright JK, Frexes ME, Pinson CW, Leach SD. 18Fluoro-deoxyglucose-positron emission tomography in the management of patients with suspected pancreatic cancer. Ann Surg 1999; 229:729–738.

73. Teefey SA, Hildeboldt CC, Dehdashti F, Siegel BA, Peters MG, Heiken JP, Brown JJ, McFarland EG, Middleton WD, Balfe DM, Ritter JH. Detection of primary hepatic malignancy in liver transplant candidates: prospective comparison of CT, MR imaging, US, and PET. Radiology 2003; 226:533–542.

74. Wudel LJ, Jr., Delbeke D, Morris D, Rice M, Washington MK, Shyr Y, Pinson CW, Chapman WC. The role of [18F]fluorodeoxyglucose positron emission tomography imaging in the evaluation of hepatocellular carcinoma. Am Surg 2003; 69:117–126.

75. Verhoef C, Valkema R, de Man RA, Krenning EP, Yzermans JN. Fluorine-18 FDG imaging in hepatocellular carcinoma using positron coincidence detection and single photon emission computed tomography. Liver 2002; 22:51–56.

76. Khan MA, Combs CS, Brunt EM, Lowe VJ, Wolverson MK, Solomon H, Collins BT, Di Bisceglie AM. Positron emission tomography scanning in the evaluation of hepatocellular carcinoma. J Hepatol 2000; 32:792–797.

77. Trojan J, Schroeder O, Raedle J, Baum RP, Herrmann G, Jacobi V, Zeuzem S. Fluorine-18 FDG positron emission tomography for imaging of hepato-cellular carcinoma. Am J Gastroenterol 1999; 94:3314–3319.

78. Schroder O, Trojan J, Zeuzem S, Baum RP. Limited value of fluorine-18-fluorodeoxyglucose PET for the differential diagnosis of focal liver lesions in patients with chronic hepatitis C virus infection. Nuklearmedizin 1998; 37:279–285.

79. Kluge R, Schmidt F, Caca K, Barthel H, Hesse S, Georgi P, Seese A, Huster D, Berr F. Positron emission tomography with [(18)F] fluoro-2-deoxy-D-glucose for diagnosis and staging of bile duct cancer. Hepatology 2001; 33:1029–1035.

80. Keiding S, Hansen SB, Rasmussen HH, Gee A, Kruse A, Roelsgaard K, Tage-Jensen U, Dahlerup JF. Detection of cholangiocarcinoma in primary

sclerosing cholangitis by positron emission tomography. Hepatology 1998; 28:700–706.

81. Skehan SJ, Fox BM, Coates G, Rawlinson J, Marcaccio M, Nahmias C, Tandan V. Investigation of biliary structures with 18F-fluorodeoxyglucose (FDG) positron emission tomography (PET): work in progress. Radiology 1999; 213(P):250.

82. Skehan SJ, Issenman R, Mernagh J, Nahmias C, Jacobson K. 18F-fluoro-deoxyglucose positron tomography in diagnosis of paediatric inflammatory bowel disease [letter]. Lancet 1999; 354:836–837.

83. Neurath MF, Vehling D, Schunk K, Holtmann M, Brockmann H, Helisch A, Orth T, Schreckenberger M, Galle PR, Bartenstein P. Noninvasive assessment of Crohn's disease activity: a comparison of 18F-fluoro-deoxyglucose positron emission tomography, hydromagnetic resonance imaging, and granulocyte scintigraphy with labeled antibodies. Am J Gastroenterol 2002; 97:1978–1985.

84. Mernagh JR, Issenman R, Thompson M, Skehan SJ, Somers S, Nahmias C. Assessment of inflammation in inflammatory bowel disease with FDG-PET during treatment. Radiology 1999; 213(P):423–423.

85. Friess H, Langhans J, Ebert M, Berger HG, Stollfuss J, Reske SN, Buchler MW. Diagnosis of pancreatic cancer by 2[18F]-fluoro-2-deoxy-D-glucose positron emission tomography. Gut 1995; 36:771–777.

86. Inokuma T, Tamaki N, Torizuka T, Magata Y, Fujii M, Yonekura Y, Kajiyama T, Ohshio G, Imamura M, Konishi J. Evaluation of pancreatic tumors with positron emission tomography and F-18 fluorodeoxyglucose: comparison with CT and US. Radiology 1995; 195:345–352.

87. Stollfuss JC, Glatting G, Friess H, Kocher F, Berger HG, Reske SN. 2-(fluorine-18)-fluoro-2-deoxy-D-glucose PET in detection of pancreatic cancer: value of quantitative image interpretation. Radiology 1995; 195: 339–344.

88. Keogan MT, Tyler D, Clark L, Branch MS, McDermott VG, DeLong DM, Coleman RE. Diagnosis of pancreatic carcinoma: role of FDG PET. AJR Am J Roentgenol 1998; 171:1565–1570.

8

Evaluation of the Small Intestine by MR Imaging

**Nicholas C. Gourtsoyiannis and
Nickolas Papanikolaou**
University Hospital of Iraklion, University of Crete
  Medical School, Iraklion Crete, Greece

INTRODUCTION

Although conventional enteroclysis (CE) is widely recognized as the most reliable method for radiological evaluation of the small bowel (1,2), it is not free of limitations. Radiation exposure, an important consideration when multiple follow-up examinations in young patients with Crohn's disease are possible, and inability to demonstrate exoenteric pathology associated with small intestinal diseases are inherent drawbacks. Computed tomography (CT) has been utilized as a complementary or alternative diagnostic approach (3), while the combination of CT and enteroclysis has recently been introduced (4) with claims that it combines the advantages of both approaches. Limited prospective data are available but suggest that the combined technique may be applicable in patients with obstructive symptoms, known or suspected malignancy, and for assessment of complicated Crohn's disease. However, poor soft tissue contrast, radiation exposure, and practical restriction to axial slices are inherent limitations of the method. Recent advances in CT technology, namely the introduction of multidetector systems, may further increase the role of CT for small bowel imaging, due to better through-plane spatial resolution and the ability to obtain multiplanar reformats (5).

Magnetic resonance imaging (MRI) has been established in diagnostic imaging for more than two decades. One of the most important limitations of MRI is its sensitivity to motion-related artifacts, which has rendered clinical application in areas subject to inherent physiological motion, like the heart or the bowel, somewhat cumbersome. However, recent technological improvements resulting in ultrafast pulse sequences have facilitated significant reduction in acquisition times and made MRI less susceptible to motion and consequently improved image quality. These technological advances have reignited research efforts in the gastrointestinal tract (6–14). MRI provides excellent soft-tissue contrast without radiation exposure, while its three-dimensional imaging capabilities are of great importance when studying tortuous organs like the small intestine. Recently, MR enteroclysis (MRE), a combined functional and morphological imaging method, was introduced in clinical practice, coupling adequate image quality with the functional benefits of a volume challenge (6). Results to date have shown that the functional information provided by MR enteroclysis equals that of conventional enteroclysis, whereas inherent advantages of the technique include detailed morphological evaluation of the bowel wall and the mesenteries.

METHODOLOGY

Examination Techniques

Two different strategies for examining the small bowel (SB) with MRI have been proposed. One is referred to as MR enteroclysis (6–8) and includes duodenal intubation and administration of a maximum amount of 2 L of contrast agent with the patient lying inside the magnet. Contrast is administered in two phases. A flow rate of 80–150 mL/min is utilized at first, until contrast reaches the terminal ileum. Subsequently, reflex atony is achieved by increasing the flow rate up to 200 mL/min. Reflex atony and administration of antiperistaltic drugs are essential to acquire images free of motion artifacts. An iso-osmotic water solution with polyethylene glycol (PEG) and electrolytes may be used as a contrast agent. Excellent distention of the bowel lumen and the capability to perform fluoroscopic evaluation of the small intestine are the major advantages of this technique (8).

Alternatively, conventional enteroclysis is initially performed using 800 mL of barium sulfate solution. A double contrast effect is then achieved following the administration of 1200 mL of methylcellulose solution mixed with a positive or negative MRI contrast medium at a proportion of 1:100

(9,10). With the later technique, adequate distention of the distal small bowel can be achieved; additional contrast medium may be administered prior to MRI examination in order to guarantee appropriate jejunal distention. This approach is combined with conventional enteroclysis, whereas MRE can be applied independently as a solitary comprehensive SB examination technique providing diagnostic information from the mucosa, the bowel wall, and extraintestinal extension or complications of SB diseases.

MR examination may also be achieved without intubation, using oral administration of 2% barium sulfate solution (11), 2.5% mannitol solution (12), iron oxide particles solution (13), or water (14). Abnormal bowel segments can be easily identified by mural thickening and contrast enhancement, but more subtle changes indicative of bowel disease will require distention of the small bowel lumen in order to be depicted (11). Additionally, oral administration of negative contrast agents may not provide homogeneous opacification of bowel segments in patients with Crohn's disease who have inflammatory stenotic lesions, because of dilution effects caused by increased intaluminal secretions (13). The use of tap water orally has been shown to result in suboptimal depiction of jejunal loops in 20% of healthy volunteers and does not provide adequate opacification of the terminal ileum in more than 30% (14).

Contrast Agents

The most important attributes of an ideal gastrointestinal (GI) contrast agent include homogeneous opacification of the entire bowel lumen, clear differentiation between the lumen and the bowel wall, no significant adverse effects, and low cost. In addition, minimal mucosal absorption and absence of artifact formation are also highly desirable. GI contrast agents are usually classified according to the signal changes they introduce on MR images: positive, negative, or biphasic. Positive contrast agents increase intraluminal signal intensity, while negative contrast agents result in decreased signal intensity of the bowel lumen (15–18). Biphasic contrast agents behave as either positive or negative agents, depending on the contrast of the sequence applied. Water solutions, including methylcellulose, mannitol, or PEG, generate low signal intensity on T1-weighted images and high signal intensity on T2-weighted images. In addition to commercially available gadolinium chelates, positive contrast agents such as ferrous ammonium citrates (15), manganese chloride (19), or iron phytate (16) have been proposed. Moreover, food products such as blueberry juice or green tea (due to their high manganese content), vegetable oil, milk or ice cream may also be used (20–22). Commercially available negative MRI contrast media include superparamagnetic iron oxide (SPIO), oral magnetic particles (OMP), and AMI-121 (9,23). Negative contrast properties of other substances such as kaolin (24), perflubron (25), barium sulfate (11), methyl cellulose (7,8), or mannitol solutions (12) have been reported also. Similarly, air or carbon dioxide may serve as negative contrast agents (26).

At present, there is no consensus on the ideal GI tract contrast agent, and only a few comparative studies have appeared in the literature so far (27). With appropriate dilution, positive, negative, or biphasic contrast media can provide homogeneous intraluminal opacification without artifact formation and/or presence of significant side effects (9).

MRI Sequences

Various sequences have proven to be of particular diagnostic value when combined with use of appropriate contrast agents (27,28). MRI examination of the small bowel usually includes T1- and T2-weighted sequences in both axial and coronal planes. Both T1- and T2-weighted sequences should be fast enough to allow comfortable breath-hold acquisition times. For T1-weighted images, most investigators use gradient echo sequences in 2D and 3D acquisition modes with or without fat saturation. For T2-weighted images, TSE and HASTE sequences are mostly employed (7,12,13). More recently, the true FISP sequence has been successfully applied in SB imaging (6), providing high-resolution images of the bowel wall (Fig. 1) and additional information from the mesenteries. Fat-suppressed TSE or STIR sequences have been also applied to assess the activity of Crohn's disease (13,29).

The combination of fat-suppressed fast gradient echo T1-weighted images, negative endoluminal contrast agents, and gadolinium DTPA enhancement has been shown to be useful for detection of small bowel wall abnormalities (23,30). Using this technique the normal wall is depicted with moderate signal intensity, while inflammatory or neoplastic pathology is conspicuous as high-intensity lesions due to gadolinium uptake. Fat exhibits low signal intensity as a result of fat suppression prepulses, while endoluminal signal is also of low intensity due to the negative contrast agents used. Acquisition of 3D FLASH T1-weighted images with fat saturation provides 2 mm slices and high spatial resolution (using a 512 matrix) (28) (Fig. 2). The major disadvantage of the 3D FLASH sequence is increased sensitivity to motion artifacts, which may cause bowel wall blurring, that can be countered by antiperistaltic drugs.

T1-weighted native sequences combined with oral administration of a positive contrast agent result in high contrast between hypointense bowel wall thickening and the high signal intensity of both intraluminal fluid and

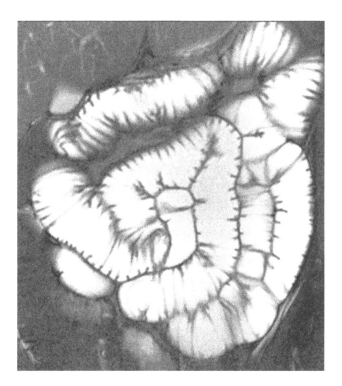

FIGURE 1   High-resolution coronal true FISP image demonstrating well-distended jejunal loops. Intraluminal iso-osmotic water solution results in homogeneous high signal intensity, whereas intestinal wall and valvulae conniventes exhibit low signal intensity.

intra-abdominal mesenteric fat. When using positive contrast agents (i.e., gadolinium solutions), 3D T1-weighted FLASH sequences with fat satura-tion provide high-resolution images of the small bowel lumen, which may be used to generate virtual endoscopic views by applying volume rendering algorithms. The acquisition of thin slices with high contrast-to-noise ratio between bowel lumen and the surrounding tissues facilitates the segmen-tation process necessary for postprocessing and results in high-quality virtual endoscopic views (31).

The HASTE sequence provides motion-free images; the normal bowel wall appears of low signal intensity (Fig. 3), while inflammatory or neoplastic lesions are of high signal intensity (Fig. 4). A limitation of the HASTE sequence is poor demonstration of the mesenteries due to k-space filtering effects. Additionally, it is sensitive to intraluminal flow artifacts

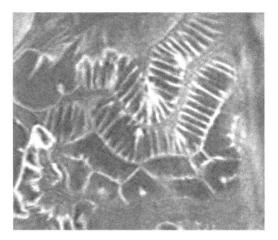

FIGURE 2   Coronal 3D FLASH sequence with fat saturation acquired 75 seconds after gadolinium injection. Homogeneous intraluminal low signal intensity results from the long T1 relaxation constant of the iso-osmotic water solution, whereas intestinal wall exhibits high signal intensity due to gadolinium uptake. Note the excellent demonstration of the valvulae conniventes.

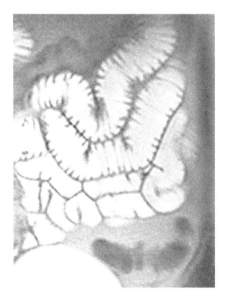

FIGURE 3   Coronal HASTE image demonstrating normal jejunal loops. Homogeneous intraluminal oppacification can be achieved only when antiperistaltic drugs are administered prior to HASTE acquisition.

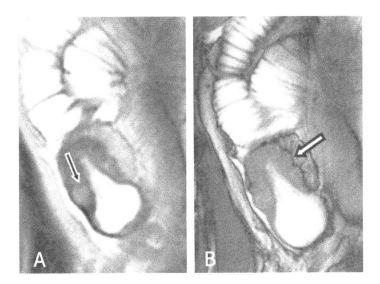

FIGURE 4   Coronal HASTE (A) and true FISP (B) images in a patient with Crohn's disease. Intramural edema (arrow) is better demonstrated against fibrotic wall thickening on HASTE imaging due to its pure T2 contrast, as opposed to the true FISP image (B), which is influenced both by T1 and T2 relaxation constants, thus providing mixed contrast. Black boundary artifacts are recognized as a black thin line in the voxels where both water and fat protons exist (white arrow) and are more pronounced on true FISP images (B).

due to peristaltic motion, and the administration of antiperistaltic drugs is recommended.

Recently, the true FISP sequence has been introduced for MR examination of the small bowel following duodenal intubation (6). Contrast in true FISP images depends on the T2:T1 ratio, and bowel wall thus exhibits indermediate signal intensity whereas fluid is of high signal intensity (Fig. 4). Motion-related artifacts are minimal on true FISP images due to short acquisition times and intraluminal flow voids are not present as a result of the flow compensated gradient scheme of the sequence in all three axes (32,33). The true FISP sequence is capable of demonstrating the mesenteries because of high contrast resolution between the bright peritoneal fat and dark vessels and lymph nodes (6).

The single shot TSE sequence results in heavily T2-weighted images and was initially introduced to visualize the pancreatobiliary tree (34). Within the context of MR enteroclysis, it is extremely helpful for monitoring the infusion process and assessing the degree of luminal distention (6). Additionally, it provides functional information (7).

MR Comprehensive Examination Protocol of the Small Intestine

A state-of-the-art MRI examination of the small intestine requires adequate bowel distention, homogeneous lumen opacification, increased conspicuity of the bowel wall, demonstration of the mesenteries, information about bowel motility, the ability to obtain dynamic postcontrast images, high-contrast resolution, sufficient spatial resolution to evaluate subtle mucosal lesions, images free from artifacts (especially motion artifacts), and rapid acquisition times. All these virtues can be intergrated in a comprehensive MRE examination protocol via small bowel intubation, administration of a biphasic contrast agent (i.e., an iso-osmotic water solution; PEG), heavily T2-weighted single shot turbo spin echo (SSTSE) images for MR fluoroscopy and for monitoring the infusion process, T2-weighted imaging employing HASTE and true FISP sequences, and dynamic T1-weighted imaging using a postgadolinium 3D FLASH sequence with fat suppression. This protocol can provide anatomic demonstration of the normal intestinal wall (true FISP, HASTE, 3D FLASH), identification of wall thickening or tumors (true FISP, HASTE, 3D FLASH), lesion characterization or evaluation of disease activity (3D FLASH, true FISP), assessment of exoenteric/mesenteric disease extension (true FISP, 3D FLASH), and information concerning intestinal motility (SSTSE).

MR enteroclysis has been primarily applied to high field strength magnets (6), although it has been proved feasible at 1.0 Tesla (7). Abdominal phased-array RF coils should be used to guarantee adequate signal-to-noise ratio, while patients are best examined in the prone position, which facilitates bowel loop separation and reduces respiratory-related artifacts (6). High-performance gradient systems are most suitable for MR enteroclysis due to the demands of the ultrafast sequences employed. MR suite examination time, when using the described protocol, may be less than 15 minutes, while the acquisition time of all MR sequences is approximately 7 minutes (6).

NORMAL APPEARANCES

Jejunum

Homogeneous opacification and good jejunal distension has been achieved using duodenal intubation combined with true FISP sequences (6). Wall conspicuity is excellent and the valvulae conniventes are clearly demonstrated on true FISP, HASTE, and postgadolinium 3D FLASH sequences (Figs. 1–3). Motion artifacts are minimal due to the short acquisition times

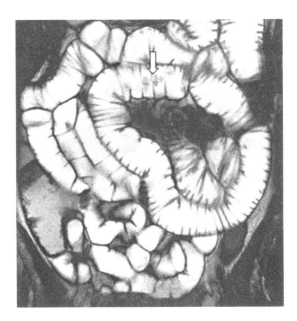

FIGURE 5   Coronal true FISP image showing typical susceptibility artifacts generated because of intraluminal air bubbles (arrow). These artifacts may be overcome
by repeating sequence acquisition.

of the true FISP and HASTE sequences ($<$ 1.5 s per slice). If gas is present,
true FISP images are prone to susceptibility artifacts that may hamper
image quality (Fig. 5), a drawback that is not shared by HASTE sequences.
Black boundary artifact is present on true FISP images (Fig. 4B) but can
be easily differentiated from mural thickening because of differences in
signal intensity.

Ileum

Duodenal intubation guarantees optimal distention of ileal loops, which
is dificult to achieve using oral administration. Furthermore, homogeneity
of opacification is excellent and tiny wall abnormalities can be detected,
especially on 3D FLASH postgadolinium high-resolution images. Adequate
demonstration of the terminal ileum is essential in clinical practice and
can be achieved consistently when combining true FISP sequences with
duodenal intubation (6). Normal bowel wall on MRE is uniformily thin
(not exceeding 2–3 mm) and exhibits moderate signal intensity on true
FISP images (Fig. 1) and high signal intensity on contrast-enhanced 3D
FLASH images (Fig. 2).

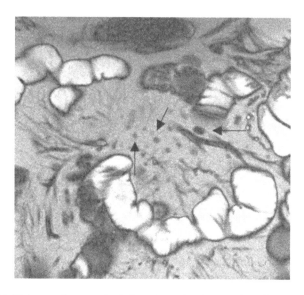

Figure 6   Multiple small mesenteric lymph nodes (arrows) and vascular branches exhibit low signal intensity on true FISP images, whereas mesenteric fat exhibits high signal intensity, resulting in superb contrast resolution of the mesenteries.

Mesenteries

Significant improvements in gradient technology and software have facilitated demonstration of the mesenteries using the true FISP sequence. Mesenteric fat appears bright, whereas lymph nodes and vessels exhibit low signal intensity, resulting in high-contrast resolution. Small lymph nodes of a few millimeters in diameter and distal vascular branches can be consistently detected without motion artifacts when short acquisition times are used (Fig. 6).

CLINICAL APPLICATIONS

Crohn's Disease

A recent study of 26 patients with Crohn's disease found that MRE was in full agreement with conventional enteroclysis for disease detection, localization, estimating the length of involved segments, assessment of mural thickening, luminal narrowing, and high-grade stenosis (35). Early, superficial lesions of Crohn's disease such as nodularity (Fig. 7) or subtle, superficial mucosal ulcerations (Fig. 8) may be depicted by MRE, although to a lesser extent than with conventional enteroclysis because of lower

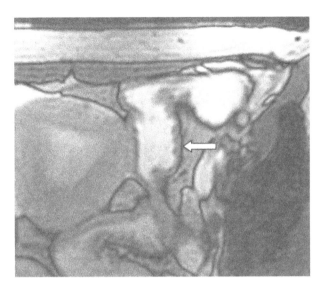

FIGURE 7 Mucosal nodularity (arrow) disclosed on an axial true FISP image in a patient with Crohn's disease. (From Ref. 39.)

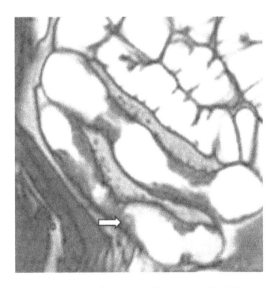

FIGURE 8 Apthous type ulcer (arrow) with the typical "volcano" appearance disclosed on a coronal true FISP image in a patient with Crohn's disease. (From Refs. 37,39.)

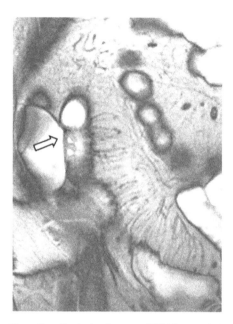

Figure 9   Patient with active Crohn's disease (CDAI = 196). Intestinal fold thickening (arrow) is demonstrated in an ileal loop on a coronal true FISP image, while high signal intensity is compatible with edema. Increased mesenteric vascularity is also shown on the mesenteric border of the involved loop. Two small lymph nodes are depicted with moderate to low signal intensity in an adjacent ileal loop.

spatial resolution. The level of agreement between MRE and CE in early disease is fair (k = 0.345) for depiction of intestinal fold distortion, moderate (k = 0.562) for detection of intestinal fold thickening (Fig. 9), and good (k = 0.73) for detection of superficial ulcers. Further improvements in spatial resolution by means of new dedicated ultrafast sequences and stronger gradients will be needed to improve visualization of these subtle, early, non-specific manifestations of the disease.

Using true FISP images, MRE can demonstrate the characteristic discrete ulceration of Crohn's disease; deep linear ulcers appear as thin lines of high signal intensity, longitudinally or transversely (fissure ulcers) oriented within the thickened bowel wall (Fig. 10) (36). The level of agreement between MRE and CE is excellent (k = 0.825) for these changes. Cobblestoning can also be appreciated on MRE, appearing as patchy areas of high signal intensity, sharply demarcated, occuring along affected small bowel segments (Fig. 11). True FISP is superior to HASTE for demonstration of linear ulcers or cobblestoning and intramural tracts, while 3D

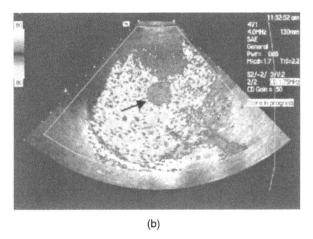

(b)

FIGURE 1 Section through the right lobe of liver in a 76-year-old man with pancreatic carcinoma. (see p. 103 for full legend)

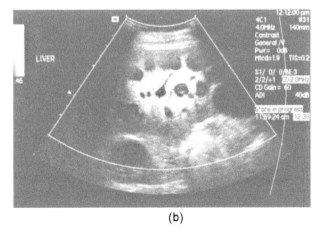

(b)

FIGURE 2 Section through the right lobe of liver in a 68-year-old man with metastatic melanoma. (see p. 104 for full legend)

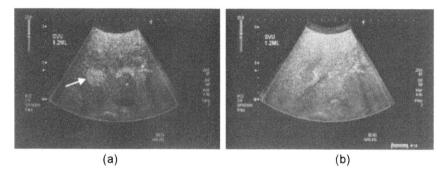

FIGURE 3 Section through the right lobe of liver. (see p. 106 for full legend)

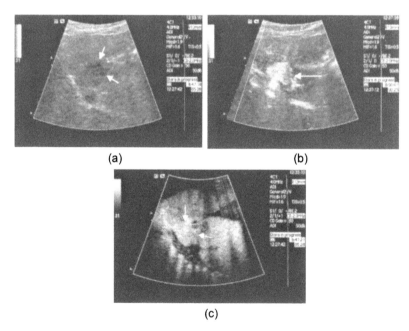

FIGURE 5 This 34-year-old man presented with abdominal pain. (see p. 111 for full legend)

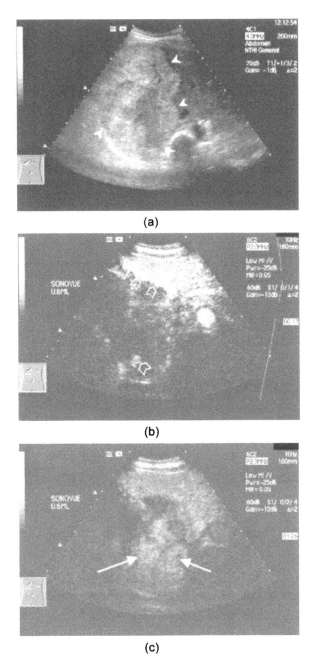

(a)

(b)

(c)

FIGURE 4　Hemangioma in a 47-year-old woman. (see p. 110 for full legend)

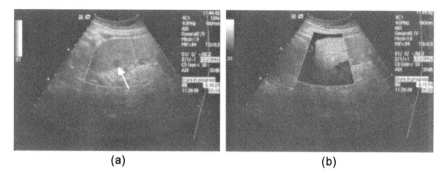

(a)   (b)

FIGURE 6   Longitudinal section through the left lobe of liver in a 76-year-old man receiving aduvant chemotherapy for colorectal carcinoma. (see p. 112 for full legend)

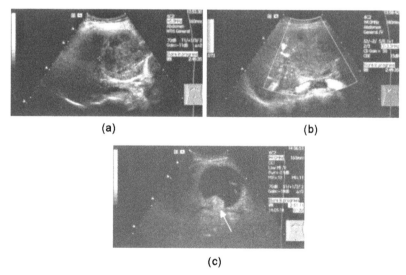

(a)   (b)

(c)

FIGURE 7   Follow-up US in a 46-year-old woman who had undergone chemo-embolization of an hepatocellular carcinoma (HCC). (see p. 113 for full legend)

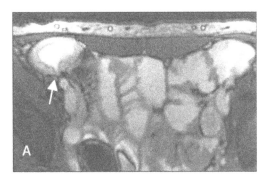

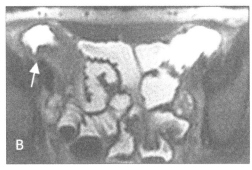

FIGURE 10 Axial true FISP (A) and HASTE (B) images demonstrating a fissure ulcer (arrow) in a patient with Crohn's disease.

FLASH is less sensitive. Wall thickening is clearly depicted by all MRE sequences provided that the SB is adequately distended, otherwise false-positive or negative results may occur (11). A thickened wall in the absence of extensive edema has a low to moderate signal intensity on true FISP and HASTE images. The thickness of bowel wall and the length of the involved segment can be accurately measured on MRE images. Intramural fat may be identified by combining information from true FISP and gadolinium-enhanced 3D FLASH images with fat saturation (Fig. 12). Discrimination between fat deposition and edema may be helpful for disease classification (37). Luminal narrowing and associated prestenotic small bowel dilatation are easily recognized with all sequences (Fig. 13), and MRE has been found equivalent to CE for diagnosis of stenosis (8).

MRE has a clear advantage over conventional enteroclysis for demonstration of exoenteric manifestations and complications of Crohn's disease (35–38). The extent of fibrofatty proliferation and its fatty or fibrotic composition can be assessed by MRE, especially on true FISP images

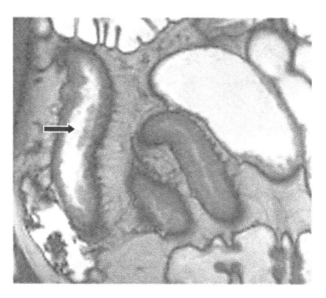

Figure 11   Intersecting longitudinal and transverse ulcers with intervening protruding edematous mucosa (arrow) shown on a coronal true FISP image in a patient with Crohn's disease. (From Ref. 36.)

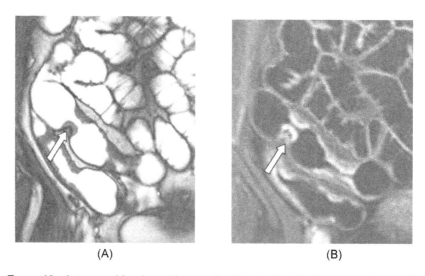

(A)   (B)

Figure 12   Intramural fat deposition can be detected by the black boundary artifact that is generated on true FISP images (arrow) (A) and the low signal intensity on 3D FLASH images with fat saturation (arrow) (B). (From Ref. 39.)

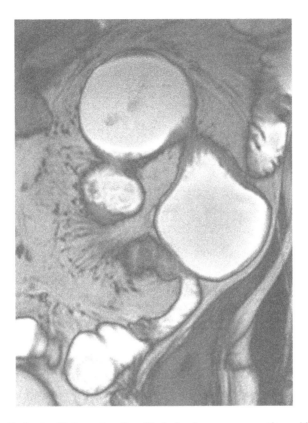

FIGURE 13 Patient with longstanding Crohn's disease presenting with symptoms of obstruction. Coronal true FISP image reveals multiple sites of high-grade stenosis with corresponding prestenotic dilatation.

(Fig. 14), while it can be only inferred on conventional enteroclysis. Fibro-fatty proliferation may simulate the characteristics of space-occupying lesions, separating and/or displacing small bowel loops. The involved mesentery may contain small lymph nodes, usually less than 8 mm in diameter and easily detected by their low signal intensity within the bright mesenteric fat on true FISP sequences. Such lymph nodes are not clearly demonstrated on HASTE images (Fig. 15), due to short T2 filtering effects, or on 3D FLASH images, due to saturation of mesenteric fat signal. Gadolinium uptake on 3D FLASH images allows identification of small inflammatory nodes (Fig. 16). Sinus tracts and fistulas (Fig. 17) are revealed by the high signal intensity of their fluid content on true FISP and HASTE images but may be overlooked on 3D FLASH images due to limited contrast

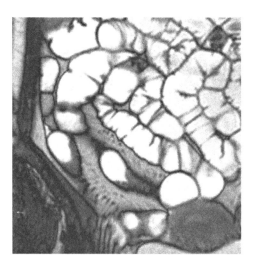

FIGURE 14 Coronal true FISP image demonstrating fibrofatty proliferation with displacement of adjacent bowel loops. (From Ref. 39.)

resolution with surrounding tissues. Abscesses can be recognized by their fluid content and enhancement of their wall postcontrast.

Disease activity can be estimated using MRE (13,29), and this may prove to be the main indication for examination in the near future. A recent study (38) compared several imaging findings and their possible combinations in patients with active Crohn's disease to a group with nonactive disease. Activity classification was based on the CDAI value (active disease, CDAI > 150). Significant differences in the presence of deep ulcers, wall thickening, and degree of gadolinium enhancement of mesenteric lymph nodes were found between active and nonactive groups (38).

The so-called comb sign, corresponding to increased mesenteric vascularity, can be easily appreciated on true FISP images (Fig. 18), adjacent to the mesenteric border of an involved segment and manifest by short, parallel, low signal intensity linear structures perpendicular to the long axis of the loop (35–38). The comb sign was found in all patients with active disease but also in some patients with inactive disease, and no significant difference in distribution was found (38). The comb sign can be demonstrated on 3D FLASH images as high signal intensity linear structures due to vascular enhancement (Fig. 18). Mural contrast uptake has long been considered the most important indicator of disease activity (13,29) and can be appreciated on T1-weighted 3D FLASH images. Wall thickening, significant mucosal enhancement, and relatively hypointense submucosal

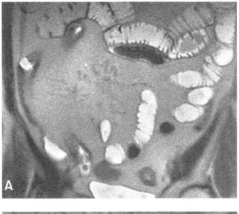

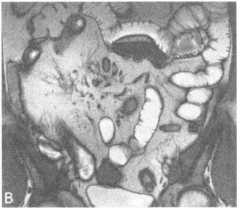

FIGURE 15   Coronal HASTE (A) and true FISP (B) images in a patient with Crohn's disease. Mesenteric lymph nodes and small vascular branches are filtered out on the HASTE sequence due to their short T2 constant.

edema have been reported as common findings on postgadolinium FLASH images in patients with active Crohn's disease (29). Disease severity can be ranked using measurements of wall thickening, the length of involved segments, and gadolinium uptake in comparison to renal cortex enhancement (29). Active disease may also be manifest by mural high signal intensity on T2-weighted images (13) (Fig. 4).

In the near future MRI may evolve into a comprehensive and thorough imaging examination of the small bowel in patients with Crohn's disease, providing anatomical and functional information and an estimate of disease activity, answering all clinical questions at one sitting (39).

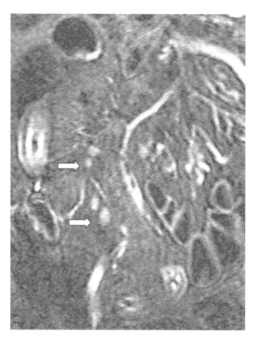

FIGURE 16   Coronal 3D FLASH with fat saturation image acquired 75 seconds after gadolinium injection. Marked contrast enhancement of mesenteric lymph nodes (arrows) is demonstrated in addition to the layered enhancement patern of the corresponding involved intestinal segment. (From Ref. 39.)

Neoplastic Bowel Disease

MRE combines the advantages of cross-sectional MRI with those of conventional enteroclysis, which is highly sensitive for detection of SB tumors. On true FISP images the high signal intensity of intraluminal fluid and mesenteric fat allows demonstration of tumors exhibiting intermediate signal intensity (Fig. 19). Small bowel neoplasms are mildly hypointense to isointense in comparison with the intestinal wall on precontrast non–fat-suppressed T1-weighted gradient echo MR images and present various enhancement patterns following gadolinium administration (30). Local extension may be demonstrated owing to the contrast difference between the tumor and surrounding high signal intensity fat (30).

Small bowel leiomyoma, leiomyosarcoma, adenocarcinoma, carcinoid tumor, and lymphoma display postcontrast enhancement that is best appreciated on fat-suppressed T1-weighted 3D FLASH images. Intense enhancement can be seen with carcinoid tumor, leiomyoma, and

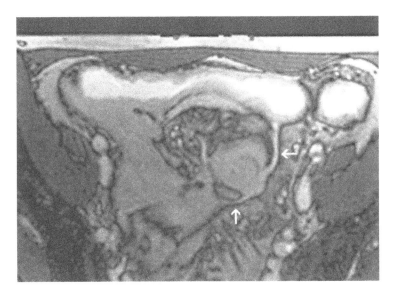

FIGURE 17 Axial true FISP image demonstrating two enteroenteric fistulas (arrows). (From Ref. 37.)

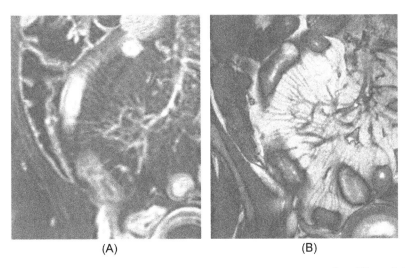

(A)   (B)

FIGURE 18 Coronal postgadolinium 3D FLASH with fat saturation (A) and true FISP (B) images in a patient with active Crohn's disease (CDAI = 257). Vascular engorgement (comb sign) is shown both on 3D FLASH and true FISP images.

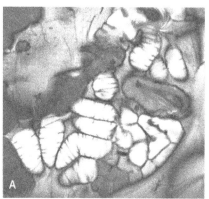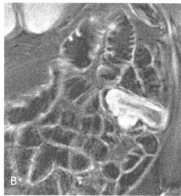

FIGURE 19   Coronal true FISP image (A) disclosing hemorrhagic foci in a jejunal stromal tumor. Marked gadolinium enhancement of the tumor is demonstrated on the 3D FLASH coronal image (B).

leiomyosarcoma. Lipomatous tumors and tumor hemorrhage can be detected on unenhanced, non–fat-suppressed 3D FLASH images, which should be acquired in addition to the MRE comprehensive imaging protocol. Distortion of small bowel loops or neoplastic invasion is depicted by all MRE sequences, while associated lymphadenopathy is well demonstrated on true FISP and 3D FLASH images.

Small Bowel Obstruction

MRE can provide anatomical and functional information identical to that provided by conventional enteroclysis in patients with SB obstruction (7). Furthermore, extraluminal causes are better illustrated using MRE (Fig. 20). MR fluoroscopy, utilizing dynamic projectional SSTSE sequences, is extremely helpful in diagnosing low-grade stenosis and in determining the level of obstruction. True FISP and postgadolinium enhanced 3D FLASH images can disclose the level and the cause of obstruction. In a recent study of 27 patients with postsurgical adhesions, cine MR imaging using the true FISP technique was found to be 87.5% sensitive and 92.5% specific (40).

Others

The role of MRI in small bowel ischemia has yet to be established. Limited reported experience indicates that bowel wall changes, vascular engorgement, and mesenteric edema can be appreciated on MRI (41). Superior

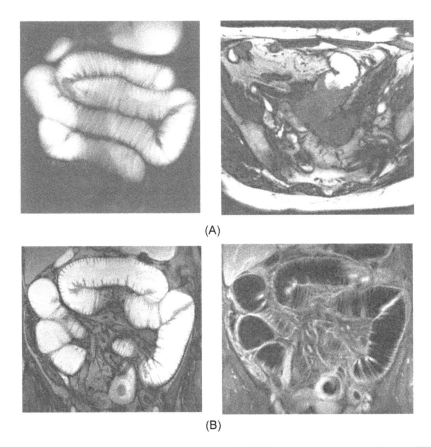

(A)

(B)

FIGURE 20 Patient with small bowel ileus. SSTSE coronal projectional image (A) disclosing the level of obstruction. On axial thin slice true FISP image (B) recurrent tumor from a previously resected sigmoid is infiltrating adjacent small bowel loops.

mesenteric artery blood flow changes in chronic mesenteric ischemia can also be studied with phase-contrast cine MRI (42). In addition, there are indications from animal studies that gastrointestinal bleeding can be diagnosed by dynamic post–contrast-enhanced 3D MR angiography using a blood pool agent (43).

CONCLUSIONS

MR imaging raises the possibility of a thorough and comprehensive evaluation of small intestinal diseases due to its superb soft tissue contrast, functional information, direct multiplanar capabilities, and lack of radiation exposure. Adequate bowel distention, homogeneous lumen opacification, fast sequences with breath-hold acquisition times, both T1- and T2-weighted imaging, and contrast enhancement are cornerstones for optimal MRI examination of the small bowel. A comprehensive MR enteroclysis imaging protocol should comprise SSTSE, true FISP, HASTE, and fat-suppressed 3D FLASH sequences. SSTSE is utilized for monitoring the contrast infusion process and performing MR fluoroscopy, whereas true FISP and HASTE are used mainly for anatomical demonstration and detection of pathology. 3D FLASH sequences following intravenous gadolinium injection may aid tissue characterization. Inflammatory or neoplastic diseases, including intestinal wall abnormalities, exoenteric disease manifestations and complications, disease activity, and, to a lesser extent, mucosal abnormalities can be appreciated on MRE.

REFERENCES

1. Dixon PM, Roulston ME, Nolan DJ. The small bowel enema: a 10-year review. Clin Radiol 1993; 4:46–48.
2. Barloon TJ, Lu CC, Honda H, et al. Does a normal small bowel enteroclysis exclude small bowel disease? A long term follow-up of concecutive normal studies. Abdom Imaging 1994; 19:113–115.
3. Gore RM, Balthazar EJ, Ghahremani GG, Miller FH. CT features of ulcerative colitis and Crohn's disease. Am J Roentgenol 1996; 167:3–15.
4. Bender GN, Maglinte DT, Kloeppel VR, Timmons JH. CT enteroclysis: a superfuous diagnostic procedure or valuable when investigating small bowel disease. AJR 1999; 172:373–378.
5. Rust GF, Holzknecht N, Olbrich D, Schopf U, Bruning R, Reiser M. Multislice computed tomography of the small intestine. Preliminary results. Radiologe 1999; 39(11):965–970.
6. Gourtsoyiannis N, Papanikolaou N, Grammatikakis J, Maris T, Prassopoulos P. Magnetic resonance imaging of the small bowel using a true-FISP sequence after enteroclysis with water solution. Invest Radiol 2000; 35(12):707–711.
7. Lomas DJ, Graves MJ. Small bowel MRI using water as a contrast medium. BJR 1999; 72:994–997.
8. Umschaden HW, Szolar D, Gasser J, Umschaden M, Haselbach H. Small-bowel disease: comparison of MR enteroclysis images with conventional enteroclysis and surgical findings. Radiology 2000; 215:717–7125.
9. Holzknecht N, Helmberger T, v. Ritter C, Gauger J, Faber S, Reiser M. Breathhold MRI of the small bowel in Crohn's disease after enteroclysis with oral magnetic particles. Radiologe 1998; 38: 29–36.
10. Rieber A, Wruk D, Nüssle K, Aschoff AJ, Reinshagen M, Adler G, Brambs H-J, Tomczak R. MRI of the abdomen in combination with enteroclysis in Crohn's disease with oral and intravenous Gd-DTPA. Radiologe 1998; 38:23–28.

11. Low RN, Francis IR. MR Imaging of gastrointestinal tract with IV Gadolinium and diluted barium oral contrast media compared with unenhanced MR imaging and CT. Am J Roentgenol 1997; 169:1051–1059.

12. Schunk K, Metzmann U, Kersjes W, Schadmann-Fischer S, Kreitner KF, Duchmann R, Protzer U, Wanitschke R, Thelen M. Serial observation in Crohn's disease: Can hydro-MRI replace follow-through examinations? Fortschr Röntgenstr 1997; 166:389–396.

13. Maccioni F, Viscido A, Broglia L, Marrollo M, Masciangelo R, Caprilli R, Rossi P. Evaluation of Crohn's disease activity with magnetic resonance imaging. Abdom Imaging 2000; 25:219–228.

14. Minowa O, Ozaki Y, Kyogoku S, Shindoh N, Sumi Y, Katayama H. MR Imaging of the small bowel using water as a contrast agent in a preliminary study with healthy volunteers. Am J Roentgenol 1999; 173:581–582.

15. Kivelitz D, Gehl HB, Heuck A, Krahe T, Taupitz M, Lodemann KP, Hamm B. Ferric ammonium citrate as a positive bowel contrast agent for MR imaging of the upper abdomen. Safety and diagnostic efficacy. Acta Radiol 1999; 40:429–435.

16. Kressel HY. Insights of an abdominal imager: What do we need for MRI enhancement? Magn Reson Med 1991; 22:314.

17. Paley MR, Ros PR. MRI of the gastrointestinal tract. Eur Radiol 1997; 7:1387.

18. Hahn PF. Advances in contrast enhanced MR imaging. Gastrointestinal contrast agents. Am J Roentgenol 1991; 156:252.

19. Small WC, DeSimone-Macchi D, Parker JR, et al. A multisite phase III study of the safety and efficacy of a new manganese choride-based gastrointestinal contrast agent for MRI of the abdomen and pelvis. JMRI 1999; 10:15–24.

20. Mirowitz SA, Susmann N. Use of a nutritional support formula as a gastrointestinal contrast agent for MRI. J Comput Assist Tomogr 1992; 16:908.

21. Karantanas A, Papanikolaou N, Kalef-Ezra J, Challa A, Gourtsoyiannis N. Blueberry juice used per os in upper abdominal MR imaging: composition and initial clinical data. Eur Radiol 2000; 10:909–913.

22. Rubin DL, Muller HH, Young SW. Formulation of radiographically detectable gastrointestinal contrast agents for magnetic resonance imaging: effects of barium sulfate additive on MR contrast agent effectiveness. Magn Reson Med 1992; 23:154.

23. Faber SC, Stehling MK, Holzknecht N, Gauger J, Helmberger T, Reiser M. Pathologic conditions in the small bowel: findings at fat-suppressed gadolinium-enhanced MR imaging with an optimized suspension of oral magnetic particles. Radiology 1997; 205:278–282.

24. Mitchell DG, Vinitski S, Mohamed FB, Mammone JF, Haidet K, Rifkin MD. Comparison of Kaopectate with barium for negative and positive enteric contrast at MR Imaging. Radiology 1991; 181:475–480.

25. Mattrey RF, Trambert MA, Brown JJ, Young SW, Bruneton JN, Wesbey GE, Balsara ZN. Perflubron as an oral contrast agent for MR imaging: results of a phase III clinical trial. Radiology 1994; 191:841–848.

26. Weinreb JC, Maravilla KR, Redman HC, Nunnally R. Improved MR imaging of the upper abdomen with glucagons and gas. J Comput Assist Tomogr 1984; 8:835–838.

27. Reiber A, Aschoff A, Nussle K, Wruk D, Tomczak R, Reinshagen M, Adler G, Brambs HJ. MRI in the diagnosis of small bowel disease: use of positive and negative oral contrast media in combination with enteroclysis. Eur Radiol 2000; 10(9):1377–1382.

28. Gourtsoyiannis N, Papanikolaou N, Grammatikakis J, Maris T, Prassopoulos P. MR Enteroclysis protocol optimization: comparison between 3D FLASH with fat saturation after intravenous gadolinium injection and true FISP sequences. Eur Radiol 2001; 11(6):908–913.

29. Schunk K, Kern A, Oberholzer K, Kalden P, Mayer I, Orth T, Wanitschke R. Hydro-MRI in Crohn's disease. Appraisal of disease activity. Invest Radiol 2000; 35:431–437.

30. Semelka RC, John G, Kelekis N, Burdeny DA, Ascher SM. Small bowel neoplastic disease: demonstration by MRI. JMRI 1996; 6:855–860.

31. Papanikolaou N, Prassopoulos P, Grammatikakis J, Maris T, Kouroumalis E, Gourtsoyiannis N. Optimization of a contrast medium suitable for conventional enteroclysis, MR enteroclysis, and virtual MR enteroscopy. Abdom Imaging 2002; 27(5):517–522.

32. Haacke M, Tkach J. Fast MR imaging: techniques and clinical applications. AJR 1990; 155:951–964.

33. Oppelt A, Graumann R, Barfuss H, Fischer H, Hertl W, Schajor W. A new fast MRI sequence. Electromed 1986; 3:15–18.

34. Laubenberger J, Buchert M, Schneider B, Blum U, Hennig J, Langer M. Breath-hold projection magnetic resonance-cholangio-pancreaticography (MRCP): a new method for the examination of the bile and pancreatic ducts. Magn Reson Med 1995; 33(1):18–23.

35. Papamastorakis G, Papanikolaou N, Prassopoulos P, Grammatikakis J, Maris T, Gourtsoyiannis N. Crohn's disease: comparison between MR enteroclysis and conventional enteroclysis. In book of abstracts; ECR 2003 B-0368, pp 208.

36. Prassopoulos P, Papanikolaou N, Grammatikakis J, Roussomoustakaki M, Maris T, Gourtsoyiannis N. MR Enteroclysis imaging findings in Crohn's disease. Radiographics 2001; 21:S161–S172.

37. Gourtsoyiannis N, Papanikolaou N, Grammatikakis J, Prassopoulos P. MR enteroclysis: technical considerations and clinical applications. Eur Radiol 2002; 12(11):2651–2658.

38. Tritou I, Papanikolaou N, Prassopoulos P, Grammatikakis I, Roussomoustakaki M, Gourtsoyiannis N. Crohn's disease activity assessment with MR enteroclysis. In book of abstracts; ECR 2003, B-0654, pp 272.

39. Gourtsoyiannis N, Papanikolaou N, Rieber A, Brambs HJ, Prassopoulos P. Evaluation of the small intestine by MR imaging. In: Gourtsoyiannis N, ed. Radiological Imaging of the Small Intestine. New York: Springer-Verlag, 2002:157–170.

40. Lienemann A, Sprenger D, Steitz HO, Korell M, Reiser M. Detection and mapping of intraabdominal adhesions by using functional cine MR imaging: preliminary results. Radiology 2000; 217:421–425.
41. Ha HK, Lee EH, Lim CH, Shin YM, Jeong YK, Yoon KH, Lee MG, Min Y, Auh YH. Application of MRI for small intestinal diseases. JMRI 1998; 8:375–383.
42. Li KCP, Whitney WS, McDonnell CH, et al. Chronic mesenteric ischemia: evaluation with phase-contrast cine MR imaging. Radiology 1994; 190: 175–179.
43. Hilfiker PR, Weishaupt D, Kacl GM, Hetzer FH, Griff MD, Ruehm SG, Debatin JF. Comparison of three dimensional magnetic resonance imaging in conjunction with a blood pool contrast agent and nuclear scintigraphy for the detection of experimentally induced gastrointestinal bleeding. Gut 1999; 45(4):581–587.

9

Multiplanar CT Enterography

Vassilios Raptopoulos
Harvard Medical School, Beth Israel Deaconess Medical Center,
  Boston, Massachusetts, U.S.A.

INTRODUCTION

Computed tomography (CT) is used in the abdomen for a wide range of indications from nonspecific abdominal pain to surgical planning or guidance for interventional procedures. Similarly, CT is used extensively in the gastrointestinal tract for a variety of indications including bowel obstruction, perforation, or ischemia, Crohn's disease, appendicitis, diverticulitis, and other inflammatory diseases, bowel tumors, and masses or fluid collections in the mesentery. Recently, speed and high resolution achieved with spiral and multislice scanning has expanded the uses of CT. The gastrointestinal tract is always imaged at abdominal CT scanning, and valuable bowel information is obtained from routine abdominal surveys. However, imaging of the bowel is challenging because of its length and orientation, the difficulty in sustaining distension and homogeneity of the oral contrast column, and variability in IV contrast enhancement. Tailoring the examination to optimize bowel detail can be done with multiplanar CT enterography. This is a minor variation on routine abdominal scanning geared towards more sustained bowel filling with oral contrast material and utilization of both axial and coronal planes. Additional small-bowel detail can be obtained with CT enteroclysis. This technique is more involved, requiring jejunal intubation and insertion of large amounts of contrast material with the use of a pump.

TECHNIQUE

The goal of small bowel CT imaging is to discriminate the small intestine from other bowel loops, distend its lumen, visualize the intestinal wall, identify vessels supplying the bowel loops, and assess the mesentery. Both multiplanar CT enterography and CT enteroclysis require gastrointestinal luminal contrast material. The use of IV contrast material is very helpful and should be encouraged. Data are acquired with volume techniques utilizing thin collimation. With single-detector row spiral scanners this may require scanning during two or three breath-holds, while the whole abdomen and pelvis can be scanned in under 15 seconds with the newer 8-row and 16-row multislice CT scanners. Prone positioning helps disperse bowel loops. Coronal reconstructions are helpful in a variety of ways, from assisting display of the images to facilitating detection of bowel or other abdominal abnormalities. Rectal contrast may be given for completion of the study in specific clinical situations.

Oral Contrast

Multiplanar CT Enterography

Conventional high-density oral contrast is given: 1600 mL of 2% barium-based or 2–2.5% water-soluble iodine-based oral contrast over 1–2 hours prior to scanning (1). This is one and a half to twice the usual dose for a standard abdominal CT examination (2). Flavoring makes the contrast more palatable. The use of a large volume of high-density oral contrast is particularly useful when collimation greater than 5 mm is used. With the advent of multislice CT and utilization of thin slice bowel detail is markedly improved. One of the original reasons for using oral contrast was to help discriminate bowel from lymph nodes and other abdominal abnormalities. This is no longer a problem as high-resolution images of bowel and mesentery help discriminate the gut easily. Currently oral contrast is primarily used to enhance evaluation of bowel wall detail and for dynamic studies. Thus, the use of higher volumes of contrast in CT enterography may not be necessary. In patients with bowel obstruction, the bowel is already distended and oral contrast may not be required or may be contraindicated (3). In suspected partial obstruction, high-density oral contrast and follow-up scanning may be required. High-density oral contrast is helpful in patients with Crohn's disease to evaluate for fistulae and sinus tracks or in those with suspected abscess. Variations to this regimen may be used, all with good results. Currently, most investigators advocate the use of approximately 1000 mL or about 4 cups of oral contrast. Wittenberg et al. (4) give a total of 600–900 mL of dilute water-soluble oral contrast at 4 hours, 2 hours, and immediately prior to scanning. We give 400–600 mL over an interval of 40–60 minutes before scanning and another 200–400 mL in the last 20 minutes (5).

Low-attenuation oral contrast such as milk or water can also be given. Low attenuation endoluminal density allows good visualization of the intestinal wall (6–8). However, IV contrast is generally needed with the use of these agents. Use of isotonic solutions has produced excellent results (7). Up to 2000 mL of flavored iso-osmotic polyethylene glycol (PEG) electrolyte balanced solution is given over a 1-hour period prior to scanning. Because PEG accelerates peristalsis, antispasmodic agents are required before scanning. Water can also be used with good effect (8,9). Water may be absorbed more readily than the other agents, but this happens mainly in the colon. A minimum of 4 glasses of water or juice is recommended. Fat density oral contrast such as flavored 12.5% corn oil emulsion provides excellent bowel distention and wall visualization but is cumbersome to produce and less palatable (6). Alternatively, 4 cups of whole milk (4% fat concentration) given within 1 hour of scanning can produce similar results (5). Compared to 2% barium suspension, the effects of milk on gastrointestinal tract distension and bowel loop discrimination are not significantly different, but milk results in significantly better mural visualization. In general, use of whole fat milk is significantly better than low fat milk, barium, water, and no oral contrast agents. Informative studies, however, can be achieved even without oral contrast provided IV contrast is given and thin collimation is used. Currently, if low attenuation contrast is required, we use a combination of 2–3 cups of water followed by 1–2 cups of whole milk. This optimizes both distal and proximal bowel distention.

CT Enteroclysis

This is done after insertion of a nasoduodenal tube just beyond the ligament of Treitz and administration of over 2000 mL of 2% diluted barium or water-soluble iodinated contrast material (10). Low-attenuation oral contrast, usually methylcellulose, or paraffin-methylcellulose suspension can also be used to distend the small bowel, as in conventional barium enteroclysis. The oral contrast is preferably delivered via an automatic pump at a rate of 60–100 mL per minute (11,12). Previous preparation of the bowel is advised. In addition, use of antiperistaltic drugs just prior to scanning is advocated as with conventional fluoroscopic or MR enteroclysis (11–13). This can be done with the use of a non-absorbable iso-osmolar solution given 6–8 hours before the examination (11). Alternatively, the patients are kept fasting of solid food for 18 hours, they are instructed to drink up to 4000 mL of fluid, and laxatives are administered (12). The issues that are considered when choosing low rather than high attenuation oral contrast material at CT enterography also apply in the selection of positive or negative oral contrast media used at CT or MR enteroclysis (14).

IV Contrast

High doses of IV contrast delivered at relatively fast injection rates produce excellent and consistent vascular and parenchymal enhancement. We inject a total of 120 or 150 mL of IV contrast depending on whether patient's weight is under or over 75 kg, respectively. Various commercial agents are available. Generally, we use 300 or 320 mg I/mL solution. The latter is used for patients who weigh over 90 kg. Nonionic contrast is preferred to avoid nausea and vomiting in patients with an already overdistended gastrointestinal tract from oral contrast. We use a biphasic injection regimen. First, 30–50 mL of IV contrast is given at 2 mL/s without the patient being scanned. After a delay of 2–3 minutes, the remainder of the IV contrast material is given: 80–100 mL is injected at a rate of 2–3 mL/s. Scanning starts 60–70 s after the beginning of the second dose of IV contrast. This biphasic injection results in optimal enhancement of the bowel wall, solid organs, mesenteric and retroperitoneal vessels, as well as the kidneys and ureters. Other regimens are quite effective as well, and one may not need to change the general IV contrast regimen used for routine abdominal scanning in the particular institution. On occasion, CT angiography may be combined with multiplanar CT enterography for specialized tests such as assessment of bowel ischemia. In these situations, low attenuation contrast is preferable to positive oral contrast media.

Scanning Techniques

We scan the abdomen and pelvis from the dome of the diaphragm to below the symphysis pubis. Volumetric scanning is important so that meaningful multiple planar reformatted (MPR) images can be obtained. With single-row spiral scanners, this may be achieved with two sequential spiral sets obtained in two breath-holds. With multislice scanners the abdomen and pelvis can be scanned during a single breath-hold. Spiral scanners allow for retrospective overlapping of axial images, while multislice scanners allow for retrospective or prospective change of slice thickness as well. The multislice scanners operate with basic detector thickness unit of either 1 mm (e.g., Siemens, Phillips, Toshiba) or 1.25 mm (e.g., General

Electric) in the z-axis. Scanning is volumetric, and final image thickness is obtained in multiples of this basic detector thickness. Most 16-detector-row scanners can divide the basic thickness by one half the original (e.g., 0.5 or 0.65 mm). In addition, slice overlapping can be helpful for smoother MPR images. In general, when deciding which collimation to use on a multislice scanner, we choose the one that will give the most body coverage within one breath-hold, with collimation as close to 1 mm as possible but not thicker than 3 mm. However, this may produce a large number (>500) of thin, grainy images. To improve image quality and decrease image glut, we use thicker images for viewing: 5 mm thick axial or MPR images, reconstructed from thin overlapping slices. The thinner the original slices, the better the final viewing hard copy images are.

Single-Detector Spiral Scanners

We use 3–5 mm slice collimation and a pitch 1.5–1.8 (1). The whole abdomen and pelvis may be scanned in two breath-holds. We avoid breath-holds longer than 20 seconds in duration. Scanning in the prone position decreases involuntary respiratory motion. Once the lower pelvis is reached, the patient can resume shallow breathing. Overlapping axial slices by one third to one half of the slice thickness improves the quality of MPR images.

Multislice 4-Detector-Row Scanners

The abdomen and pelvis can be scanned at 2 or 2.5 mm collimation in a single breath-hold. Alternatively, 1 or 1.25 mm collimation can be used, but this would require two breath-holds. Hard copy film or PACS viewing is done using 5 mm axial and MPR slices reconstructed from the thinner slices.

Multislice 8- and 16-Detector-Row Scanners

The speed of these scanners allows for single-breath scanning with 1 or 1.25 mm collimation. The 16-row scanners can utilize submillimeter collimation. This results in isotropic or near isotropic voxels allowing for high-resolution axial or multiplanar images and volume renderings that are of anatomical atlas quality.

Multiplanar Reformations

Coronal views are increasingly helpful as axial slice collimation decreases and quality of MPRs improves. We use average-density 5 mm images reconstructed from thin slices. This can be done either prospectively or retrospectively. We are becoming increasingly dependent on coronal images reconstructed from 1 or 1.25 mm axial collimation. Comparing the various scanners, we found that coronal MPR images from single slice spiral scanners confirmed abnormalities seen on axial images in the majority of cases and in some cases allowed better understanding of the abnormality in question. Consequently, MPR images with single-detector spiral CT studies of patients with Crohn's disease improved the confidence of overall interpretation, assessment of wall thickening, and extent of disease (1). In addition, MPR images have been shown to be helpful in assessing intestinal obstruction (15). In our experience, coronal MPR images from 4-detector-row multislice scanners improve understanding of an abnormality in the majority of cases. Even better, the MPR image quality obtained from 8-detector-row-multislice scanners approaches the quality of the axial images. We have seen abnormalities on MPR not initially appreciated on axial scans in many cases, a significant improvement over both single and 4-detector-row scanners. Currently, the quality of MPRs achieved is such that we consider coronal images to be as complementary to the axial scans as the axial images are to the coronal. In addition to average-density MPR, thick slab (10–20 mm) coronal maximum intensity projection (MIP) images may be helpful, especially in following the course of bowel loops, mesenteric vessels, and ureters. Volume renderings may also be helpful, especiatcutlly in cancer staging.

Exam Display Strategies

Whichever collimation is chosen, multislice multiplanar CT enterography will result in a large number of images to be viewed. This image glut may create not only eye fatigue for the reader, but also confusion in case presentation and frustration for independent clinical staff reviewing the studies. The communication burden can be counterproductive in patient management and health care economics. Ironically, superb and utterly helpful images may be buried in the multiplicity of choices. In addition, storage problems in film or electronic memory (PACS) may create logistical and financial concerns. Because of the infinite number of projections available, operators and technologists may become confused as to how to finally display the studies. To alleviate this problem we use the following protocol: biphasic IV contrast injection with scanning during the second phase only, with as thin collimation as possible. For viewing, we reconstruct 5 mm thick axial and coronal average-density images and 20 mm thick MIP images. This protocol produces about 120–140 images, which are stored in PACS or filmed on six to seven sheets of film in a 20-on-1 format. Additional image processing is obtained only in special circumstances.

MULTIPLANAR CT ENTEROGRAPHY VS.
CT ENTEROCLYSIS

As with conventional fluoroscopic enteroclysis, CT enteroclysis provides a high degree of consistent small bowel distension. The resultant studies are of superb quality and can provide fine mucosal and luminal detail on a par with conventional double contrast fluoroscopic enteroclysis (10,16,17). Although the examination is very helpful in patients with partial small bowel obstruction and Crohn's disease, it is contraindicated in patients with suspected bowel perforation and high-grade obstruction. Despite the superb images, CT enteroclysis may be uncomfortable for the patient and expense is increased compared with CT enterography because of the need for the tubing and pump and longer utilization of the CT room. The risk of complication is also increased because bowel distension is performed blind in contrast to fluoroscopic techniques. The additional information provided by CT enteroclysis may not be worth the added effort in the majority of cases. In the past few years, MR enteroclysis techniques have provided high-resolution images as an alternative to CT enteroclysis (13,14,18,19). In addition, MR enteroclysis can provide real-time functional information allowing assessment of peristalsis.

Although multiplanar CT enterography provides less distension of the small intestine, the degree of bowel distension may be more physiological than the unnaturally distended small bowel achieved with enteroclysis. Furthermore, the examination is more comfortable for patients and requires less preparation and room utilization. Although fine anatomical detail is not achieved to the same extent as with fluoroscopic studies, other signs that may help characterize small bowel disease are available, including abnormalities in wall enhancement patterns, extraluminal abnormalities, and assessment of the mesentery (1,4). We prefer CT enterography to other techniques described and use it as our routine protocol for CT evaluation of suspected gastrointestinal abnormalities, including acute abdominal pain.

CLINICAL APPLICATIONS

Evaluation of bowel is difficult because of its length (about 7 m of small intestine), convoluted course, and physiological peristaltic motion. Even with the relatively short colon ($\sim$1.5 m), which has a predictable course from right lower quadrant to rectum, variations exist as to the location of the cecum, the ileocecal valve, and the appendix and the undulation of the hepatic and splenic flexures and sigmoid colon. Multiplanar CT enterography can help recognize individual bowel components, localize abnormalities, and show the extent of disease (1). Stomach distention is variable. Gastric folds are well seen and an increase in thickness and/or disruption seen on MPR images should be considered abnormal. The duodenum has very active peristalsis. Milk reduces duodenal peristalsis and appears to be particularly helpful in evaluation the pancreas and duodenum. The jejunum is rich in folds and normal plicae circularis may give the appearance of a thickened wall, especially if nondistended or only moderately distended (Fig. 1). The ileum has less internal architecture with a relatively smooth wall and occasional folds (5). Normal small bowel loops should be similar in appearance to the adjacent small bowel loops and appear pliable. In thin patients with little

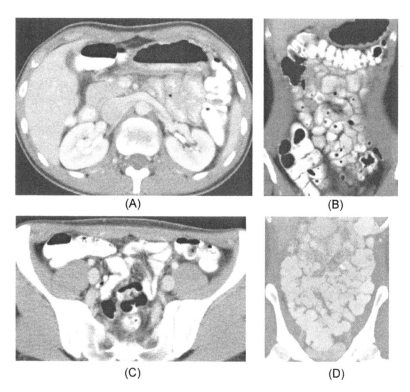

(A)   (B)

(C)   (D)

Figure 1 Normal multiplanar CT enterography: axial image (A) shows normal jejunum with the feathery appearance of its wall caused by plicae. The ileum in the pelvis (B) shows an absence of intrinsic wall architecture. Average-density coronal reformation (C) shows normal distribution of the small bowel and ascending colon. MIP coronal reformation (D) of another patient shows good filling of the GI tract with oral contrast and a good overview of the small bowel.

or no mesenteric fat, the small bowel loops are closely applied to one another and their shape appears interdependent, while in patients with more mesenteric fat, the loops separate and appear round or oval. In contrast, abnormal bowel with wall thickening will appear stiff with loss of the normal contour and undulation.

The terminal ileum and ileocecal valve are always seen at multiplanar CT enterography. Evaluation of the colon may be hindered by the presence of fecal material and, if not distended, may appear abnormal. If doubt arises, 100–300 mL of rectal contrast (water or 2% barium suspension or water-soluble iodinated solution) may be helpful. Most often, however, an abnormal colon will be associated with other findings in the adjacent mesentery, making the use of a contrast enema rarely necessary. Interactive multiplanar viewing is helpful in differentiating normal structures from bowel abnormalities (Fig. 2). In the postoperative bowel the addition of MPR images helps to detect sites of anastomoses, to evaluate neoterminal ileum, and to assess extent of diseases.

Increased bowel wall thickness is a nonspecific but important finding. Because of peristalsis, considerable variation in bowel wall thickness exists. Normal distended small bowel wall is 1–2 mm thick while non-distended bowel may be as thick as 4 mm, especially the jejunum (2,20). Patterns of attenuation and IV contrast enhancement of the wall may help in the differential diagnosis. Wittenberg et al. (4) described five such patterns: (a) homogeneous bright enhancement (white) may be seen in shock bowel, ischemia, inflammatory bowel disease, adhesions and tumor (uncommon); (b) hypoenhancing (gray) wall may be seen in inflammatory bowel disease and tumor; (c) water attenuation (water halo or target pattern) is seen in ischemia, inflammatory bowel disease, acute infection, radiation, and tumor (uncommon); (d) fat attenuation (fat halo) is seen in inflammatory bowel disease (usually chronic disease) such as Crohn's or ulcerative colitis, and chronic radiation enteritis; and (e) pneumatosis can be seen in blunt or iatrogenic trauma, ischemia, and acute infection (Table 1).

Crohn's Disease

CT may demonstrate nonspecific wall thickening along with extramural complications of Crohn's disease. Multiplanar CT enterography provides high-quality images that can be used for diagnosis as well as monitoring disease progression and detection of complications. Compared with fluoroscopic studies, CT may not depict aphthous or linear ulceration, but it is superior in showing wall thickening, edema, fistulae, and all extraluminal abnormalities (1,10). Nodular thickening of the wall and mural sinuses may be seen (Figs. 3 and 4). The degree of intestinal wall enhancement

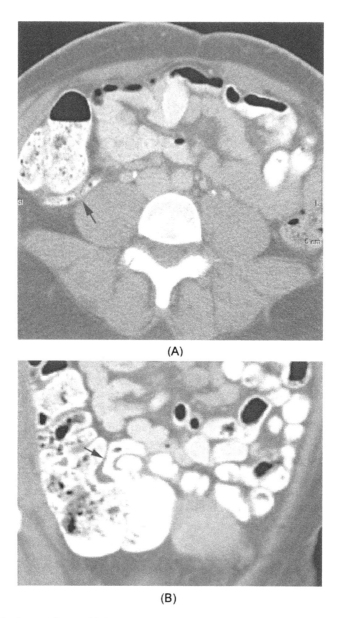

(A)

(B)

FIGURE 2   Interactive multiplanar viewing. Because of their orientation, the normal appendix (arrow) in this patient is seen on axial image (A), while the terminal ileum (arrow) is best identified on coronal image (B).

TABLE 1 Common Enhancement Patterns of Bowel Wall Abnormalities

Homogeneous enhancement (white)	Hypoattenuation	Water density (water halo or target)	Fat density (fat halo)	Pneumatosis
Shock bowel				Trauma
Ischemia		Ischemia		Ischemia
IBD	IBD	IBD	IBD (usually chronic)	
Adhesion				
Tumor (uncommon)	Tumor	Tumor (uncommon)		
		Acute infection		Acute infection
		Radiation	Radiation (chronic)	

Source: Adapted from Ref. 4.

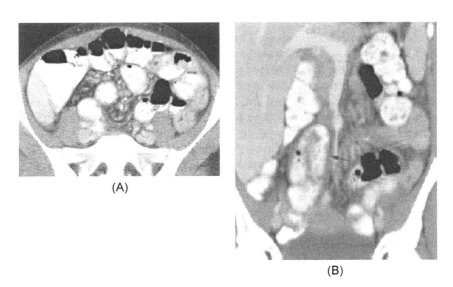

(A)

(B)

FIGURE 3 Axial (A) and coronal (B) images of patient with Crohn's disease. There is nodular thickening of the wall of the distal ileum (arrow), better appreciated on the coronal image. Lymph node prominence is better appreciated on the axial image.

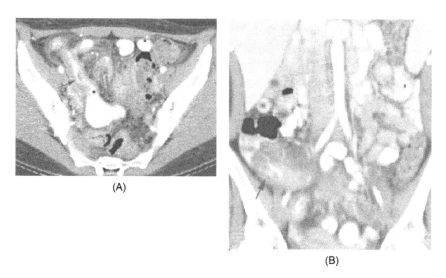

(A)

(B)

FIGURE 4   Wall thickening in the terminal ileum and intramural sinus (arrow) in patient with Crohn's disease and recurrent symptoms. The scan was performed using a 4-detector-row multislice scanner. Although the axial image (A) is of high quality, the coronal reformat (B) lags behind in quality as it is obtained from data acquired in the axial plane with 2.5 mm collimation.

may be related to disease activity. This also applies to increased and prominent vascularity (comb sign) and fibro fatty proliferation of both the mesentery and anti mesenteric fat (Fig. 5). Lee et al. (21) found that increased bowel wall vascularity is related to clinically active disease in that it may require more aggressive treatment. They also found that increased bowel wall vascularity was associated with increased mucosal ulceration and a greater length of affected bowel on conventional barium studies. Other signs indicating activity have been described on MR imaging and can be extrapolated to CT. These include bowel thickening of more than 4 mm, abnormal wall enhancement (ratio with normal bowel of 1.3:1), layered enhancement, and increased mesenteric vascularity (22). Fistulas may be seen as well as bowel loop adherence. Although motility cannot be assessed by static images, adherent bowel loops associated with fibrous tissue, often with a stellate mesenteric fibrosis, indicates fixation of the bowel (Fig. 6). This is commonly associated with fistula formation. Strictures are associated with dense wall thickening with little enhancement and varying degree of proximal bowel dilatation. Compared with barium studies, we found that multiplanar CT enterography with single-detector spiral CT provided more information in 4 of 19 patients and equal information in 14 of

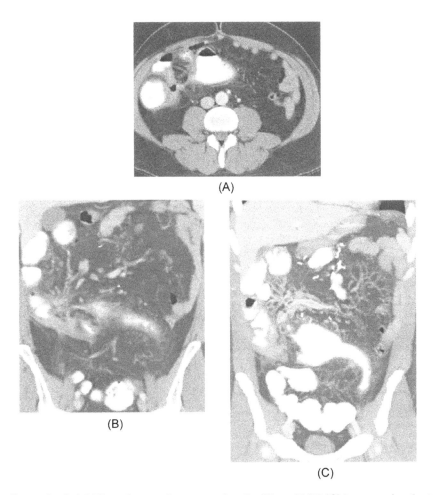

(A)

(B)

(C)

FIGURE 5   Axial (A) and coronal average-density (B) and MIP (C) images of patient with acute exacerbation of Crohn's disease. There is bowel wall thickening associated with increased vascularity and fibro-fatty proliferation, a comb sign, distal to which the ileum is dilated with subsequent stricture formation with adherence and fistulae to other bowel loops at the ileocecal juncture. There is increased mesenteric vascularity and prominent mesenteric lymph nodes.

19 patients studied (1). The addition of MPR images improves disease detection and assessment of bowel involvement. Strictures may be occasionally confused with peristalsis. Although tube enteroclysis is contraindicated in complete obstruction, in partial obstruction it reportedly shows areas of bowel narrowing more reliably (10,11,16,17). Multiplanar

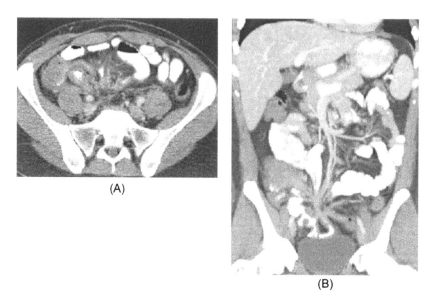

(A)

(B)

FIGURE 6   Axial (A) and coronal (B) images of patient with Crohn's disease in relative remission. In the right lower quadrant the bowel loops are thick walled and are matted together, but there is little mesenteric reaction.

imaging is helpful in assessing postoperative complications or progress of disease in the remaining bowel (Fig. 7).

Acute Abdominal Pain

The impact of CT on diagnosis and management of patients with acute abdominal pain has been shown (23). CT is especially helpful in patients without previous history of abdominal disease. In these patients the sensitivity of CT was 90% compared with a sensitivity of 47% for initial clinical assessment, and CT changed management plans in 37% of 59 patients (24). We found multiplanar CT enterography helpful in identifying the normal appendix. An abnormal appendix is usually readily seen on axial CT images, but in many cases visualization of a normal appendix is difficult. Because appendicitis cannot be definitively excluded if the appendix is not seen, interactive multiplanar imaging may increase confidence of excluding the disease. Similarly, the addition of MPR images facilitates visualization of the uterus and ovaries. Diagnosis of other conditions including cholecystitis, ulcerative colitis, diverticulitis and abdominal abscess is also enhanced using the multiplanar CTE technique (Figs. 8–11).

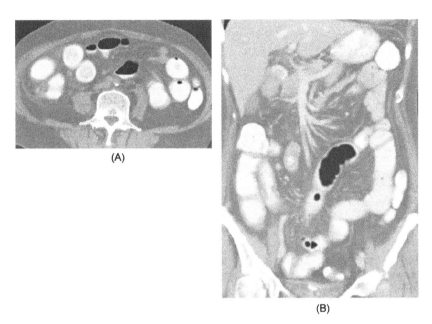

(A)

(B)

FIGURE 7 Axial (A) and coronal (B) images of patient with Crohn's disease. There has been previous resection of the terminal ileum and recurrence at the neo-terminal ileum as manifested by bowel wall thickening.

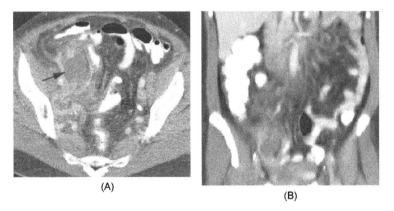

(A)

(B)

FIGURE 8 Appendiceal abscess (arrow) seen on an axial image (A). The coronal reformat (B) generated from axial images obtained with 5 mm collimation is significantly inferior in image quality compared with the axial view. Nevertheless, it is a useful image because it helps confirm the diagnosis and gives a different perspective of the relationship of the abscess with the uterus, bladder, and colon.

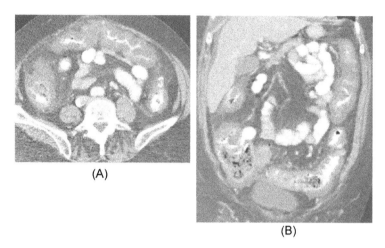

FIGURE 9 Psudomembranous colitis involving the entire colon. Marked wall thickening with narrowing of the lumen (accordion sign) is seen on both axial (A) and coronal (B) views.

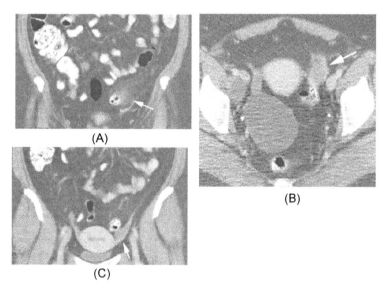

FIGURE 10 Mild acute diverticulitis of the sigmoid colon as seen on CT with minimal stranding of fat (arrow) around the sigmoid colon (A). On the axial image (B) a possible small abscess (arrow) is noted on the left adjacent to the sigmoid. On another coronal reformation (C), this was shown to be normal left ovary (arrow). There is a large ovarian cyst on the right.

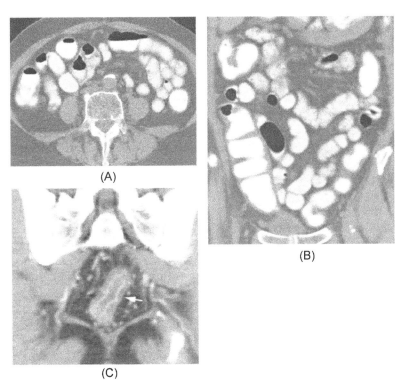

FIGURE 11 Axial (A) and coronal (B) images of a patient with ulcerative colitis. The wall thickening is more conspicuous on the coronal image compared with the axial view. Coronal reformation of the pelvis (C) shows water density enhancement pattern (arrow) of the wall of the rectum (target pattern).

Bowel Obstruction

CT is accurate in demonstrating small bowel obstruction with reported sensitivities of 80–100% (3). Because peristalsis cannot be assessed, the CT diagnosis of bowel obstruction relies on changes in bowel caliber and identification of a transitional zone (20). In these circumstances, MPR images may contribute more to establishing the diagnosis than the type or amount of oral contrast ingested (15). A transition point can be demonstrated and the cause of obstruction identified. The small bowel is considered dilated if its caliber is greater than 2.5 cm (25). The difficulty lies in differentiating obstruction from focal or generalized adynamic ileus. Oral contrast may be contraindicated if the patient is vomiting or overly distended. Conversely, if oral contrast can be tolerated, it may not reach the site of obstruction for hours. Scanning 1 hour after oral contrast ingestion will provide the diagnosis in most cases. In the remaining cases, follow-up scanning after a 4- to 6-hour delay may be required.

Causes of bowel obstruction are many. In the small bowel, the most common cause is adhesions, followed by hernia (3,26). Interactive viewing of axial and coronal images helps to detect the point of transition, and the actual adhesion may be seen as an enhancing band (Fig. 12). Similar evaluation may be helpful in closed loop obstruction. Imaging findings in closed loop obstruction include a C- or U-shaped loop of dilated bowel, adjacent collapsed loops, convergence of mesenteric vessels, and beak or whirl signs (26,27). The latter three signs are nicely demonstrated on cine-viewing on PACS or MPR images. Similarly, MPR images are helpful in the evaluation of cecal or sigmoid volvulus.

After adhesions, hernias are the next most frequent cause of obstruction. These are divided into external (through the abdominal wall) and internal (through bowel mesentery or peritoneal bands). Hernias may be spontaneous or traumatic, including iatrogenic (e.g., incisional). The diagnosis of external hernia is easy with CT and, depending on the

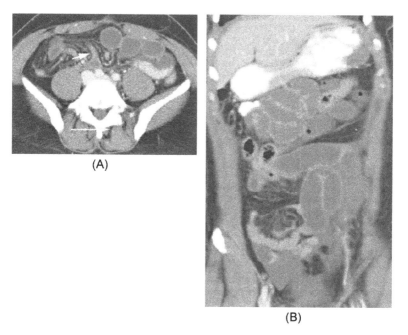

(A)

(B)

Figure 12 Small bowel obstruction due to adhesion (arrow), seen well on an axial image (A). Coronal reformation (B) shows the transition from dilated to collapsed small bowel loops.

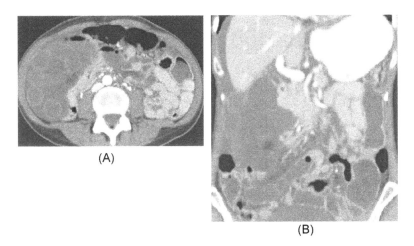

(A)

(B)

FIGURE 13 Internal hernia with dilated small bowel loops in the right upper abdomen. Axial (A) and coronal (B) images show dilated loops with mild wall enhancement. There is edema in the mesentery of the herniated bowel, suggesting vascular compromise. An incarcerated internal hernia through a hole in the omentum with moderate ischemia was found at surgery.

orientation of the hernial sac, MPR images may be helpful. Internal hernias are less obvious and should be suspected when bowel loops are identified in unconventional locations (28). These include the lesser sac, to the right of the duodenum, and lateral to the ascending or descending colon, or if large portion of jejunum appears on the right side of the abdominal cavity without other evidence of malrotation (Fig. 13). For all other causes of obstruction, multiplanar CT enterography may enhance the diagnostic confidence. These include intrinsic or extrinsic tumors, abscess and hematomas, inflammatory lesions, radiation or ischemic enteritis, trauma, intussusceptions, foreign bodies, including bezoars or gallstones ileus. Obstruction may be caused by or may cause ischemia. On multiplanar CT enterography of strangulating (ischemic) obstruction, a combination of findings relating to obstruction and ischemia may be seen, including a transition zone with proximal bowel dilation, hyper- or hypoenhancement of the bowel wall, pneumatosis, edema, and fluid in the mesentery (29).

Tumors

Small bowel tumors are uncommon. Because of the liquid nature of small bowel content, obstruction occurs late and when the masses are large. Most

CT signs of small bowel tumors have been interpolated from barium studies. A mass greater than 3 cm suggests a neoplasm (30). Stromal tumors are usually large, located in the upper GI tract, homogeneous on unenhanced images, with variable enhancement following IV contrast.

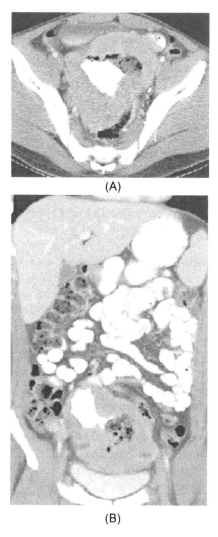

(A)

(B)

FIGURE 14   Small bowel lymphoma. A large mass is demonstrated in the pelvis with a central cavity containing oral contrast (A). On coronal reformation (B) the small bowel origin of the mass becomes more apparent.

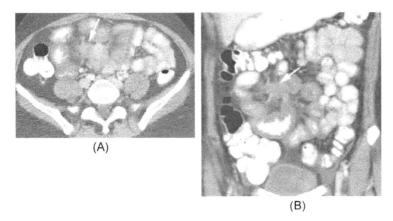

FIGURE 15 Carcinoid tumor (arrow) with desmoplastic reaction in the mesentery and nodular thickening of the bowel wall.

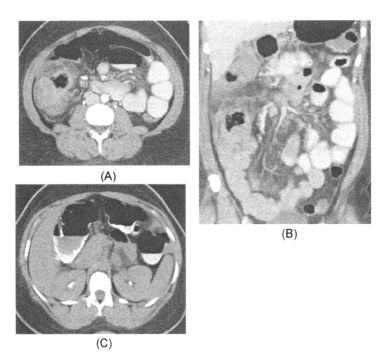

FIGURE 16 Large mass in the cecum with small bowel dilation (A). Coronal reformation helps localize the mass to the cecum (B). A delayed scan 3 hours later (C) shows passage of contrast distal to the mass.

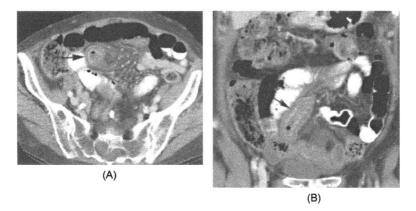

(A)

(B)

FIGURE 17   Small bowel ischemia. Thick edematous small bowel wall (arrow) is seen on axial (A) and coronal (B) images. In addition to wall thickening, there are other secondary signs of ischemia, including engorgement of the mesenteric vessels and edema, better appreciated on the coronal image.

A little less than one half of GI stromal tumors are found in the stomach and about one half in the small bowel (31). Small bowel lymphomas are usually large, ulcerated masses, located more distally in the small bowel (Fig. 14). Carcinoid tumors may produce mesenteric retraction (Fig. 15). Colon cancer is the most common cause of large bowel obstruction (Fig. 16). CT diagnosis and staging of colon cancer is improving with high-resolution fast imaging (32,33). Signs of ischemia may be seen proximal to the tumor (34). Multiplanar images are useful for treatment planning and detection of extracolonic extension of tumor and can be used in conjunction with a metastatic survey of the abdomen. The actual mass and presence of pericolic extension, lymphadenopathy, and distant metastasis to liver and peritoneum can be evaluated.

Ischemia

The larger mesenteric arteries and veins are well opacified at CT, and vascular occlusion or thrombus can be seen as well as secondary changes in the bowel wall and mesentery (35,36). Nonocclusive ischemia is more common than ischemia secondary to major vessel occlusion (Fig. 17). The degree of mural enhancement or lack of enhancement plays an important role in diagnosis. The wall of the bowel may be either hyper- or hypoenhancing (37,38). Indirect signs of ischemia include bowel wall thickening, mural enhancement abnormalities, engorgement, haziness and obliteration of the mesenteric vessels, localized fluid or hemorrhage, and pneumatosis (39,40). Pneumatosis in the mesenteric vessels suggests transmural infarction (41).

REFERENCES

1. Raptopoulos V, Schwartz RK, McNicholas MMJ, Movson J, Pearlman J, Joffe N. Multiplanar helical CT enterography in patients with Crohn's disease. AJR 1997; 169:1545–1550.
2. Raptopoulos V. Technical principles in CT evaluation of the gut. Radiol Clin North Am 1989; 27(4):631–651.
3. Furukawa A, Yamasak M, Furuich K, Yokoyama K, Nagata T, Takahashi M, Murata K, Sakamoto T. Helical CT in the diagnosis of small bowel obstruction. Radiographics 2001; 21:341–355.
4. Wittenberg J, Harisinghani MG, Jhaver Ki, Varghese J, Mueller PR. Algorithmic approach to CT diagnosis of the abnormal bowel wall. Radiographics 2002; 22:1093–1109.
5. Thompson SE, Raptopoulos V, Sheiman RG, McNicholas MMJ, Prassopoulos P. Abdominal helical CT: milk as a low-attenuation oral contrast agent. Radiology 1999; 211:870–875.
6. Raptopoulos V, Davis MA, Davidoff A, Karellas A, Heys D, D'Orsi C, Smith EH. Fat-density oral contrast agent for abdominal CT. Radiology 1987; 164:653–665.
7. Mazzeo S, Caramella D, Battola L, et al. Crohn disease of the small bowel: spiral CT evaluation after oral hyperhydration with isotonic solution. J Comput Assist Tomogr 2001; 25:612–616.
8. Horton KM, Eng J, Fishman EK. Normal enhancement of the small bowel wall: evaluation with spiral CT. J Comput Assist Tomogr 2000; 24:67–71.
9. Winter TC, Ager JD, Nghiem HV, et al. Upper gastrointestinal tract and abdomen: water as an orally administered contrast agent for helical CT. Radiology 1996; 201:365–370.
10. Makó EK, Mester ÁR, Tarján Z, Karlinger K, Toth G. Enteroclysis and spiral CT examination in diagnosis and evaluation of small bowel Crohn's disease. Eur J Radiol 2000; 35:168–175.
11. Rolandi GA, Biscaldi E, Scettro M. CT and MRI enteroclysis: how I do it. Abdominal Radiology Course 2002. Society of Gastrointestinal Radiologists and European Society of Gastrointestinal and Abdominal Radiologists, Orlando, F1, pp 338–339.
12. Rust GF, Spiekermann A, Daum F, et al. New developments in imaging the small bowel with multislice computed tomography and negative contrast medium. In: Reiser MF, Takahashi M, Modic M, Bruening R, eds. Multislice CT. Heidleberg: Springer, 2002: 51–60.
13. Prassopoulos P, Papanikolaou N, Grammatikakis J, Rousomoustakaki M, Maris T, Gourtsoyiannis N. MR enteroclysis imaging of Crohn disease. Radiographics 2001; 21:S161–S172.

14. Rieber A, Aschoff A, Nüssle K, et al. MRI in the diagnosis of small bowel disease: use of positive and negative oral contrast media in combination with enteroclysis. Eur Radiol 2000; 10:1377–1382.

15. Caoili EM, Paulson EK. CT of small-bowel obstruction: another perspective using multiplanar reformations. AJR 2000; 174:993–998.

16. Rolandi GA, Curone PF, Biscaldi E, et al. Spiral CT of the abdomen after distension of small bowel loops with transparent enema in patients with Crohn's disease. Abdom Imag 1999; 24:544–549.

17. Bender GN, Maglinte DDT, Koppel R, et al. CT enteroclysis: a superfluous diagnostic procedure or valuable when investigating small bowel disease? AJR 1999; 172:373–378.

18. Gourtsoyiannis N, Papanikolaou N, Grammatikakis J, Maris T, Prassopoulos P. MR imaging of the small bowel with a true-FISP sequence after enteroclysis with water solution. Invest Radiol 2000; 35:707–711.

19. Maglinte DDT, Siegelman ES, Kelvin FM. MR Enteroclysis: the future of small bowel imaging? Radiology 2000; 215:639–641.

20. Balthazar EJ. CT of the gastrointestinal tract: principles and interpretation. AJR Am J Roentgenol 1991; 156:23–32.

21. Lee SS, Ha HK, Yang S-K, et al. CT of prominent pericolic or perienteric vasculature in patients with Crohn's disease: correlation with clinical disease activity and findings on barium studies. AJR 2002; 179:1029–1033.

22. Koh DM, Miao Y, Chinn RJS, Amin Z, Zeegen R, Westaby D, Healy JC. MR imaging evaluation of the activity of Crohn's disease. AJR 2001; 177: 1325–1332.

23. Rosen MP, Siewert B, Sands DZ, Bromberg R, Edlow J, Raptopoulos V. Value of abdominal CT in the emergency department for patients with abdominal pain. Eur Radiol 2003; 13:418–424.

24. Siewert B, Raptopoulos VD, Mueller MF, Rosen MP, Steer M. Impact of CT on diagnosis and management of patients having acute abdomen initially treated without surgery. AJR 1997; 168:173–178.

25. Fukuya T, Hawes D, Lu C, et al. CT diagnosis of small-bowel obstruction: efficacy in 60 patients. AJR Am J Roentgenol 1992; 158:765–769.

26. Balthazar EJ. CT of small-bowel obstruction. AJR 1994; 162:255–261.

27. Balthazar EJ, Birnbaum BA, Megibow AJ, et al. Closed-loop and strangulating intestinal obstruction: CT signs. Radiology 1992; 185:769–775.

28. Blachar A, Federle MP, Brancatelli G, Peterson MS, Oliver JH, Li W. Radiologist performance in the diagnosis of internal hernia by using specific CT findings with emphasis on transmesenteric hernia. Radiology 2001; 221:422–428.

29. Balthazar EJ, Liebeskind ME, Macari M. Intestinal ischemia in patients in whom small bowel obstruction is suspected: evaluation of accuracy limitations, and clinical implications of CT in diagnosis. Radiology 1997; 205: 519–522.

30. Macari M, Balthazar EJ. CT of bowel wall thickening: significance and pitfalls of interpretation. AJR 2001; 176:1105–1116.

31. Burkill GJ, Badran M, Al-Mueris O, et al. Malignant gastrointestinal stromal tumors: distribution, imaging features, and pattern of metastatic spread. Radiology 2003; 226:527–532.

32. Hundt W, Braunschweig R, Reiser M. Evaluation of spiral CT in staging of colon and rectum carcinoma. Eur Radiol 1999; 9:78–84.

33. Horton KM, Abrams RA, Fishman EK. Spiral CT of colon cancer: imaging features and role in management. Radiographics 2000; 20:419–430.

34. Koh DM, Miao Y, Chinn RJS, Amin Z, Zeegen R, Westaby D, Healy JC. MR imaging evaluation of the activity of Crohn's disease. AJR 2001; 177: 1325–1332.

35. Horton KM, Eng J, Fishman EK. Multi–detector row CT of mesenteric ischemia: can it be done? Radiographics 2001; 21:1463–1473.

36. Wiesner W, Khurana B, Ji H, Ros PR. CT of acute bowel ischemia. Radiology published online January 15, 2003, 10.1148/radiol.2263011540.

37. Chou CK. CT manifestations of bowel ischemia. Am J Roentgenol 2002; 178:87–91.

38. Rha SE, Ha HK, Lee SH, et al. CT and MR imaging findings of bowel ischemia from various primary causes. Radiographics 2000; 20:29–42.

39. Taourel PG, Fabre JM, Prafel JA, et al. Value of CT in the diagnosis and management of patients with suspected acute small-bowel obstruction. Am J Roentgenol 1995; 165:1187–1192.

40. Frager D, Baer JW, Medwid SW, et al. Detection of intestinal ischemia in patients with acute small-bowel obstruction due to adhesion or hernia: efficacy of CT. Am J Roentgenol 1996; 166:67–71.

41. Kernagis LY, Levine MS, Jacobs JE. Pneumatosis intestinalis in patients with ischemia: correlation of CT findings with viability of the bowel. Am J Roentgenol 2003; 180:733–736.

10

Radiofrequency Ablation of Liver Disease

David J. Breen and Brian Stedman
Southampton University Hospitals NHS Trust, Southampton, England

INTRODUCTION

The use of targeted energy for the destruction of solid organ neoplasms has been in evolution over the last three to four decades. The most extensive experience has been gained in the use of cryotherapy in order to achieve focal tissue destruction by means of a "freeze-thaw" cycle. Similarly, laser thermal ablation was reported in 1983 by Bown (1) but has been hindered by limited treatment volumes achievable within living tissue and the costs of the initial equipment set-up. More recently there have been increasing reports of small-diameter coaxial microwave systems being used to create spheres of thermal destruction within the liver (2). Of all these forms of "thermotherapy," however, it is radiofrequency ablation (RFA) that has established itself as a robust interventional tool for the treatment of solid organ neoplasms.

Primary malignant or metastatic disease within the liver is the cause of death in many disease processes owing to overwhelming tumor burden. In particular, approximately half of those patients with colorectal cancer will present at some stage with metastatic liver disease (3). Cytotoxic chemotherapy, while often debulking disease, has achieved only modest slight improvements in the median survival rate to 15–20 months, and 5-year survival still falls short of 5% (4). It is surgery, with resection of limited metastatic disease, which has undoubtedly had most impact in

255

raising the 5-year survival to 20–46% (5). However, given the age and frequent comorbidity of these patients and the technical limitations of even the most ambitious metastectomy, at best only 10–20% of patients can be offered surgical resection (6). Other disease processes, such as metastatic neuroendocrine tumors and primary malignancy arising within cirrhotic liver, also benefit from cytoreduction, and it is against this background that interstitial therapies have gradually come to the fore. These techniques aim to ablate small volume neoplasms without incurring the significant morbidity of surgical hepatic resection. Interstitial therapies have also evolved by virtue of improvements in radiological targeting modalities such as tissue harmonic ultrasound, fluoroscopic real-time CT, and open MR imaging.

RFA uses alternating current to heat tissues to the point of denaturation. Initially, probes generated only small ablative volumes and were therefore used to treat aberrant cardiac conduction pathways. However, recent developments in multiple electrode and expandable RFA probe arrays have enabled the targeting of larger lesions. Additional modifications such as perfused or cooled electrodes as well as "wet electrodes" have expanded the sphere of tissue destruction and reduced the time required to achieve complete ablation, adding to the scope of this interventional tool. RFA is currently used in the treatment of small volume disease in the liver, kidney, adrenal, bone, and lung.

This chapter will focus on the use of RFA in the treatment of focal liver lesions, notably hepatocellular carcinoma (HCC), colorectal metastasis (CRC), and neuroendocrine metastases (NEM), and will outline the current level of clinical and scientific knowledge relating to its use.

PHYSICS

The application of heat to coagulate living tissue and remove tumors is by no means new. The Edwin Smith papyrus dating from 3000 B.C. described the use of thermal cautery for tumors and ulcers of the breast (Fig. 1). D'Arsonval is credited with the first documented research into radiofrequency waves in the body, titled "Physiological Actions of Alternating Current," published in 1891 (7). His initial article showed that radiofrequency waves passing through living tissue elevated tissue temperatures without causing neuromuscular excitation. This work resulted in the rapid development of clinical applications, with Beer of New York pioneering the use of electrosurgical techniques in the destruction of urinary bladder tumors through a cystoscope in 1908 (8). Clark, a histopathologist, described the changes seen with electocautery in 1924 (9); "the cells shrunken and shrivelled and their nuclei mummified,"

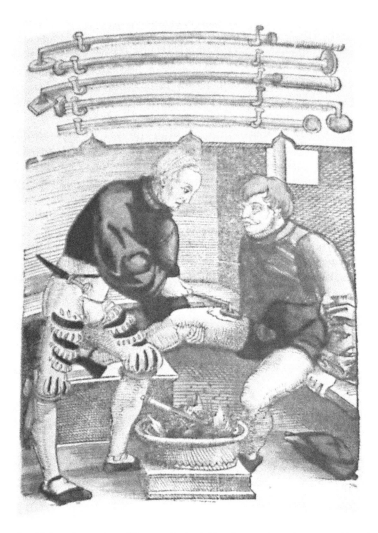

FIGURE 1   Sixteenth century lithograph depicting thermal cautery, used to staunch bleeding and treat superficial tumors.

changes he called desiccation. Over the following 20 years the use of electrocautery in surgery became widely popularized by the Davis-Bovie knife (Liebel Florsheim, Cincinnati, OH) (10).

Radiofrequency ablation works by converting electromagnetic energy into thermal injury within the target tissues. The term radiofrequency relates to the alternating frequency (200–1200 kHz) at which the current flows from the uninsulated probe tip. A closed serial loop is formed by the generator, targeting electrode, patient, and large grounding pads (Fig. 2). The alternating electrical field within the patient causes marked ionic agitation, which is focused in the tissue immediately adjacent to the targeting electrode. The discrepancy in surface areas between the large grounding pads and the small targeting electrode results in focused frictional heating of the target tissue.

In 1976 Organ demonstrated that at low power settings, alternating electricity results in ionic agitation and heating, with conduction into adjacent tissues. However, at higher power settings the immediate tissues are quickly destroyed, with tissue desiccation and vaporization. Modern RFA probes attempt to maximize the former and minimize the latter. It is this "peri-probe" vaporization and desiccation that confounded many earlier versions of locally applied thermal energy.

The nature of the thermal damage caused by RFA will be determined by the temperature achieved in the target tissue and by the duration of heating. Heating tissues to 50–55°C for 5 minutes results in irreversible

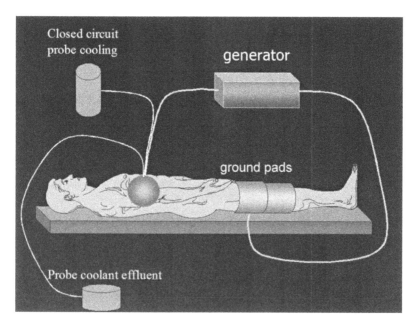

FIGURE 2 Basic arrangement of apparatus for radiofrequency ablation. Tissue destruction occurs in a sphere around the tip of the uninsulated monopolar probe. This diagram also includes a separate closed circuit for probe coolant, as utilized by some manufacturers.

necrosis, while temperatures from 60 to 100°C cause immediate coagulation. Tissue carbonization and vaporization at 100–110°C promotes gas production, which serves as an insulator and prevents further electrical and heat conduction into the tissues with a limitation of overall treatment volume. Within living perfused tissue it has been noted that a single uninsulated monopolar probe can only induce a 16 mm diameter necrotic ovoid without adjuvant maneuvers (11). To achieve adequate tumor necrosis, the entire tumor volume must be subjected to cytotoxic temperatures. This can be achieved by heating the tumor and a surrounding cuff of 1 cm of normal liver to 50–100°C for 5 minutes. In practice the slow thermal conduction to the periphery of the target volume may require prolonged treatment times in briskly perfused tissues.

The overall prediction of an adequate treatment sphere is further compromised by the inherent inhomogeneity of living tissue where calcification or cystic degeneration within tumors may result in variable tissue heating. This can only be overcome by maintaining adequate tissue temperatures for a finite time period. In particular, flowing vessels of greater than 3 mm passing through the target tissue zone are known to compromise tissue heating. Anecdotally this has been shown to result in small areas of perivascular tumor-sparing, and evolving treatment strategies are set to address this issue.

PROBE DESIGN

The main limitation of RFA is the size and reproducibility of the thermal lesion created. With a single uncooled electrode, the lesion produced is ovoid and only 16 mm in diameter, enabling only a 5 mm lesion with 5 mm margins to be treated in a single session. As most lesions in clinical practice are rounded in nature and in excess of this size at presentation, the initial focus of development by electrode manufacturers has been to increase the size of the thermal ablation. This was initially achieved by increasing the effective size of the treatment electrode via use of expandable arrays such as the LeVeen electrode (Radiotherapeutics, Boston-Scientific Corporation, Watertown, MA) (Fig. 3A) or the RITA needle (RITA Medical Systems, Mountainview, CA) (Fig. 3C). Cluster probe arrays have also been developed (Fig. 3B) and their effectiveness compounded by closed-circuit perfusion of electrode tip with coolant (Tyco-Radionics, Burlington, MA). This improved the thermal profile around the uninsulated tip and thereby increased the overall volume of tissue destruction. More recently manufacturers have been revisiting the concept of the "wet electrode," which aims to enhance tissue ionicity around the electrode tip in a controlled fashion and, therefore, the overall lesion size.

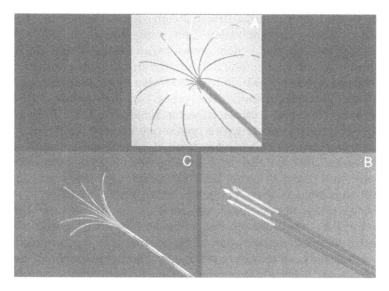

FIGURE 3   Radiofrequency probe arrays from the three main manufacturers. (A) The expandable umbrella-shaped Le Veen electrode from Radiotherapeutics. (B) The "cool-tip" cluster electrode from Tyco-Radionics. The three uninsulated tips are actively cooled during treatment. (C) The expandable RITA starburst needle. This deploys nine retractable tines into the tissue target.

The Radiotherapeutics probe (Fig. 3A) utilizes a 14-gauge needle housing 10 solid retractable "tines." The tines are available in variable lengths (2–3.5 cm). However, the 3.5 cm device is most widely used. In use the tines are fully deployed before application of the 100 W generator (480 kHz). The generator initiates current and thereby energy deposition at 30 W, increasing by 10 W every 60 seconds until a peak energy of 90 W is attained. The device is kept at the peak power for 15 minutes or until a rapid rise in impedance is detected. If impedance rises, the generator switches off for 30 seconds "impedance-regulated" before restarting at maximum power.

Tyco-Radionics have developed single needle probes and three 17-gauge needles mounted in a triangular "cluster" with a common hub (Fig. 3B). To maintain the correct geometry of the cluster, a guidance thimble is utilized. The insulated needles have a hollow shaft with two internal channels, which allow the needle to be perfused with chilled water or saline. This reduces rate-limiting tissue desiccation around the electrode tip and helps maximize overall tissue heating. The needle tip is closed and contains a thermocouple for recording the temperature of adjacent tissues, allowing current reduction if tissue impedance starts to rise. The generator provided with the cooled-tip radiofrequency needles is the most powerful of the three commercially available generators, with a peak output of 200 W, and is operated at 480 Hz. It is, however, modulations of the energy deposition algorithm that enhance the overall effectiveness, and not simply a more powerful generator. Most workers utilize a 12-minute cycle and gradually increase the power to a peak of 180–200 W. According to the generator settings, this power output is maintained until critical impedance rises are noted by the generator, and it cuts out for a short period before recommencing operation. This is "impedance control mode." Otherwise the generator can be controlled manually. Successful ablation usually aims to increase the temperature of the ablated tissues to above 60°C for a finite period of time.

RITA (Fig. 3C) expandable needle electrodes (model 70 and model 90 Starburst XL Needles; RITA Medical Systems, Mountainview, CA) consist of 14- or 15-gauge insulated outer needles that house seven or nine retractable, curved electrode tines. By gradual deployment, these create a large composite sphere of ablated tissue. Four of the electrodes are hollow and contain thermocouples in their tips that permit measurement of tissue temperatures towards the margin of the ablative lesion. The tip of the needle is advanced into the desired location, and the tines are then deployed to approximately two thirds of their length. Generators of 50 and 150 W are available, both operating at 460 kHz. The generator starts at 25 W and gradually increases the wattage to a maximum in 30–120 seconds. The thermocouples monitor tissue temperature and feedback to reduce current when temperatures above 95°C are attained. The operator monitors the temperatures, and once adequate tumoricidal temperatures have been attained, the tines are slowly advanced to full deployment while maintaining target temperatures. The recommended timing for the smaller probe is given as 8–12 minutes, and 25 minutes for the larger probe. After the cycle is complete, a temperature reading of over 50°C at 1 minute postprocedure is believed to indicate adequate tumor ablation.

DISEASE PROCESSES

Colorectal Cancer

Colorectal cancer (CRC) is one of the most common solid tumors in the western world, responsible for approximately 10% of all cancer deaths. The liver is the most common site of distant metastasis, and half of all patients with colonic cancer ultimately develop liver disease (3). Colonic cancer is somewhat unique among the common solid tumors in that surgical resection of distant metastatic disease can result in long-term survival and even "cure". Until recently surgery represented the only hope of cure in this group of patients, with 5-year survival rates of up to 46% being achieved (5). Unfortunately, only 10–20% of patients with CRC and liver metastasis are deemed suitable for hepatic resection (6), and systemic chemotherapy produces only a modest increase in survival. An additional problem for conventional surgery is that following apparently curative resection, recurrent tumor develops in 60% of patients, with repeat surgery compromised by reduced liver volume and additional risks related to surgical adhesions. Surgical data demonstrate that the number of metastases is not the paramount consideration in determining long-term survival. Rather, complete excision with tumor-free margins has been shown to be essential. If this can be achieved, then survival after resection of up to eight metastases is similar to that after resection of a solitary metastasis.

RFA of CRC metastases has yielded some promising results but has been limited by local recurrence rates of 10–40% (12,13). CRC metastases tend to exhibit an ill-defined margin with irregular permeative tumor growth and occasionally budding and tumor microsatellites in the adjacent liver parenchyma. Hence, if the necrosis volume produced by RFA treatment is only equivalent to that of the visible native lesion, tumor recurrence caused by microscopic rests of tumor along the boundary is likely to result in local recurrence. Therefore, when treating CRC metastasis, a safety margin of coagulative necrosis in the liver parenchyma of at least 5 mm and preferably 10 mm is required. This has led many workers to reduce the size of target CRC metastases that they are prepared to treat to 3.5–4.0 cm or less in order to ensure a reasonable chance of disease eradication.

Hepatocellular Carcinoma

Hepatocellular carcinoma (HCC), although relatively uncommon in western countries, is probably one of the most common solid organ cancers on a global basis, with an annual incidence estimated to be between one half and one million new patients per annum. Few patients affected by hepatocellular carcinoma are ideal candidates for surgical resection because of comorbidity, age at time of diagnosis, and often concurrent advanced cirrhosis with compromised synthetic function. Moreover, the 5-year recurrence rate after surgery is about 80%. Therefore, in those patients not amenable to surgery or transplant, novel approaches are required. RFA is suited to the treatment of HCC as by virtue of parenchymal sparing there is minimal disruption to synthetic function. The characteristics of the tumor are also favorable to RFA. The encapsulated nature of many HCC nodules can result in the "oven effect," as described by Livraghi. This relates to the improved current flux and tumoricidal temperatures obtained within the encapsulated malignant nodule. Hepatocellular carcinoma, where paucinodular, represents a relatively soft tumor within the substrate of a firm cirrhotic liver. Consequently, larger well-defined tumors up to 5–7 cm in diameter, can be effectively treated anecdotally with a considerably reduced risk of local recurrence when compared with CRC metastases.

Neuroendocrine Liver Metastases

Neuroendocrine liver metastases (NEM) display distinct biological and clinical features that render their management challenging. Since their initial description by Paul Langerhans in 1869, neuroendocrine cells have been a constant focus of interest due to their unique histological and cytological features and the complex nature of the pathologies to which they give rise.

Liver metastases develop in fewer than 5% of patients with carcinoid tumor, 10% of patients with insulinoma, 25–90% with gastrinoma, and in 75% with glucagonoma (14). The metastatic neuroendocrine tumors may have an indolent course, complicated in some cases by hormonal secretion. However, the 5-year survival with metastatic neuroendocrine liver metastases is still only 25%, and it is overall tumor burden that is the ultimate cause of death. Although surgical resection is the gold standard, curative resection is only possible in 10% of patients, and chemotherapy has limited value (15). The long indolent course and the need for symptom control, and perhaps more importantly reduction of tumor load, has led to the use of RFA as a "cytoreductive therapy" in an attempt to improve quality of life and prolong survival.

Extrahepatic metastatic gastrointestinal tumors have also been treated in the lungs with survival benefit (16). There are increasing reports of technical success in the treatment of solid nodular disease within the lungs (17). In particular, the high impedance encountered during treatments is due to the target being surrounded by aerated lung. As long as the probe is in contact with the nodule, this favorable treatment environment facilitates complete tumor destruction. To date most successful treatments have been of smaller peripheral malignancies where the pneumothorax risk is reduced and there is less chance of heat-sumping or critical thermal injury to larger perihilar vessels.

PROCEDURAL CONSIDERATIONS

RFA should be performed percutaneously whenever possible. This reduces morbidity, and treatments can be performed as day cases or on an overnight stay basis under either general anesthesia or conscious sedation. The percutaneous route allows repeat procedures and is relatively inexpensive. Advocates of laparoscopic RFA claim that additional information can be gained with the use of laparoscopic high-frequency ultrasound and via direct visualization of the peritoneal surface of the liver. Detection of unexpected peritoneal disease can terminate a planned RFA treatment. An additional benefit of laparoscopic and operative RFA is the ability to perform a "pringle maneuver," with temporary occlusion to hepatic perfusion. This may decrease heat loss and enable greater treatment volumes (18,19). However, experience of laparoscopic RFA is limited, and added invasiveness and complexity, along with increased costs, have limited its use. Open, operative RFA attracts the associated morbidity and mortality of laparotomy and general anesthesia, along with increased recovery periods. However, it may improve the targeting and isolation of problematic lesions, for example, adjacent to the gallbladder, diaphragm, or bowel, and is increasingly used as an adjunct to hepatic resection.

Early experience also demonstrates the feasibility and safety of performing RFA on synchronous metastatic liver tumors in conjunction with primary colorectal cancer resection. In this setting any added morbidity is low and additional disease control may improve survival. This chapter will focus on the percutaneous applications of RFA.

PREPROCEDURAL CHECKS

An outpatient assessment the week before treatment presents the operator with an invaluable chance to review all the available imaging. An up-to-date assessment of the number and size of lesions and their relationship to surrounding structures is vital. The likely approach can be ascertained and the targeting modality chosen. If ultrasound is to be used, hepatic sonography should be performed to determine tumor conspicuity and to identify a safe passage to the lesion. This time also allows for patient counseling, with particular attention to the possibility of postprocedural liver hemorrhage, adjacent thermal gut injury, and the chance of local disease recurrence, while bearing in mind the size of the target lesions at the outset. On this visit baseline hematology tests with a coagulation profile should be obtained in addition to biochemistry with α-fetoprotein and carcinoembryonic antigen levels as appropriate. Coagulopathy should be corrected prior to RFA, especially given the relatively large needle size and the occasional necessity for multiple transhepatic punctures.

ANESTHESIA

The majority of percutaneous RFA procedures are performed on an overnight stay basis, although uneventful treatments in fit patients can be carried out as day cases. Treatment is usually performed under conscious sedation (neuroleptanalgesia). This has the advantage of allowing for patient cooperation with breathing and positioning prior to heavier sedation for the actual treatment itself. It is notable that as RF treatments have become more ambitious, there has been a gradual drift among practitioners towards general anesthesia.

Having fasted for 6 hours, the patient is prepared with peripheral intravenous access and cardiovascular and respiratory monitoring. The planned puncture site is prepared for a sterile procedure, and the puncture site is anesthetized with 1% lidocaine hydrochloride (Xylocaine, AstraZeneca). An intercostal approach is favored for right lobe lesions, while lesions in the left lobe are best approached with a subcostal approach. If anesthetic support is not available, then a qualified nurse should monitor the patient's vital signs during the procedure. Traditional sedation with a fast-acting opiate (Fentnyl, Janssen-Cilag, Beerse, Belgium) and a short-acting benzodiazepine (Midazolam, Dormicum, Hoffmann-La Roche, Basel, Switzerland) has proved adequate for the majority of straightforward procedures.

Ablation of peripheral lesions close to the liver capsule causes significantly more pain than parenchymal RFA, and in this setting premedication with an anti-inflammatory (Voltarol 100 mg PR) or the use of postprocedure patient-controlled analgesia (PCA) pump may be warranted. Pain is usually experienced for about 3 hours postprocedure, and most patients require simple analgesia for this time.

Routine prophylactic antibiotics use is advocated by some workers, although there is no consensus on their use, especially since infective complications of RFA treatment are uncommon. If prophylactic antibiotics are to be used, then a broad-spectrum cephalosporin may be considered. Many practitioners have reported an increased risk of abscess formation in the setting of a biliary stent or choledocho-enteric anastomosis. This is evolving as a relative contraindication but, if undertaken, should certainly be covered by medium-term antibiotic prophylaxis. The Italian Multicentre Collaborative experience highlighted an increased risk of abscess formation in diabetics and those patients with pneumobilia following previous surgical biliary bypass or stenting (20).

GUIDING MODALITIES

Adequate targeting of the lesion is the key to successful ablation. RFA needle probes can be placed under ultrasound, CT, or MR guidance using a percutaneous approach (Fig. 4). The guiding modality will be determined by target conspicuity. However, ultrasound guidance offers the most robust technique with real-time visualization and multiplanar

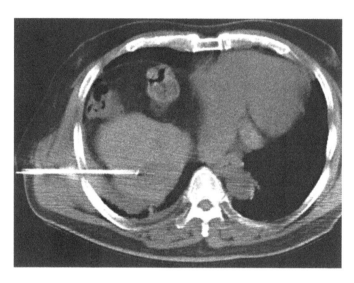

Figure 4   A small-volume hepatocellular carcinoma undergoing CT-guided RFA due to problems with visualization of the high right hemiliver at ultrasound.

assessment, along with advantages of availability and cost. The primary disadvantage of ultrasound is its limited ability to assess the effectiveness of ablation and the gradual obscuration of the target by microbubble formation during the RF process (Fig. 5). Not only can this compromise immediate assessment of treatment adequacy, it can also impair targeting of subsequent lesions to be treated at the same session. It is always the authors' practice to target smaller, deeper lesions first, followed by larger more superficial disease. By waiting for 5–8 minutes between treatments of individual nodules, there is considerable clearing of diffuse bubble-mediated echogenicity from the liver parenchyma, and this pause can facilitate secondary targeting. Undoubtedly the newer ultrasound contrast media will have a role to play in improved visualization, in particular of "chemo-modulated" disease, which remains problematic. The authors have noted that if preprocedural particulate embolization has been employed (poly-vinyl alcohol, PVA) within the preceeding 48 hours, as in the case of HCC, the lesion is often highlighted by a retained "PVA twinkle," which can aid lesion targeting in the setting of the nodular cirrhotic liver (Fig. 6).

Lesions that are poorly visualized on ultrasound may be visualized by either CT fluoroscopy or real-time MR imaging. However, practicing radiologists will appreciate the difficulties of targeting small volume disease at unenhanced CT fluoroscopy, where the temporal window for probe placement during contrast enhanced CT is inadequate. Similarly,

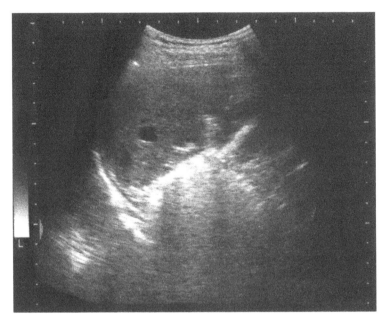

FIGURE 5 Following RFA of a hepatocellular carcinoma in a cirrhotic liver, the treated nodule is obscured by a veil of microbubbles. This can impair secondary needle placement within the same lesion.

MR imaging remains limited by spatial resolution, although some authors have highlighted the use of T1-thermometry for an enhanced appreciation of treatment adequacy (21). When planning an individual patient's suitability for treatment, not only should lesion size be taken into account, but also their position and number. Multiple colorectal metastatic nodules may be ablated over a number of sessions. In the authors' experience, the chances of inadequate treatment increase considerably if more than three lesions are treated at any one sitting. In addition, these lesions should ideally be less than 4 cm in diameter in order to ensure tumor eradication. Larger hepatocellular cancer nodules up to 6 cm can be treated with the expectation of complete ablation. Caution should be taken when treating peri-hilar lesions as there have been occasional reports of critical proximal bile duct injury. Furthermore, residual disease seems highly likely in the setting of large perihilar vessels. In addition, treatments within segment 6 of the right lobe and on the underside of segment 3 should be carried out with due consideration of the risk of adjacent thermal gut injury in the closed patient (Fig. 7). It may be that these would be better treated by RFA during open laparotomy, building a team approach with surgeons for the

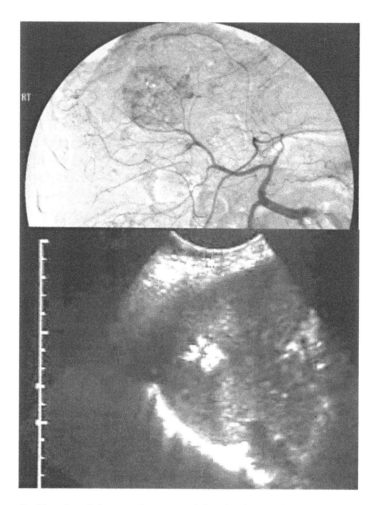

FIGURE 6 Hepatocellular carcinoma nodules in the setting of cirrhosis. These nodules have been previously embolized with particulate material resulting in a "PVA twinkle," which enhances targeting for RFA.

management and ablation of these diseases. The operator should also be aware that treatment close to the diaphragm can cause significant pain and/or hiccoughs and also risks pleural effusion or even fistulation.

TREATMENT ENDPOINTS

The commercially available generators define treatment endpoints on physical parameters. The Radionics and Radiotherapeutics generators

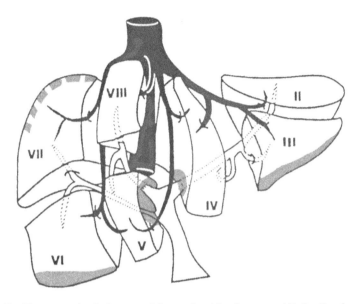

FIGURE 7   The grey-shaded areas at the underside of segment 3, the tip of segment 6, and the perihilar liver should be approached with caution. There is a risk of thermal injury adjacent to the lesser curve of the stomach or to the hepatic flexure of the colon, particularly in those who have had previous surgery. Lesions are likely to remain undertreated with a risk of biliary injury at the liver hilum. Treatments close to the diaphragm (hatched) may incur pain and diaphragmatic irritation.

both use impedance rises to define the end of the treatment cycle, while RITA generators monitor tumor temperatures, with a final temperature 1 minute after treatment above 50°C described as reflecting adequate treatment. Morphological endpoints on imaging criteria have proved disappointing. Acute postprocedure contrast-enhanced CT often results in misleading and ill-defined peripheral enhancement due to an acute hyperaemic parenchymal response. The use of contrast-enhanced ultrasound has been described for detection of viable residual tumor, but experience is currently limited (22). It is the authors' practice to assess posttreatment response via contrast-enhanced CT performed between 72 hours and 30 days, at which point the RF lesion is much more crisply defined and residual untreated disease is usually more apparent (Fig. 8).

COMPLICATIONS

Percutaneous RFA is a relatively new technique, and only interim data are available relating to its efficacy and use in the treatment of focal liver

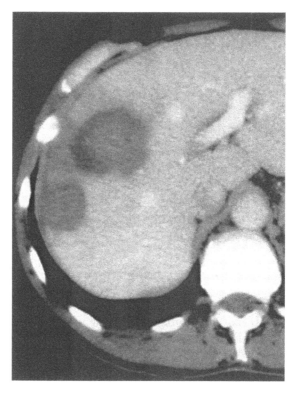

Figure 8 Two colorectal metastases following RFA. The posttreatment thermal injuries are crisply delineated at 72 hours after treatment. (For posttreatment image interpretation, see later.)

lesions. All published data currently indicates a low complication rate. The largest reported experience to date is from the Italian Collaborative group (20): 2320 patients (3554 lesions, 3.1 ± 1.1 cm) were treated between July 1995 and January 2001 in 41 centers using similar RFA protocols. Of these, 1620 were cases of hepatocellular carcinoma in the setting of chronic liver disease, and 683 patients had metastatic disease, mostly colorectal carcinoma. When considering the results, we should bear in mind the currently reported 4% mortality for surgical liver resection combined with a 16–27% major complication rate (23,24). In contrast, mortality in the Italian study was 0.25%, representing 6 patients. Two of the deaths were attributed to faeculent peritonitis as a result of RF-induced thermal colonic injury. Surgical adhesions and the close proximity of the target liver lesion to the colonic wall have been implicated as possible risk factors. Thermal damage with a biliary stricture was implicated in one death following treatment of a perihiliar lesion. A superficial HCC ruptured following treatment, causing massive peritoneal hemorrhage and subsequent hepatic coma. Two further deaths were reported, although the exact causality remains unclear.

Major Complications

The Italian series reported a 2.1% major complication rate that included 12 cases (0.5%) of intraperitoneal haemorrhage requiring treatment, of which the majority were HCC patients with an elevated INR. Six cases (0.25%) of intrahepatic abscess were identified, the majority responding to intravenous antibiotics and/or percutaneous drainage. Colonic perforations occurred in 5 cases with a close association with previous colonic resection noted, presumably related to adhesions attaching the liver to the gastrointestinal tract. Other reported complications included a biloma, one biliary stricture, and three cases of hemothorax requiring drainage. Neoplastic seeding was noted 4–18 months later in 12 patients (0.5%). The majority were from superficial lesions. However, a few deep poorly differentiated HCC were also found to seed despite RF heating of the electrode tract, a process known as "hot withdrawal" or "track ablation."

Minor Complications

Minor complications occurred in 4.1% of cases. Peri-procedural pain was noted in superficial lesions and in those close to the liver hilium. This is likely to reflect the somatic innervation of Gleeson's capsule. The pain is most pronounced during high-energy RF delivery at the beginning of the procedure. The majority of patients experience minimal pain during the weeks following RFA. However, the aggressive treatment of peripheral and especially subdiaphragmatic lesions occasionally results in significant pain. In this setting premedication and post-procedural pain relief with a nonsteroidal anti-inflammatory (Voltarol 100 mg PR) or the use of PCA may be warranted. Postablation pyrexia is often noted, analogous to the postembolization syndrome.

TARGET TISSUE MODULATION

Effective ablation of diseased tissue has been approached from two angles. The probe manufacturers have striven to make RF probes more effective by various means, including increased power output, expandable, cooled, and perfused electrodes, and pulsed energy-delivery algorithms. Living tissues, both those diseased and the background parenchyma, can confound effective RF ablation as they may be electrically inhomogeneous, close to temperature-sensitive structures, or heating to lethal temperatures may be compromised by overall tissue perfusion. Many clinicians are in the process of devising adjunctive interventional maneuvers by which these rate-limiting steps can be overcome.

Perfusion-mediated cooling has been particularly problematic, and animal experiments have clearly shown that the volume of the ablated tissue can be significantly increased by decreasing overall tissue perfusion (18). Similarly, anecdotal experience has shown that vessels of 3 mm and above often remain patent through the margins of a sphere of otherwise effective tissue necrosis. This vessel preservation is likely due to heat loss to the flowing vessel, a phenomenon termed "heat-sumping." By implication there must be a cuff of viable cells around these vessels, and certainly anecdotal experience has suggested that perivascular disease recurrence does occur adjacent to flowing vessels towards the margin of an RF lesion. Patterson et al. have shown that the sphere of tissue destruction can be enhanced by performing a pringle maneuver (occlusion of the hepatic artery and portal vein) during RFA in anesthetized pigs (18). Similarly, Curley et al. reported use of the LeVeen monopolar electrode in the treatment of 169 tumors in 123 patients (75 metastasis, 48 HCC) (19). Approximately three quarters of these procedures were performed intraoperatively and with 2–3 minutes of vascular inflow occlusion. The authors attributed their low rate of recurrence (1.8%; 3 of 169) to the pringle maneuver. In this series metastatic disease progressed at other sites in 34 patients (27.6%).

Hepatic artery balloon occlusion has also been reported to have a possible role in the treatment of HCC. The dominant and hypervascular arterial supply of nodular hepatoma may compromise heat-mediated cellular destruction. While the nodular HCC in the cirrhotic liver undoubtedly lends itself to RFA, for physical reasons already discussed, it appears that larger hepatomas can be effectively treated following temporary hepatic arterial balloon occlusion (25) or particulate embolization. Many anecdotal reports now suggest that diminishing tissue perfusion by these means, and even possibly chemotherapy, may help to enhance the overall effectiveness of RFA. Other workers have sought to improve overall heat deposition by increasing target tissue ionicity and thereby its conductivity by infusing hypertonic saline into the area to be ablated. Livraghi et al. reported both ex vivo and in vivo animal experience as well as preliminary human studies utilising saline-augmentation of RFA (26). Both bolus (1–20 mL) and continuous infusion (1 mL/min) enhanced the overall zone of necrosis, but the authors noted that the treatment zones were often irregular and difficult to predict. The uncertainty of bolus-injected hypertonic saline has reduced its usage more recently. One manufacturer (RITA, Mountainview, CA) has, however, produced a very slow, impedance-regulated perfused probe with the aim of inducing more controlled tissue destruction. Vessel mediated tissue cooling can also be problematic where disease abuts major veins. De Baere et al. have recently reported transhepatic temporary balloon occlusion of hepatic veins as a means to reduce perivenular recurrence (27).

Target tissue chemo-sensitization is a further strategy. Early experience suggests that there may be not just an additive but a compounding effect where chemotherapy and RFA are used in close conjunction with one another. It is already clear that the pretreatment with chemotherapy results in a decrease in the temperature required to cause cell death. Work by Goldberg et al. has also shown that intralesional instillation of doxorubicin results in an augmentation of the tumoricidal effects of RFA, which may be progressive after the treatment (28): clearly further work is needed to evaluate the benefits and timing of such adjuvant treatments.

IMAGING FOLLOW-UP

Most of the current methods used for interstitial tissue ablation result in obscuration of the target during treatment (Fig. 5). As such, it has been difficult to accurately assess treatment completion at the time of the procedure. Some success has been reported using T1-thermometry at MR imaging (21) and with contrast-enhanced ultrasound following clearance over the coarser "RF-bubble shower," within minutes of treatment cessation. It is widely accepted, however, that such peri-procedural assessments can be inaccurate and even underestimate the treatment volume because greater areas of tissue necrosis are confirmed by other modalities a few days later. Many workers in the field now aim to treat as adequately as possible and reserve imaging assessment as an outpatient procedure at 3–30 days. By 3 days the RF lesion is more clearly defined at CT and MR imaging and demonstrates a number of characteristic features (29,30).

The unenhanced CT image frequently demonstrates ill-defined high attenuation within the central ablated zone. This reflects hemorrhage within the area of coagulative necrosis (Fig. 9A). The ablated area shows no enhancement with contrast, but in the late arterial, and perhaps moreso in the portal venous phase, demonstrates a thin rind of enhancement of a few millimeters in diameter (Fig. 9B, C). This penumbral zone of thermal injury response is only approximately 2 mm thick and marks the transition from coagulated tissue to adjacent viable parenchyma. Of note, contrast is often retained in this penumbral zone on postequilibrium imaging (Fig. 9 D). This hyperemic zone tends to resolve over the course of 4 weeks or so and should not be mistaken for residual tumor. Some authors have argued that postprocedural imaging may be better carried out following complete resolution of this thermal injury response, which usually occurs

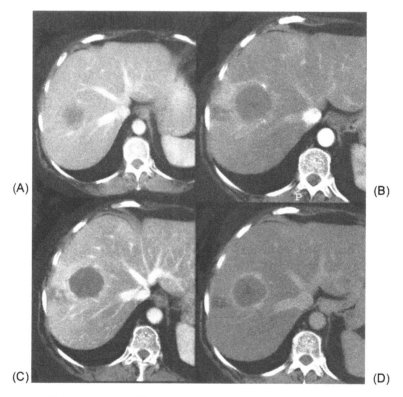

FIGURE 9   (A) Pretreatment CT of colorectal carcinoma deposit. (B) Arterial phase CT demonstrating thin enhancing line of perilesional response to thermal injury. Subtending arterioportal shunt is also noted and should not be misinterpreted as residual disease. This lesion was pretreated with 15 mL of hypertonic saline. Some of this has caused a peripheral patch of necrosis presumably where it has passed into an occluded biliary radicle. (C) Portal venous phase CT image again demonstrates perilesional thermal injury response and subtended high attenuation. (D) Contrast persists in the penumbral zone of thermal injury in the post equilibrium phase, likely due to defective contrast clearance.

by about one month (31). The interpreting radiologist should also be aware of arterioportal shunting, which may declare itself in the subtended liver parenchyma and again should not be misinterpreted as disease recurrence (30) (Fig. 10).

While no absolute consensus regarding follow-up scheduling has been reached, this should be guided by the natural history of the treated tumor. Most protocols recommend imaging at 3 months and then every 6 months. Clearly a colorectal metastasis can be expected to develop local recurrence earlier than a subtotally treated indolent carcinoid deposit. Of note, Solbiati et al. reported the follow-up of 117 patients with 179 colorectal metastases and noted that 54 of 70 (70%) local recurrences were apparent within 6 months of the initial treatment (12).

RF lesions tend to demonstrate crisp margins and slow involution in the months following treatment. Any ill definition or expansion usually

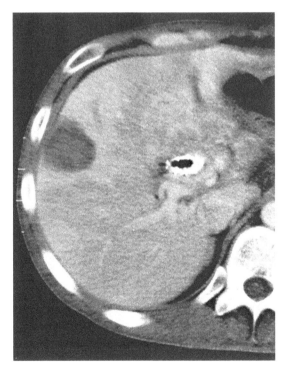

FIGURE 10 Large enhancing segmental arterioportal shunt around a treated colorectal metastasis. This is frequently encountered and clearly should not be misinterpreted as perilesional tumor recurrence. The presence of biliary-enteric bypass or a stent should be regarded as a relative contraindication.

represents locally recurrent disease. Patterns of recurrence appear to fall into a number of typical patterns. Hepatocellular carcinoma, particularly encapsulated disease, frequently demonstrates peripheral nodular recurrences. As with the original disease, this is usually best demonstrated on a high-dose late arterial phase CT study (Fig. 11). HCC can also recur as a contiguous but usually nodular outgrowth from the treated lesion (32). Recurrent colorectal disease usually declares itself within 6 months as eccentric nodular disease at the margin of the RF lesion, or simply as an expanding RF lesion following treatment, the "halo" recurrence (Fig. 12).

CLINICAL RESULTS

Although RF ablation is becoming widely adopted, it still remains a relatively new technique. Only recently have larger series and longer-term results in HCC, CRC metastatic, and, to a lesser extent, metastatic

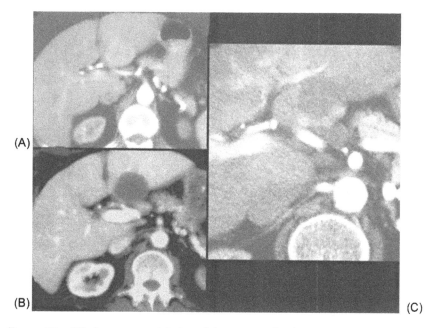

FIGURE 11   (A) An encapsulated and hypervascular hepatoma is seen at the posterior aspect of segment 3. (B) Following treatment this appears entirely ablated with no evidence of enhancement in the late arterial phase. (C) At 6 months follow-up there is a small "chain" of nodular recurrence at the deep aspect of the treated hepatoma—"peripheral nodular recurrence."

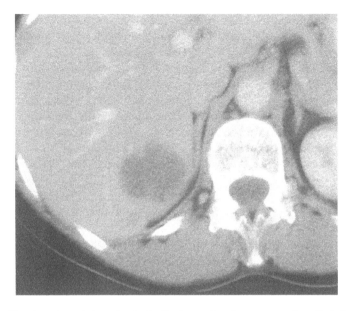

FIGURE 12   A colorectal metastasis that previously appeared well defined and adequately treated at 3 months now expresses enlargement and an ill-defined border at 6-month CT. This is a typical, expanding, or "halo" recurrence.

neuroendocrine disease been published. Earlier series were from mixed populations with heterogeneous inclusion criteria, techniques, and outcome measures. Due to the rapidly evolving nature of RF, useful 5-year survival data are still awaited. Initial clinical experience from the mid-1990s was aimed at assessing local therapeutic efficacy and safety.

To date the largest experience has been acquired in the treatment of hepatocellular carcinoma. In 1995 Rossi et al. reported immediate outcome in 24 patients with 25 HCCs of 3 cm or less, with complete tumor destruction in 23 out of 25 lesions (33). In a subsequent series the same group had treated 50 patients, 39 with 41 small hepatomas (< 3.5 cm in diameter) and 11 with 13 metastases (34). This series is notable for the high number of treatment sessions per patient of 3.3. The hepatoma cohort was followed for a mean of 22.6 months with a median survival of 44 months. Only 2 (5%) of this group developed local recurrence. In the 11 metastatic patients the mean follow-up was 11 months, with 2 patients proceeding to surgery within 1 month of RFA. Of these 11 patients, 2 developed local recurrence under follow-up. Two publications by Livraghi et al. serve to highlight some pertinent points regarding the RFA of HCC (36,36): (a) the increased effectiveness of RFA compared with percutaneous ethanol installation for treatment of small (< 3 cm) HCC; (b), that smaller HCCs tend to be treated effectively when compared to larger nodules, with complex infiltrative morphology, and (c) that size greater than 5 cm is significantly predictive of treatment failure. Livraghi et al. (36) noted that encapsulated hepatomas appeared to be treated very effectively even if the ablation zone conformed neatly to the encapsulated nodule. Experience suggests an "oven effect," with the surrounding cirrhotic liver parenchyma serving to concentrate current flux and heat deposition within the encapsulated hepatoma.

More recently Buscarini et al. have reported 101 hepatocellular carcinomas treated in 88 patients with a mean follow-up of 34 months (37). They achieved complete posttreatment tumor necrosis by imaging assessment in all cases, with a local recurrence rate of 22% and a 5-year survival of 33%.

As discussed earlier, animal work (18) and anecdotal surgical experience (19) indicates that diminished hepatic vascular inflow increases the volume of RF-induced necrosis in the liver. Subsequently, a multicenter trial set out to assess this premise (38). A consecutive series of 62 patients with unifocal HCC of 3.5–8.5 cm (mean 4.7 cm) underwent RFA following either hepatic artery balloon occlusion or preembolization with gelatin sponge. The balloon occlusion was either at the time of RFA ($n = 40$), immediately following embolization ($n = 13$), or in the following 2–5 days ($n = 9$). Complete tumor eradication at postprocedure imaging was deemed to have been achieved in 56 of 62 patients (90%); subtotal treatments occurred in 6 of 62 patients (10%) who subsequently underwent secondary RFA to complete tumor destruction. Two patients proceeded to liver resection, but the 60 remaining were followed for a mean of 12 months (range 3–36 months) with local recurrence detected in 11 of 60 (18%). This means that of these larger problematic lesions, some 49 of 60 (82%) had no local recurrence but 18 of 60 patients demonstrated new intrahepatic disease. Thirty-one of 60 (52%) remained disease-free during the follow-up period.

Colorectal carcinoma has proved more resistant to treatment by RFA. Necessarily many patients that might be good candidates for RFA are referred for surgical resection with local ablation tending to be reserved for those believed unfit for surgery. Results to date also suggest that the infiltrative margin of colorectal metastases greater than 3 cm must be thoroughly treated in order to avoid high rates of local recurrence. Solbiati et al. reported their experience in the treatment of 179 metachronous colorectal metastases in 117 patients between July 1995 and October 1999 (12). The follow-up ranged from 6 to 52 months with an estimated median survival for all patients of 36 months. Survival analysis yielded estimated

1-, 2-, and 3-year survival rates of 93, 69, and 46%, respectively. These figures are a substantial improvement on those currently achievable with systemic chemotherapy alone (48% at 1 year, 21% at 2 years, and 3% at 3 years). Local recurrence occurred in 70 of 179 (39%) of lesions following RFA. As described earlier, 54 of these were seen by 6 months and 67 by 1 year. De Baere, et al. reported the treatment of 121 metastases in 68 patients (13); 33 metastases (5–20 mm) were treated intraoperatively and 88 (10–42 mm) at percutaneous RFA. Of 100 metastases closely followed between 4 and 23 months (mean 14 months), 91% demonstrated complete local eradication. Tumor control was equivalent between intraoperative (94%) and percutaneous (90%) RFA.

The surgical community has also reported promising results in the use of intraoperative RFA including that under laparoscopic guidance and in combination with surgical resection. Curley et al. treated 169 lesions (48 HCC, 75 metastases) in 123 patients with a mean diameter of 3.4 cm (19). Approximately one third of these were treated percutaneously and two thirds intraoperatively. They reported a local recurrence rate of 1.8% during a median follow-up of 15 months. Progressive metastatic disease was, however, noted in 34 (28%) patients. Siperstein treated 250 primary and secondary hepatic tumors in 66 patients under laparoscopic guidance (39). Of these lesions, 178 appeared adequately treated at initial post-procedure assessment and 156 of 178 (88%) demonstrated progressive resolution when followed for at least 3 months. There were 22 (12%) local recurrences, of which 17 were apparent by 6 months. Favorable outcomes have also been reported in the treatment of metastatic neuroendocrine tumors.

Hellman et al. treated 43 neuroendocrine liver metastases in 21 patients (12 midgut carcinoids, 4 nonfunctional endocrine pancreatic tumors, 1 VIPoma, 1 glucagonoma, 1 gastrinoma, and 2 adrenal carcinoma) (40). Of these 21 there was intention-to-cure in 14 by RF alone or RF plus surgery in 1. At a mean follow-up of 2.1 years (range 3 months to 4 years), two lesions had developed signs of further growth, yielding a local recurrence rate of 4.6%. Four of the 15 patients treated with curative intent remained disease-free under follow-up. Other series indicate a clear role for RFA in an overall cytoreductive approach to metastatic neuroendocrine disease alongside surgery and long-acting somatostatin analogues (41,42).

SUMMARY

Accruing experience clearly demonstrates a role for percutaneous thermal ablation and particularly RFA in the treatment of small to intermediate-volume malignant liver disease. Recent large series have confirmed the overall safety and low morbidity of the technique. Results suggest a central role for the treatment of hepatocellular carcinoma and an adjunctive role for colorectal carcinoma and metastatic neuroendocrine disease alongside surgery and chemotherapy. Above all, this is an in situ, image-guided technique in which radiologists are central to accurate implementation and careful follow-up. Further implementation will require the radiology community to adopt a pivotal role in the dissemination of good practice and the accrual of valuable data through experience in multiple centers.

REFERENCES

1. Bown SG. Phototherapy in tumors. World J Surg 1983; 7(6):700–709.
2. Tabuse Y, Tabuse K, Mori K, Nagai Y, Kobayashi Y, Egawa H, Noguchi H, Yamaue H, Katsumi M, Nagasaki Y. Percutaneous microwave tissue coagulation in liver biopsy: experimental and clinical studies. Nippon Geka Hokan 1986; 55(3):381–392.
3. Landis SH, Murray T, Bolden S, Wingo PA. Cancer statistics, 1999. CA Cancer J Clin 1999; 49(1):8–31.
4. Wagner JS, Adson MA, Van Heerden JA, Adson MH, Ilstrup DM. The natural history of hepatic metastases from colorectal cancer. A comparison with resective treatment. Ann Surg 1984; 199(5):502–508.
5. Harmon KE, Ryan JA Jr, Biehl TR, Lee FT. Benefits and safety of hepatic resection for colorectal metastases. Am J Surg 1999; 177(5):402–404.
6. Scheele J, Stangl R, Altendorf-Hofmann A. Hepatic metastases from colorectal carcinoma: impact of surgical resection on the natural history. Br J Surg 1990; 77(11):1241–1246.
7. D' Arsonval MA. Action physiologique des courants alternatifs. CR Soc Biol 1891; 43:283–293.
8. Beer E. Removal of neoplasms of the urinary bladder: a new method employing high frequency (oudin) currents through a cauterizing cystoscope. JAMA 1910; 54:1768–1769.
9. Clark WL, Morgan JD, Asnia EJ. Electrothermic methods in treatment of neoplasms and other lesions with clinical and histological observations. Radiology 1924; 2:233–246.
10. Cushing H, Bovie WT. Electro-surgery as an aid to the removal of intracranial tumors. Surg Gynecol Obstet 1928; 47:751–784.
11. Goldberg SN, Gazelle GS, Solbiati L, Livraghi T, Tanabe KK, Hahn PF, Mueller PR. Ablation of liver tumors using percutaneous RF therapy. AJR Am J Roentgenol 1998; 170(4):1023–1028.
12. Solbiati L, Livraghi T, Goldberg SN, Ierace T, Meloni F, Dellanoce M, Cova L, Halpern EF, Gazelle GS. Percutaneous radio-frequency ablation of hepatic

metastases from colorectal cancer: long-term results in 117 patients. Radiology 2001; 221(1):159–166.

13. de Baere T, Elias D, Dromain C, Din MG, Kuoch V, Ducreux M, Boige V, Lassau N, Marteau V, Lasser P, Roche A. Radiofrequency ablation of 100 hepatic metastases with a mean follow-up of more than 1 year. AJR Am J Roentgenol 2000; 175(6):1619–1625.

14. Siperstein AE, Berber E. Cryoablation, percutaneous alcohol injection, and radiofrequency ablation for treatment of neuroendocrine liver metastases. World J Surg 2001; 25(6):693–696.

15. Oberg K. The use of chemotherapy in the management of neuroendocrine tumors. Endocrinol Metab Clin North Am 1993; 22(4):941–952.

16. Sakamoto T, Tsubota N, Iwanaga K, Yuki T, Matsuoka H, Yoshimura M Pulmonary resection for metastases from colorectal cancer. Chest 2001; 119(4):1069–1072.

17. Highland AM, Mack P, Breen DJ. Radiofrequency thermal ablation of a metastatic lung nodule. Eur Radiol 2002; 12(suppl 4): S166–170.

18. Patterson EJ, Scudamore CH, Owen DA, Nagy AG, Buczkowski AK. Radio-frequency ablation of porcine liver in vivo: effects of blood flow and treatment time on lesion size. Ann Surg 1998; 227(4):559–565.

19. Curley SA, Izzo F, Delrio P, Ellis LM, Granchi J, Vallone P, Fiore F, Pignata S, Daniele B, Cremona F. Radiofrequency ablation of unresectable primary and metastatic hepatic malignancies: results in 123 patients. Ann Surg 1999; 230(1):1–8.

20. Livraghi T, Solbiati L, Meloni MF, Gazelle GS, Halpern EF, Goldberg SN. Treatment of focal liver tumors with percutaneous radio-frequency ablation: complications encountered in a multicentre study. Radiology 2003; 226: 441–451.

21. Dick EA, Joarder R, De Jobe M, Taylor-Robinson SD, Thomas HC, Foster GR, Gedroyc WM. MR-guided laser thermal ablation of primary and secondary liver tumors. Clin Radiol 2003; 58:112–120.

22. Solbiati L, Goldberg SN, Ierace T, Dellanoce M, Livraghi T, Gazelle GS. Radio-frequency ablation of hepatic metastases: Postprocedural assessment with a US microbubble contrast agent-early experience. Radiology 1999; 211:643–649.

23. Cunningham JD, Fong Y, Shriver C, Melendez J, Marx WL, Blumgart LH. One hundred consecutive hepatic resections. Blood loss, transfusion, and operative technique. Arch Surg 1994; 129(10):1050–1056.

24. Melendez JA, Arslan V, Fischer ME, Wuest D, Jarnagin WR, Fong Y, Blumgart LH. Perioperative outcomes of major hepatic resections under low central venous pressure anesthesia: blood loss, blood transfusion, and the risk of postoperative renal dysfunction. J Am Coll Surg 1998; 187(6): 620–625.

25. Lencioni R, Cioni D, Donati F, Bartolozzi C. Combination of interventional therapies in hepatocellular carcinoma. Hepato-Gastroentrology 2001; 48:8–14.

26. Livraghi T, Goldberg SN, Monti F, et al. Saline-enhanced radio-frequency tissue ablation in the treament of liver metastases. Radiology 1997; 202:205–210.

27. de Baere T, Bessoud B, Dromain C. Percutaneous radiofrequency ablation of hepatic tumors during temporary venous occlusion. AJR 2002; 178:53–59.

28. Goldberg SN, Girnan GD, Lukyanov AN. Percutaneous tumor ablation; increased necrosis with combined radiofrequency ablation and intravenous liposomal doxorubicin in a rat breast tumor model. Radiology 2002; 222:797–804.

29. Goldberg SN, Gazelle GS, Compton CC, Mueller PR, Tanabe KK. Treatment of intrahepatic malignancy with radiofrequency ablation: radiologic-pathologic corrolation. Cancer 2000; 88:2452–2463.

30. Breen DJ, Puri S, Maraveyas A, Nonson J. Early multiphasic CT appearances of metastatic liver disease following radiofrequency ablation. RSNA 2001:1246.

31. Mc Gahan JP, Dodd III GD. Radiofrequency ablation of the liver: current status. AJR Am J Roentgenol 2001; 176:3–16.

32. Catalano O, Lobianco R, Esposito M, Siani A. Hepatocellular carcinoma recurrence after percutaneous ablation therapy: helical CT patterns. Abdom Imag 2001; 26:375–383.

33. Rossi S, Distasi M, Buscarini E, et al. Percutaneous radiofrequency interstitial thermal ablation in the treatment of small hepatocellular carcinoma. Cancer J Sci Am 1995; 210:655–661.

34. Rossi S, Distasi M, Buscarini E, et al. Percutaneous RF interstitial thermal ablation in the treatment of hepatic cancer. AJR 1996; 167:759–768.

35. Livraghi T, Goldberg SN, Lazzaroni S, Meloni F, Solbiati L, Gazelle GS. Small hepatocellular carcinoma: treatment with radiofrequency ablation versus ethanol injection. Radiology 1998; 210:655–661.

36. Livraghi T, Meloni F, Goldberg SN, Lazzaroni S, Solbiati L, Gazelle GS. Hepatocellular carcinoma: radio-frequency ablation of medium and large lesions. Radiology 2000; 214:761–768.

37. Buscarini L, Buscarini E, Di Stasi M. Percutaneous radiofrequency ablation of small hepatocellular carcinoma: long term results. Eur Radiol 2001; 11:914–921.

38. Rossi S, Garbagnati F, Lencioni R et al. Percutaneous radiofrequency thermal ablation of non-resectable hepatocellular carcinoma after occlusion of tumor blood supply. Radiology 2000; 217:119–126.

39. Siperstein A, Garland A, Engle K. Local recurrence after laparoscopic radio-frequency thermal ablation of hepatic tumors. Ann Surg Onco 2000; 7: 106–113.

40. Hellman P, Ladjevardi S, Skogseid B, Akerstrom G, Elvin A. Radiofrequency tissue ablation using cooled tip for liver metastases of endocrine tumors. World J Surg 2002; 26:1052.

41. Gulec SA, Mountcastle TS, Frey D, Cundiff JD, Mathews E, Anthony L, O'Leary JP, Boudreaux JP. Cytoreductive surgery in patients with advanced-stage carcinoid tumors. Am Surg 2002; 68:667–671.

42. Chung MH, Pisegna J, Spirt M, Giuliano AE, Ye W, Ramming KP, Bilchik AJ. Hepatic cytoreduction followed by a long-acting somatostatin analogue: a paradigm for intractable neuroendocrine tumours metastatic to the liver. Surgery 2001; 130:954–962.

11

Endoscopic Ultrasound

S. Ashley Roberts
University Hospital of Wales, Cardiff, Wales

INTRODUCTION

Endoscopic ultrasound (EUS) is a marriage between ultrasound and endoscopy. Cross-sectional images of the gut wall and adjacent structures are obtained by passing an ultrasound probe into the gastrointestinal (GI) tract. The technique originated just after the second world war, when newly obsolete naval ultrasound equipment became available. Wild and Reid modified the equipment and developed a mechanical ultrasound transducer, which they inserted into the rectum of several healthy volunteers in order to obtain endoluminal ultrasound images of the rectal wall (1). The upper gastrointestinal tract was first examined by Rasmussen and colleagues (2), who passed an ultrasound catheter probe down the biopsy channel of an early endoscope. They were able to measure the thickness of the stomach wall with this technology.

Endoscopic ultrasound only became a useful clinical tool in the early 1980s with the development of dedicated endoscopes (3). These early echoendoscopes contained a rotating ultrasound transducer at their tip, which produced a 360 degree radial image perpendicular to the long axis of the endoscope insertion tube. They were first used for staging upper gastrointestinal tract cancer, particularly in the esophagus. While EUS still has a crucial role in the management of esophageal cancer (4), the indications for EUS have widened enormously. In particular, the development of linear echoendoscopes has precipitated the new field of interventional EUS. Using linear EUS, the ultrasound beam is parallel to the long axis of the endoscope and thus is in line with the biopsy channel rather than perpendicular to the long axis. When a needle is passed out of the endoscope, it remains in the ultrasound beam throughout its length, greatly enhancing visualization. It can be guided through the bowel wall into adjacent structures such as the pancreas and lymph nodes with a high degree of accuracy.

This chapter will discuss the clinical role of radial and linear EUS in the upper gastrointestinal tract, with particular reference to the new development of interventional EUS.

EQUIPMENT AND TECHNIQUES

Radial Echoendoscopes

Mechanical radial echoendoscopes are produced by Olympus and, despite relying on the same basic ultrasound technology developed by Wild and Reid, they remain the most widely used. The orientation of the ultrasound beam allows accurate staging of GI tract tumors because 360 degrees of the gut wall can be seen on any particular section. The entire esophagus and adjacent structures can be examined by simply passing the endoscope up and down throughout its length. In addition to the more usual echo-endoscopes, which provide a video or fiberoptic endoscopic image, Olympus also produces a narrow diameter echoendoscope specifically designed for staging esophageal cancer. This has no endoscopic image, which allows the reduction in diameter, and it is introduced over a guide wire rather than by direct vision. This modification can safely traverse tight strictures while facilitating highly accurate staging in what would otherwise be a difficult situation (5).

More recently, Pentax/Hitachi have produced an electronic radial echoendoscope, which produces a 270 degree image perpendicular to the long axis of the endoscope. This remains under evaluation, but initial experience is encouraging. This endoscope has excellent image quality, particularly in the near field, and the added advantage of color Doppler.

Catheter or "mini probe" transducers, which can be passed down the biopsy channel of conventional endoscopes, also provide radial images. They are usually of high frequency and therefore have limited penetration. This makes assessment of resectability of esophageal cancer difficult, although more recently Fujinon produced a more penetrating 7.5 MHz probe specifically for this purpose.

As described above, radial EUS does have significant limitations when guiding EUS interventional procedures because of the relationship between the ultrasound beam and biopsy needle. If a needle is passed out of the biopsy channel, it will tangentially cross the ultrasound beam and appear only as a localized dot on the image. There is therefore no information about the position of the needle tip within a lesion (Fig. 1). Although interventional EUS has been attempted with radial echoendoscopes (6), it is widely accepted that accurate interventional EUS requires a linear echoendoscope.

Linear Echoendoscopes

The first linear echoendoscope was developed by Pentax/Hitachi in the late 1980s. The linear assembly uses an electronic array of transducers, which are sequentially activated to produce a sector ultrasound beam parallel to the long axis of the endoscope. In contrast to the radial system, the full length of the needle can be tracked in real-time into a lesion (Fig. 2). This electronic curvilinear array assembly is the echoendoscope of choice for performing interventional procedures. A mechanical linear echoendosope (Olympus GF-UM30P) is available with the Olympus radial scanning processor and is therefore less expensive than the electronic linear counterparts, while retaining benefits of the correct orientation. Image quality is poorer, however, and there is no Doppler capability. Reasonable results have been achieved with this endoscope (7), but it is generally accepted that electronic echoendoscopes are preferable if finance allows.

Olympus/Aloka (GF-UC30P), Pentax/Hitachi (FG-32UA, FG-36UA, and FG-38UA), and Toshiba (PEF-703FA) produce electronic curvilinear array echoendoscopes for interventional EUS. The diameter of the biopsy channel varies between the endoscopes, with some allowing the use of larger biopsy needles and stents. Some also have an elevator device, which can alter the direction of needle puncture. In terms of image quality, however, there is little to choose between them, particularly when they are used with a state-of-the-art ultrasound processor.

Needle Biopsy Assembly for EUS-Guided Biopsy

The needle biopsy assembly allows needle deployment without damaging the biopsy channel of the endoscope. The needle is approximately 140 cm long and is surrounded by a metal spiral sheath, which protects the biopsy channel. The needle must be withdrawn into this sheath when the assembly is passed through the channel. A handle at the proximal end of the needle assembly can be Luer-locked to the biopsy channel inlet and allows the needle to be advanced out of the metal spiral sheath into a lesion by manually pushing a "plunger" (Fig. 3). The needle also contains a stylet that prevents contamination of the sample with mucous or epithelial cells from the gut wall mucosa.

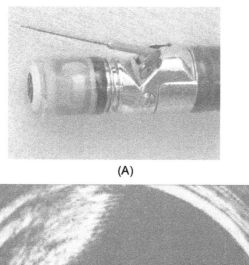

(A)

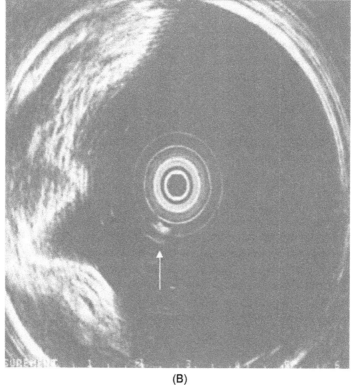

(B)

FIGURE 1 (A) Tip of the Olympus UM-20 mechanical radial echoendoscope. A Cook EUS biopsy needle has been passed down the working channel. (B) Subsequent image of a phantom, where the needle is only seen as a dot (arrow) as it crosses the radial ultrasound beam.

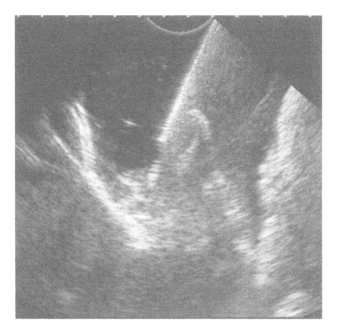

FIGURE 2   Image of the same phantom as in Figure 1B with the Toshiba linear scope. The Cook needle has been passed out of the biopsy channel and is seen throughout its length due to the orientation of the ultrasound beam.

The two most widely used needle systems are the Hancke-Villman (GIP, Grassau, Germany) and Wilson-Cook (Letchworth, Hertfordshire, UK) assemblies. The Wilson-Cook needle is single use, whereas the GIP needle assembly handle and metal spiral sheath can be reused after autoclaving. A comparison of the two needle types (8) in focal pancreatic lesions showed no significant difference in their handling. However, more inadequate samples were obtained with the GIP needle, although more technical problems (breakage of the outer sheath and inability to reinsert the central stylet) were encountered using the Wilson-Cook device.

EUS-Guided Biopsy Technique

The author's preferred image display locates the cranial aspect on the right side of the image screen, which is opposite to the system used for conventional transabdominal ultrasound. The needle, therefore, enters the image at top right. Once the lesion for biopsy has been identified, the needle assembly is introduced into the biopsy channel with the needle withdrawn into the metal spiral sheath. The handle is then locked into position. With

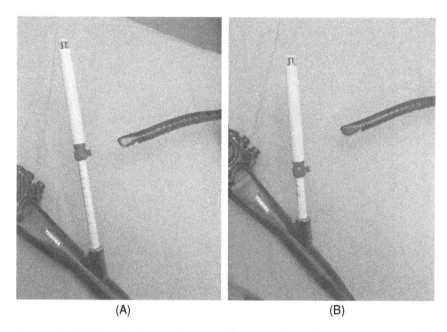

(A)   (B)

FIGURE 3   (A) The Cook needle assembly handle is locked onto the top of the biopsy channel of the Toshiba linear echoendoscope. The metal sheath is just seen protruding from the biopsy channel exit near the ultrasound transducer. (B) The "plunger" on the handle has been pushed in, and the needle has advanced out of the metal sheath.

the transducer against the bowel wall to maintain optimal visualization of the lesion, the needle is advanced into it. The stylet is completely withdrawn and suction applied using a primed syringe: 50 mL for pancreatic lesions and 10 mL for lymph nodes. Approximately 5–10 to-and-fro movements of the needle-tip within the lesion are required to obtain an adequate aspirate. The negative pressure is then released and the whole assembly withdrawn. Material is expelled onto glass slides, either with a syringe or by reintroducing the stylet. Small cores of tissue are often seen and may be placed in formalin for histological assessment. During subsequent passes the amount of suction can be varied depending on the aspirates obtained—more if the sample is scanty, less if bloody. Occasionally no suction is required, as advocated in a recent comparative study of different techniques for EUS-FNA of lymph nodes (9).

The average number of passes required is lesion-dependent. Typically, solid pancreatic lesions require five or more passes, three passes for lymph nodes; cystic lesions should be aspirated only once in order to minimize any risk of infection. Ideally, a cytopathologist should be available in the room, but this is not always feasible.

ANATOMICAL CONSIDERATIONS AND
TNM TUMOR CLASSIFICATION

At frequencies of between 5 and 12 MHz, the gastrointestinal wall is usually resolved as a five-layered structure of alternating hyper- and hypoechoic bands (Fig. 4), which show good correlation with the corresponding histological layers (10). The fourth (hypoechoic) layer represents the muscularis propria. At higher frequencies, the muscularis propria is split into longitudinal and circular muscle, producing seven layers in total, but this is of little clinical significance. Importantly, the muscularis propria is the key layer for histological staging of gastrointestinal tumors according to the TNM classification (Table 1). By defining the relationship of gut wall tumors to these histological layers, a preoperative T stage can be established, which influences patient management. EUS is almost unique in providing this information compared with other preoperative imaging modalities.

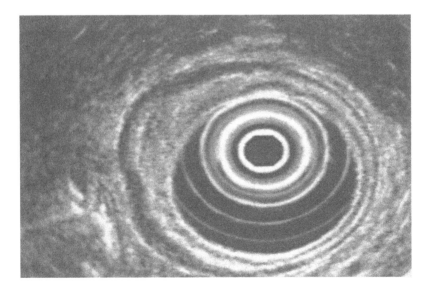

FIGURE 4 Radial EUS image of the distal stomach. From 12 o'clock through to 8 o'clock the normal five-layered structure with alternating hyper- and hypoechoic bands is seen. At 10 o'clock there is a hypoechoic mass, which does not breach the muscularis propria. This is a T1 gastric cancer.

TABLE 1   TNM Classification for Local Staging of Gut Wall Tumors

T stage	Definition
T1	Tumor involves the mucosa/submucosa
T2	Tumor involves the muscularis propria
T3	Tumor extends beyond the muscularis propria
T4	Tumor invades contiguous structures and organs

Involvement of regional lymph nodes (N), and distant lymph node metastases (M1a) in esophageal cancer can also be determined by EUS. The following criteria are suggestive of malignant lymph nodes: hypoechoic structure, sharply demarcated borders, rounded contour, and size greater than 10 mm (Fig. 5). If all four features are present, the positive predictive value for nodal involvement is 80—100% (11,12). Because reactive nodes can occasionally mimic malignant nodes, confirmation with EUS-FNA is usually performed if the lymph node site is considered metastatic, rather than regional.

Limited information regarding metastatic disease (M staging) can be obtained with EUS since only certain local structures can be assessed: left adrenal, liver segments I–VI, mediastinal and abdominal lymph nodes (M1a). CT is therefore still required to adequately exclude distant metastases.

CLINICAL APPLICATIONS OF EUS

Esophageal Cancer

Preoperative staging of esophageal cancer remains the most common indication for EUS, and radial echoendoscopes are the most widely used due to easier anatomical orientation in the mediastinum. The relationship of tumor to the esophageal wall layers and adjacent structures provides preoperative T staging (Fig. 6) and, in particular, may determine whether a tumor is technically resectable or not (Fig. 7). Local (N) and metastatic (M1a) lymph node involvement can be also assessed. Comparative studies with CT have consistently demonstrated superior T and N staging accuracy, and the development of helical CT (13) has had little impact on the role of EUS in this disease. These studies have been systematically reviewed by Harris et al.(4), who found that T and N staging accuracy of EUS approaches 90% and 80%, respectively. EUS has its greatest impact with advanced, nonresectable tumors by preventing open and closed thoracotomy. In patients with T4 esophageal cancer on preoperative EUS, two

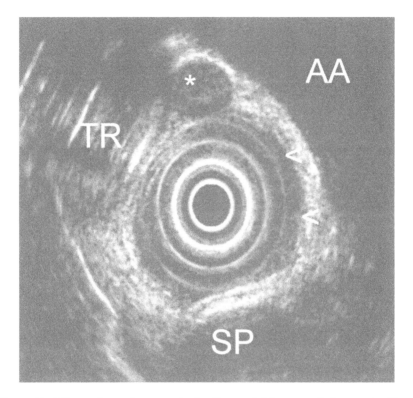

FIGURE 5   T3 esophageal cancer (<) with no visible muscularis propria. Tumor abuts the aortic arch (AA), but there is no evidence of direct invasion. A hypo-echoic left paratracheal lymph node with well-defined margins is seen at 12 o'clock(*). This has the typical appearance of a malignant node. TR = trachea, SP = spine.

studies have demonstrated that surgery has no impact on survival compared to nonsurgical controls (14,15). EUS can also guide the use of neoadjuvant chemotherapy or radio-chemotherapy and assess the response to treatment prior to surgery (16,17).

The site and number of lymph nodes identified preoperatively in esophageal cancer are closely related to eventual prognosis (18). In particular, involved celiac nodes and proximal mediastinal nodes in distal esophageal carcinoma are considered metastatic. It is therefore important to know with certainty if a lymph node is malignant or not as its presence may deny a patient potentially curative surgery. However, even when the specific endosonographic features described above are present, accuracy for predicting malignant invasion may be only 80% (11). It is therefore desirable

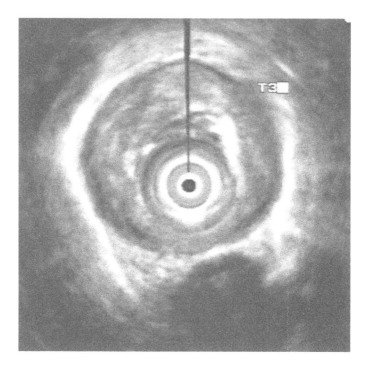

FIGURE 6 Esophageal adenocarcinoma. The muscularis propria is seen as a hypoechoic layer and is largely intact. At 2 o'clock, the tumor breaches this layer and is therefore T3.

to perform EUS-FNA of lymph nodes that may be metastatic in order to reduce any uncertainty (Fig. 8). Previous studies have shown that this strategy influences patient management and is safe (19,20).

Gastric Cancer

The clinical impact of EUS in gastric adenocarcinoma is less well defined than for esophageal cancer. This is perhaps due to lower staging accuracy (21) and the increased role of laparoscopy in gastric cancer. CT equipment and techniques have also improved. EUS has a role in confirming the diagnosis of gastric linitis plastica, which is characterized by thickening of the submucosa and/or the muscularis propria in a poorly distensible stomach. Other features such as lymphadenopathy and ascites may also be seen (Fig. 9).

Adenocarcinoma at the gastroesophageal junction should be considered separately, however, and there has been a marked increase in the

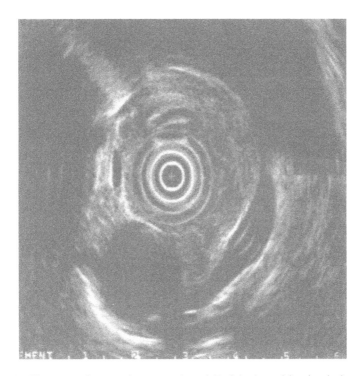

FIGURE 7   The aorta is seen between 6 and 7 o'clock and is clearly invaded by this esophageal squamous cell carcinoma, with tumor extending into the aortic lumen.

incidence of this disease over the past few years. Siewert's classification of these tumors into Types I, II, and III has gained widespread acceptance (22,23). Carcinoma of the distal esophagus (Type I), true carcinoma of the cardia (Type II), and subcardial gastric carcinoma (Type III) may all involve the gastroesophageal junction, but they require a different surgical strategy. In general terms, Type I requires esophagectomy, whereas Types II and III require gastrectomy. EUS can define the proximal extent of disease in the distal esophagus, particularly if there is submucosal extension. This can determine if an abdominal approach alone will enable complete resection of Type II and III junctional tumors (Fig. 10).

EUS influences the management of gastric MALT (mucosa-associated lymphoid tissue) lymphoma. In the majority of patients, disease is confined to the mucosa and usually responds to *Helicobacter* eradication therapy. However, where there is extension into the submucosa and beyond on EUS, patients will not respond to *Helicobacter* eradication therapy alone (24).

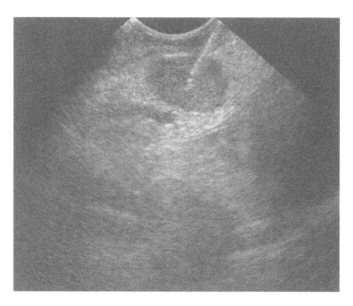

FIGURE 8   Malignant looking 1 cm paraesophageal lymph node in the proximal mediastinum in a patient with adenocarcinoma of the gastroesophageal junction. Transesophageal EUS-FNA confirmed adenocarcinoma. The needle is clearly seen in the center of the node.

Gastrointestinal Submucosal Lesions

At endoscopy, submucosal lesions produce a visible bulge, and EUS can distinguish a true submucosal lesion from an extrinsic mass such as a pancreatic pseudocyst or a normal structure such as gallbladder or spleen. Submucosal lesions are better demonstrated with EUS than CT (25), and the layer of origin can help narrow the differential diagnosis. Gastrointestinal submucosal lesions include lipomas (submucosa), pancreatic rests (submucosa), and gastrointestinal stromal cell tumors (muscularis propria/subserosa). The beam orientation of the linear echoendoscope is well suited to the assessment of submucosal lesions as normal gut wall can be seen merging with the abnormal region (Fig. 11). EUS-FNA is therefore simple to perform, since there is no need to change endoscopes, although the diagnostic yield of EUS-FNA in gut wall lesions is relatively low. In a series of 12 patients with submucosal lesions, only 50% of the samples were diagnostic and the one case of leiomyosarcoma was missed (26). Although it is not possible to reliably differentiate leiomyomas from leiomyosarcomas on cytology, EUS features such as size, margins, cystic changes, and the presence/absence of locoregional nodes may be helpful (27). Higher

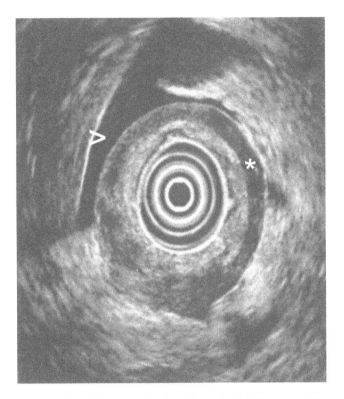

FIGURE 9 Radial EUS of the gastric body with marked thickening of the muscularis propria (*), and submucosa, which is typical of linitis plastica. Ascites is also demonstrated (>).

yields have been reported from gastrointestinal wall lesions using EUS guidance (28,29), particularly where a submucosal mass is due to lymphoma or adenocarcinoma. The author avoids EUS-FNA of cystic lesions when possible, due to the potentially increased risk of infective complications (30).

Pancreatic Tumors

Early comparative studies demonstrated that EUS was more accurate than CT and MRI for detection and staging of pancreatic cancer (31,32), but with improvements in CT technology this gap is now closing. For example, Legmann et al. have shown spiral CT and EUS have similar staging accuracy (33). EUS is still used where a pancreatic tumor is suspected but no mass is visible on CT and to clarify equivocal CT staging. EUS-FNA may also provide a tissue diagnosis (Fig. 12).

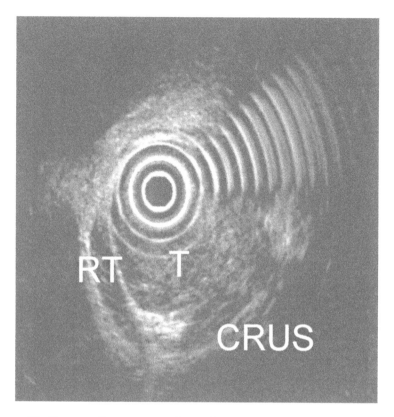

FIGURE 10   Tumor at the gastroesophageal junction (T) invades the left crus of the diaphragm (CRUS). The right crus (RT) is separated from the tumor by an echogenic interface.

A comparative assessment of the linear and radial EUS systems found no significant difference in staging accuracy (34). However, with the linear system, EUS-FNA of the pancreatic tumor, lymph node, or liver metastases is an option and is therefore the author's echoendoscope of choice. The linear system also permits the addition of EUS-guided celiac plexus neurolysis for pain relief if clinically indicated.

Sensitivities and specificities of up to 92% and 100%, respectively, have been reported for EUS-FNA of solid pancreatic masses (26,35,36). The presence of a cytopathologist at the time of the procedure decreases the number of needle passes required, but if this is not available, five or more passes are suggested (37). The pancreatic head is biopsied from the duodenum, and the body and tail from the stomach. An advantage of

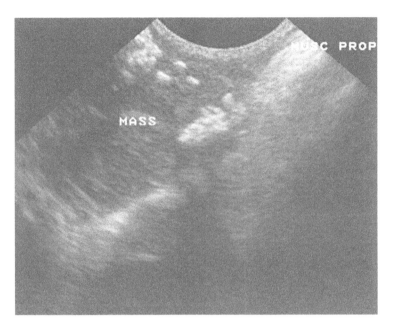

FIGURE 11   Esophageal leiomyoma. The linear echoendoscope is well suited for demonstrating the layer of origin. This partially calcified lesion is seen merging with the normal muscularis propria.

transduodenal EUS-FNA of the pancreatic head is that the needle track will be excised at the time of pancreatico-duodenectomy. There is therefore no theoretical risk of seeding, which is of particular value when assessing masses associated with chronic pancreatitis.

Cystic pancreatic lesions can pose a diagnostic dilemma. If pancreatic cysts are simple, with thin walls or thin septa, then it is reasonable to assume they are nonneoplastic (38). EUS as a positive predictor of malignancy is less reliable, however. Although thick-walled, complex cysts with solid components are thought to make malignancy more likely, these signs are unreliable. In a blinded review of the original endosonographic images, 61% of benign lesions were thought to have a solid component (39). In particular, pseudocysts cannot be easily distinguished from mucinous cystadenomas (40).

Aspiration of pancreatic cysts can therefore be used to narrow the differential diagnosis. EUS-FNA is ideally suited for this purpose due to the close proximity of the pancreas to the stomach and duodenum. A single pass technique is advocated due to the higher complication rates associated with EUS-FNA of cystic pancreatic lesions (41,42). Cytology

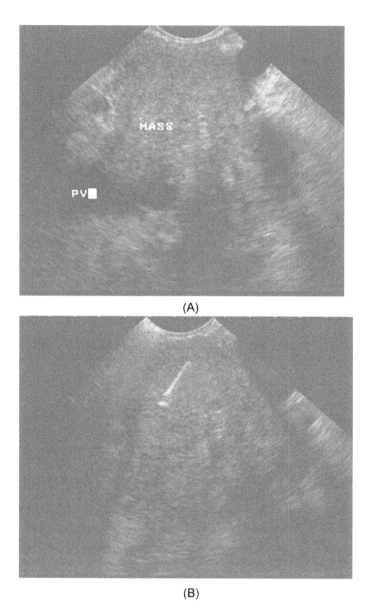

(A)

(B)

FIGURE 12   (A) 3 cm pancreatic head mass directly invades the portal vein (PV). (B) During the same procedure transduodenal EUS-FNA confirmed adeno-carcinoma. The needle is clearly seen within the lesion.

alone is fairly insensitive but can be improved by additional assessment of tumor markers such as CEA, CA125, CA19–9, and CA72–4 (marker for mucinous tumors) (43–45). Assessment of the amylase level is also useful as this is raised where lesions communicate with the ductal system (pseudocysts and side-branch intraductal papillary mucinous tumors, for example) and lowered in serous cystadenomas. CEA values are uniformly low in serous cystadenomas, higher in mucinous lesions, and markedly elevated in mucinous cystadenocarcinomas.

Pancreatic neuroendocrine tumors are clearly demonstrated by EUS as hypoechoic, vascular lesions, often with posterior acoustic enhancement. EUS is particularly useful where patients have biochemical evidence of a functioning tumor but other imaging modalities have failed to detect any lesion. While EUS is sensitive for detection of both insulinoma and gastrinoma (93% and 79%, respectively), somatostatin receptor scintigraphy is only sensitive in gastrinoma (86% vs. 14% in insulinoma) (46,47). EUS-FNA can confirm the nature of a neuroendocrine tumor, but accuracy rates are lower than for ductal adenocarcinoma (48). This is of only limited significance, as the primary role of imaging is localization since the diagnosis will usually have been made biochemically beforehand.

Gallstones and Acute Pancreatitis

The role of EUS in gallstone disease was first explored in the 1980s (49), and early comparative studies, with ERCP as the gold standard, demonstrated that EUS was far superior to other noninvasive tests. In particular, EUS was shown to have a negative predictive value of 97% for common bile duct stones (50). With the development of laparoscopic cholecystectomy, non-invasive preoperative imaging became even more important and EUS provided high accuracy (51). In these patients with suspected CBD stones, ERCP with its associated complications could be avoided by a negative EUS examination.

While it is no longer acceptable to perform ERCP primarily as a diagnostic test for CBD stones, what is the role of EUS in the era of MR cholangiography? The answer to this question depends upon the clinical circumstances. Comparative studies of MR cholangiography versus EUS indicate similar accuracy for large stones, but the sensitivity of MR cholangiography declines significantly with smaller stones (52,53). A positive result with MR cholangiography can therefore define the need for ERCP, but a negative result leads to uncertainty. Small stones can be a potent cause of acute pancreatitis, and EUS therefore retains a prominent role in defining the etiology of acute pancreatitis.

If there is evidence of gallbladder or bile duct stones on transabdominal ultrasound, it is reasonable to proceed to ERCP, assuming a diagnosis
of gallstone pancreatitis. If there are no gallstones and there is no other
clear etiology for the acute pancreatitis then EUS has a role. In a study
from Hong Kong, gallstones were detected by EUS in 14 of 18 patients
who had been wrongly classified as having idiopathic pancreatitis by
conventional examinations such as ultrasound, CT, and ERCP (54). Subsequent larger studies confirm that idiopathic pancreatitis should not be
diagnosed unless EUS has been performed to exclude biliary microlithiasis
and "missed" gall stones (55,56) (Fig. 13). In patients with gallstone pancreatitis, some authors have suggested that the presence of bile duct stones
on EUS may better select those who should undergo ERCP (57,58)
(Fig. 14). However, larger studies are needed to confirm the superiority of

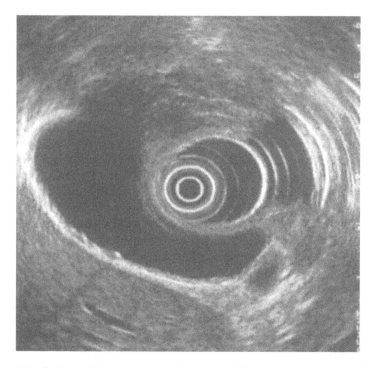

FIGURE 13   Patient with recurrent acute pancreatitis and normal transabdominal
ultrasound on two separate occasions. EUS demonstrates a tiny calculus in the
body of the gall bladder with typical acoustic shadowing. Cholecystectomy
confirmed the findings and there were no further episodes of pancreatitis on
follow-up.

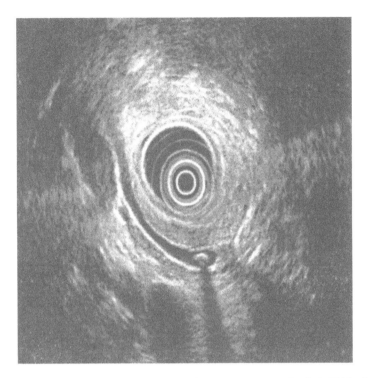

FIGURE 14   Recurrent pancreatitis postcholecystectomy. Radial EUS demonstrates a 3 mm stone at 6 o'clock in a nondilated bile duct. These findings were subsequently confirmed following endoscopic sphincterotomy.

this strategy compared with ERCP alone for the management of biliary pancreatitis.

Chronic Pancreatitis

EUS in chronic pancreatitis was first described in 1986, defining some morphological features of the disease by correlation with histopathology (59). More recently, the criteria for making the diagnosis of chronic pancreatitis on EUS have been refined and are classified into parenchymal and ductal changes. Parenchymal changes include echogenic foci (calcification), prominent interlobular septae (fibrosis), small cystic cavities (edema), lobulated outer gland margin (fibrosis/atrophy), and heterogeneous parenchyma. Ductal changes include dilation, irregularity, echogenic wall (fibrosis), side-branch ectasia, and echogenic foci (stones). Furthermore, there is good interobserver agreement among experienced endosonographers when using these criteria (60) (Fig. 15).

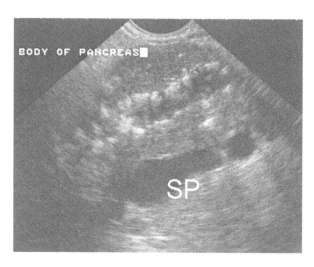

FIGURE 15   Chronic pancreatitis. Linear EUS of the pancreatic body demonstrates
a dilated, irregular pancreatic duct with echogenic walls and ductal calculi.
Echogenic foci are seen in the pancreatic parenchyma. SP = splenic vein.

In an early comparative study of EUS versus ERCP, EUS demonstrated inflammatory changes in almost all patients in whom ERCP suggested chronic pancreatitis. EUS was also positive in a considerable
number of cases with a normal pancreatogram but a probable clinical epi-
sode of pancreatic inflammation. Due to the absence of a histological gold
standard in the majority of patients, it was not certain whether EUS was
oversensitive or ERCP undersensitive for diagnosis of early chronic pancreatitis (61). Does EUS-FNA help answer this question? When using
ERCP as the gold standard, Hollerbach et al. found that EUS morphological features had a sensitivity of 97%, a specificity of 60%, positive predictive value of 94%, and negative predictive value of 75% for diagnosis of
chronic pancreatitis (62). The addition of EUS-FNA increased the negative
predictive value to 100%, and negative EUS-FNA findings therefore effectively ruled out chronic pancreatitis. In this study EUS-FNA did not
improve the specificity of EUS findings when positive for chronic pancreatitis, and the question remained unanswered. More recently, however, it has
become clear that ERCP is no longer the gold standard for early chronic
pancreatitis and EUS appears to be more sensitive. In a prospective,
follow-up study of 130 patients thought to have chronic pancreatitis,
those with ERCP changes of chronic pancreatitis also had changes on EUS
(63). However, in 38 patients, the pancreatogram was normal, but EUS

suggested chronic pancreatitis in 32 of these. During follow-up, chronic pancreatitis was subsequently confirmed by repeat ERCP in 22 of these 32 patients (68.8%), suggesting that EUS was the better predictor of disease. On the basis of these follow-up data, the sensitivities of EUS and endoscopic retrograde pancreatography at the time of the first examination were, respectively, 100% and 80% (63). EUS should therefore be used to make the diagnosis of chronic pancreatitis before ERCP, particularly given the much higher complication rate of ERCP.

EUS-Guided Celiac Plexus Neurolysis

EUS-guided celiac plexus neurolysis (EUS-CPN) can be used for the palliation of intractable abdominal pain, usually in patients with inoperable pancreatic carcinoma but also in chronic pancreatitis (64–67). Injection of the celiac plexus is possible due to its constant relationship to the celiac axis, which can be clearly visualized on EUS (Fig. 16). A combination of a

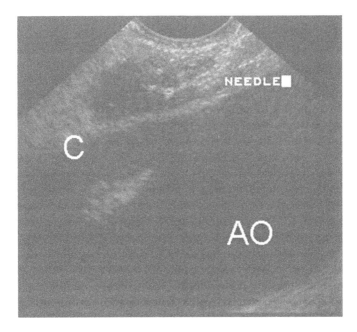

FIGURE 16 EUS guided celiac plexus neurolysis. A needle has been passed into the presumed position of the celiac plexus just above the celiac axis origin (C) from the aorta (AO). Following local anesthetic, absolute alcohol is injected producing an echogenic cloud.

long-acting local anesthetic such as bupivacaine and absolute alcohol is used in malignant disease. Steroids such as triamcinolone have been used in chronic pancreatitis.

EUS-CPN is more successful in patients with pancreatic carcinoma compared to chronic pancreatitis. In the largest reported series to date, pain scores declined in 45 of 58 (78%) patients with pain from inoperable malignancy, and there were no significant complications (67). There is no theoretical risk of causing paraplegia from inadvertent injection into the artery of Adamkiewicz, because the celiac plexus is accessed via an anterior transgastric approach: there is a 1% risk of paraplegia with the posterior percutaneous approach. There are no comparative studies of EUS-CPN and CT-guided CPN in malignant disease to the author's knowledge. In chronic pancreatitis, however, a higher proportion of patients remain pain-free for a longer period of time with EUS CPN, compared to CT-guided CPN (66). In the same study, Gress et al. demonstrated, that EUS-CPN was preferred by patients (66).

EUS-CPN for malignant disease is a relatively simple, safe, and effective method of pain relief. It is less effective in chronic pancreatitis (65), and further data are needed to clarify any role in this group of patients, who are often very difficult to manage effectively by any means.

Pancreatic Pseudocyst Drainage

Pancreatic pseudocysts require intervention if local pressure causes symptoms of pain or gastric outlet obstruction or there are complications such as infection. They can be treated by endoscopic pancreatic stent insertion if the cyst communicates with the main pancreatic duct, but this is not always the case. They can be drained radiologically, surgically, or endoscopically by the creation of a cystgastrostomy or cystduodenostomy. Although endoscopic management is less invasive than surgery, it is not possible in all cases as it relies on a visible bulge to determine the appropriate puncture site. EUS is playing an increasing role in guiding the endoscopic drainage of pseudocysts for several reasons (68,69). Using EUS, a visible bulge becomes less crucial and the optimal puncture site can be chosen so the distance between the pseudocyst and bowel wall is less than 1 cm. Hemorrhage can be a major complication of the technique, and linear EUS augmented by color Doppler helps avoid vascular structures. Drainage may also be "EUS-assisted" where the optimal puncture site is marked with biopsy forceps down the echoendoscope. The stent is then inserted into the cyst using a large channel ERCP scope under fluoroscopic guidance. The development of large channel echoendoscopes that will accommodate 8–10 French stents has allowed single step "EUS-directed" procedures without the need for fluoroscopy (70). Several studies have demonstrated that these techniques are safe and effective (68–70).

Mediastinal Lymphadenopathy and Lung Cancer

The accurate detection of mediastinal lymph nodes in esophageal cancer had obvious implications for staging patients with lung cancer, and EUS in lung cancer was first described in Japan in 1988 (71). Comparative studies with CT have since confirmed the superior staging accuracy of EUS for this disease (72,73). Further improvements in the sensitivity and specificity of EUS have been achieved with the addition of EUS-FNA (74,75). In particular, EUS can detect mediastinal disease in more than one third of patients whose mediastinal CT is normal.

EUS-FNA can provide cytological staging of mediastinal nodes in all nodal stations except the anterior mediastinum due to the position of the trachea. In particular, the subcarinal, aortopulmonary, para-tracheal, and para-esophageal regions are readily accessible (Fig. 17), regions that are not easily accessed by mediastinoscopy. A small comparative study

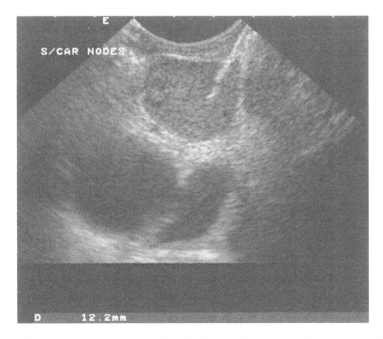

FIGURE 17 Lung cancer staging. EUS-FNA of a 12 mm subcarinal node confirmed non-small-cell carcinoma.

suggested that EUS-FNA and mediastinoscopy are complementary—mediastinoscopy for the anterior mediastinum and EUS-FNA for the remainder (76). There are also data suggesting that EUS-FNA is more cost-effective than mediastinoscopy: $1,975 vs. $7,795 (77). Also, staging of lung cancer using EUS is not confined to the mediastinum. Excellent views of the left adrenal gland, the left lobe of the liver, and the majority of the right lobe can be obtained. Any abnormalities seen can then undergo transgastric EUS-FNA. Some authors therefore advocate routine use of EUS with EUS-FNA in lung cancer staging algorithms, with CT and mediastinoscopy only if required (74,75). EUS-FNA can also provide the primary histological diagnosis in lung cancer. In one series, EUS-FNA of mediastinal nodes provided the diagnosis and cytological classification in 25 of 26 patients in whom previous bronchoscopic biopsy had failed (78).

There is also a role in establishing the cause of lymphadenopathy in benign conditions such as sarcoidosis and tuberculosis. Fritscher-Ravens et al. found a sensitivity of 94% and specificity of 100% in establishing the presence of epithelioid granulomata, suggesting the diagnosis of sarcoidosis (79). The author has previously described the problem-solving role of subcarinal EUS-FNA in a range of benign and malignant conditions (80).

OTHER APPLICATIONS FOR INTERVENTIONAL EUS

Liver

Percutaneous core biopsy of liver lesions is the preferred method for obtaining a tissue diagnosis. However, focal lesions are occasionally encountered using EUS, which have not been detected on US or CT, and EUS-FNA can then be performed (Fig. 18). Nguyen et al. (81) described 574 patients who underwent EUS for the staging of pulmonary or gastrointestinal malignancy, of whom 14 were found to have liver lesions, in only 3 patients were lesions detected on CT. Diagnostic tissue was obtained in all the EUS-FNA samples without complication. In the author's practice, when staging esophageal, lung, and, in particular, pancreatic cancer, the liver is carefully assessed as far as possible. All but segments VII and VIII can be examined, and if focal lesions are seen, EUS-FNA is performed. The yield from focal liver lesions is greater than from the frequently fibrotic primary pancreatic tumor.

Adrenal Glands

Excellent transgastric views of the left adrenal gland can be obtained, and EUS-FNA of lesions as small as 1 cm is relatively straightforward. Chang et al.(82) reported that the left adrenal gland was visualized on EUS in

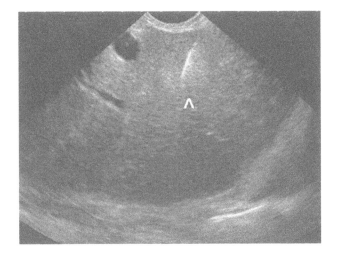

FIGURE 18   Patient with pancreatic mass but normal liver on three phase CT. Transgastric EUS-FNA of 1 cm echogenic lesion in liver (^) confirmed adenocarcinoma.

30 out of 31 patients and positive cytology was obtained in one case by EUS-FNA where CT-guided biopsy had been unsuccessful. When assessing mediastinal lymph node status in lung cancer, the author therefore routinely assesses the left adrenal. Although MRI is increasingly used to characterize adrenal lesions, EUS should be considered as an alternative method for tissue diagnosis (Fig. 19).

Thoracocentesis and Paracentesis

EUS may detect pleural or ascitic fluid not identified on other imaging modalities (83), and EUS-guided aspiration of this fluid can be performed successfully and safely. In a study of 85 patients with ascites detected incidentally on EUS (84), initial staging CT detected ascites in only 14 out of 79 patients with upper gastrointestinal malignancy. Thirty-one patients went on to have this fluid aspirated without complication, and 5 patients had malignant cytology. Volumes aspirated are inevitably small (mean volume 7.5 mL in thoracocentesis and 7.9 mL in paracentesis), but positive cytology for malignancy helps to avoid unnecessary surgery.

Botulinum Injection for Achalasia

Achalasia can be treated by balloon dilatation of the lower esophageal sphincter or by surgical myotomy. Alternatively, endoscopic injection of

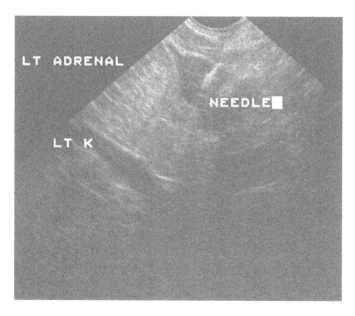

FIGURE 19   EUS-FNA of 1 cm left adrenal mass noted during EUS staging of lung cancer. Cytology confirmed squamous cell carcinoma.

botulinum toxin into the sphincter produces a good initial symptomatic response in 90%. However, 42% relapse at 6 months, requiring further injection (85). More precise injection into the sphincter using EUS for guidance may produce better long-term results. The lower esphageal sphincter is a hypoechoic structure on EUS and is thickened in achalasia. Small studies suggest the relapse rate may be reduced (86,87), with all patients symptom-free over a study period of 13 months, although results are still preliminary.

EUS-Guided Cholangiopancreatography

EUS-guided puncture of the common bile (CBD) and/or pancreatic duct (PD) following an unsuccessful ERCP has been described (88,89). The CBD is usually punctured via the first or second part of the duodenum and the PD via the stomach. Until recently, application of this technique has been limited by the inability to perform a therapeutic procedure at the same sitting. However, Giovannini et al. have described entero-biliary stent insertion guided by EUS (90).

It has been argued that EUS/EUS-FNA should be performed prior to ERCP in the investigation of patients with obstructive jaundice. Erickson et al. (91) found that when performing EUS/EUS-FNA first, only 53% of the 147 patients subsequently required ERCP, an approach that resulted in considerable cost savings of between $1,007 and $1,313 per patient.

COMPLICATIONS

Complications occur with any endoscopic procedure and include perforation, aspiration, and cardio-respiratory events related to sedation. Perforation was a problem in the early years of EUS, with dilatation of stenotic esophageal cancer required if large echoendoscopes were to traverse tight strictures. Indeed, in one study the perforation rate was as high as 24% (92). Happily, with refinements in EUS equipment and narrow diameter probes, perforation is now unusual. The author has described successful EUS staging of 100 consecutive cases of esophageal cancer with no perforations, probably as the direct result of a narrow diameter probe (5). The author has since performed over 500 cases with this probe with no morbidity.

EUS-FNA brings additional complications, but the complication rates are generally low, particularly when compared with ERCP. Two large series report complication rates for interventional EUS. In a multicentre study, Wiersema et al.(26) reported complication rates following EUS-FNA for a wide variety of mediastinal and abdominal lesions. There were only five complications associated with EUS-FNA of 554 lesions; two were endoscopy-related perforations (duodenal cap perforation and perforation following dilatation of esophageal carcinoma), and three were directly related to EUS-FNA. All three latter complications occurred with EUS-FNA of cystic pancreatic lesions (fever, hemorrhage), and two of these patients required surgery. The overall complication rate in that study was 1.1%. O'Toole et al. (41) reported five complications following EUS-FNA in 322 consecutive patients (345 lesions) ; four of these occurred in cystic pancreatic lesions, (self-limiting acute pancreatitis in 3, aspiration pneumonia in 1), and one patient developed aspiration pneumonia following EUS-FNA of a stromal cell tumor. The overall complication rate in that series was 1.6%. There have been no reported complications of EUS-FNA of peri-intestinal lymph nodes in the mediastinum or abdomen, or indeed solid pancreatic masses. EUS-FNA is therefore a safe procedure, but caution is needed with cystic pancreatic lesions. Based on these studies (26,41), there is a consensus among EUS users to administer antibiotic prophylaxis and only to perform a single needle pass when dealing with cystic pancreatic lesions in order to minimize the risk of complications.

CONCLUSION

EUS has an important role for the staging of upper gastrointestinal and lung cancer. In particular, accurate preoperative staging of esophageal cancer has made a significant impact on the morbidity of this disease by preventing unnecessary surgery. Open and closed thoracotomy is now an unusual occurrence in the author's practice. While EUS is almost synonymous with esophageal cancer, the technique demonstrably has an important role in other conditions. The more recent development of EUS-FNA has allowed tissue to be obtained from a variety of structures, with mediastinal lymph nodes and small pancreatic tumors forming the majority of the interventional EUS workload. The technique can allow a tissue diagnosis from small (< 1 cm) lesions in areas that are otherwise difficult or impossible to access, such as the posterior mediastinum. EUS-FNA is performed as a day case using only conscious sedation, which has clear economic advantages when compared with more invasive alternatives. EUS can guide therapeutic interventions such as pancreatic pseudocyst drainage and celiac plexus neurolysis, and the indications for interventional EUS continue to widen.

REFERENCES

1. Wild JJ, Reid JM. In: Kelly E (ed.), Ultrasound in Biology and Medicine. American Institute of Biological Sciences 1957; 1:30–45.
2. Rasmussen SN, Riis P, Northeved A. Ultrasonographic measurements of the rectal and gastric wall thickness. Scand J Gastroenterol 1975; 10(suppl 34):25.
3. DiMagno EP, Buxton JL, Regan PT, Hattery RR, Wilson DA, Suarez JR, et al. Ultrasonic endoscope. Lancet 1980; 1(8169):629–631.
4. Harris KM, Kelly S, Berry E, Hutton J, Roderick P, Cullingworth J, et al. Systematic review of endoscopic ultrasound in gastro-oesophageal cancer. Health Technol Assess 1998; 2(18):i–134.
5. Bowrey DJ, Clark GW, Roberts SA, Maughan TS, Hawthorne AB, Williams GT, et al. Endosonographic staging of 100 consecutive patients with esophageal carcinoma: introduction of the 8-mm esophagoprobe. Dis Esophagus 1999; 12(4):258–263.
6. Gress FG, Hawes RH, Savides TJ, Ikenberry SO, Lehman GA. Endoscopic ultrasound-guided fine-needle aspiration biopsy using linear array and radial scanning endosonography. Gastrointest Endosc 1997; 45(3):243–250.
7. Sahai AV, Schembre D, Stevens PD, Chak A, Isenberg G, Lightdale CJ, et al. A multicenter U.S. experience with EUS-guided fine-needle aspiration using the Olympus GF-UM30P echoendoscope: safety and effectiveness. Gastrointest Endosc 1999; 50(6):792–796.
8. Fritscher-Ravens A, Topalidis T, Bobrowski C, Krause C, Thonke E, Jackle S, et al. Endoscopic ultrasound-guided fine-needle aspiration in focal pancreatic

lesions: a prospective intraindividual comparison of two needle assemblies. Endoscopy 2001; 33(6):484–490.

9. Wallace MB, Kennedy T, Durkalski V, Eloubeidi MA, Etamad R, Matsuda K, et al. Randomized controlled trial of EUS-guided fine needle aspiration techniques for the detection of malignant lymphadenopathy. Gastrointest Endosc 2001; 54(4):441–447.

10. Kimmey MB, Martin RW, Haggitt RC, Wang KY, Franklin DW, Silverstein FE. Histologic correlates of gastrointestinal ultrasound images. Gastroenterology 1989; 96(2 Pt 1):433–441.

11. Bhutani MS, Hawes RH, Hoffman BJ. A comparison of the accuracy of echo features during endoscopic ultrasound (EUS) and EUS-guided fine-needle aspiration for diagnosis of malignant lymph node invasion. Gastrointest Endosc 1997; 45(6):474–479.

12. Catalano MF, Sivak MV, Jr., Rice T, Gragg LA, Van Dam J. Endosonographic features predictive of lymph node metastasis. Gastrointest Endosc 1994; 40(4):442–446.

13. Romagnuolo J, Scott J, Hawes RH, Hoffman BJ, Reed CE, Aithal GP, et al. Helical CT versus EUS with fine needle aspiration for celiac nodal assessment in patients with esophageal cancer. Gastrointest Endosc 2002; 55(6):648–654.

14. Chak A, Canto M, Gerdes H, Lightdale CJ, Hawes RH, Wiersema MJ, et al. Prognosis of esophageal cancers preoperatively staged to be locally invasive (T4) by endoscopic ultrasound (EUS): a multicenter retrospective cohort study. Gastrointest Endosc 1995; 42(6):501–506.

15. Fockens P, Kisman K, Merkus MP, van Lanschot JJ, Obertop H, Tytgat GN. The prognosis of esophageal carcinoma staged irresectable (T4) by endosonography. J Am Coll Surg 1998; 186(1):17–23.

16. Bowrey DJ, Clark GW, Roberts SA, Hawthorne AB, Maughan TS, Williams GT, et al. Serial endoscopic ultrasound in the assessment of response to chemoradiotherapy for carcinoma of the esophagus. J Gastrointest Surg 1999; 3(5):462–467.

17. Chak A, Canto MI, Cooper GS, Isenberg G, Willis J, Levitan N, et al. Endosonographic assessment of multimodality therapy predicts survival of esophageal carcinoma patients. Cancer 2000; 88(8):1788–1795.

18. Eloubeidi MA, Wallace MB, Reed CE, Hadzijahic N, Lewin DN, Van Velse A, et al. The utility of EUS and EUS-guided fine needle aspiration in detecting celiac lymph node metastasis in patients with esophageal cancer: a single-center experience. Gastrointest Endosc 2001; 54(6):714–719.

19. Giovannini M, Monges G, Seitz JF, Moutardier V, Bernardini D, Thomas P, et al. Distant lymph node metastases in esophageal cancer: impact of endoscopic ultrasound-guided biopsy. Endoscopy 1999; 31(7):536–540.

20. Wallace MB, Hawes RH, Sahai AV, Van Velse A, Hoffman BJ. Dilation of malignant esophageal stenosis to allow EUS guided fine-needle aspiration: safety and effect on patient management. Gastrointest Endosc 2000; 51(3):309–313.

21. Rosch T, Lorenz R, Zenker K, von Wichert A, Dancygier H, Hofler H, et al. Local staging and assessment of resectability in carcinoma of the esophagus,

stomach, and duodenum by endoscopic ultrasonography. Gastrointest Endosc 1992; 38(4):460–467.

22. Holscher AH, Bollschweiler E, Siewert JR. Carcinoma of the gastric cardia. Ann Chir Gynaecol 1995; 84(2):185–192.

23. Stein HJ, Feith M, Siewert JR. Cancer of the esophagogastric junction. Surg Oncol 2000; 9(1):35–41.

24. Nakamura S, Matsumoto T, Suekane H, Takeshita M, Hizawa K, Kawasaki M, et al. Predictive value of endoscopic ultrasonography for regression of gastric low grade and high grade MALT lymphomas after eradication of Helicobacter pylori. Gut 2001; 48(4):454–460.

25. Rosch T, Lorenz R, Dancygier H, von Wickert A, Classen M. Endosono-graphic diagnosis of submucosal upper gastrointestinal tract tumors. Scand J Gastroenterol 1992; 27(1):1–8.

26. Wiersema MJ, Vilmann P, Giovannini M, Chang KJ, Wiersema LM. Endo-sonography-guided fine-needle aspiration biopsy: diagnostic accuracy and complication assessment. Gastroenterology 1997; 112(4):1087–1095.

27. Palazzo L, Landi B, Cellier C, Cuillerier E, Roseau G, Barbier JP. Endosono-graphic features predictive of benign and malignant gastrointestinal stromal cell tumours. Gut 2000; 46(1):88–92.

28. Caletti GC, Brocchi E, Ferrari A, Bonora G, Santini D, Mazzoleni G, et al. Guillotine needle biopsy as a supplement to endosonography in the diagnosis of gastric submucosal tumors. Endoscopy 1991; 23(5):251–254.

29. Wegener M, Adamek RJ, Wedmann B, Pfaffenbach B. Endosonographically guided fine-needle aspiration puncture of paraesophagogastric mass lesions: preliminary results. Endoscopy 1994; 26(7):586–591.

30. Ryan AG, Zamvar V, Roberts SA. Iatrogenic candidal infection of a media-stinal foregut cyst following endoscopic ultrasound-guided fine-needle aspiration. Endoscopy 2002; 34(10):838–839.

31. Muller MF, Meyenberger C, Bertschinger P, Schaer R, Marincek B. Pancreatic tumors: evaluation with endoscopic US, CT, and MR imaging. Radiology 1994; 190(3):745–751.

32. Palazzo L, Roseau G, Gayet B, Vilgrain V, Belghiti J, Fekete F, et al. Endoscopic ultrasonography in the diagnosis and staging of pancreatic adeno-carcinoma. Results of a prospective study with comparison to ultrasonography and CT scan. Endoscopy 1993; 25(2):143–150.

33. Legmann P, Vignaux O, Dousset B, Baraza AJ, Palazzo L, Dumontier I, et al. Pancreatic tumors: comparison of dual-phase helical CT and endoscopic sonography. AJR Am J Roentgenol 1998; 170(5):1315–1322.

34. Gress F, Savides T, Cummings O, Sherman S, Lehman G, Zaidi S, et al. Radial scanning and linear array endosonography for staging pancreatic cancer: a prospective randomized comparison. Gastrointest Endosc 1997; 45(2):138–142.

35. Chang KJ, Nguyen P, Erickson RA, Durbin TE, Katz KD. The clinical utility of endoscopic ultrasound-guided fine-needle aspiration in the diagnosis and staging of pancreatic carcinoma. Gastrointest Endosc 1997; 45(5):387–393.

36. Williams DB, Sahai AV, Aabakken L, Penman ID, Van Velse A, Webb J, et al. Endoscopic ultrasound guided fine needle aspiration biopsy: a large single centre experience. Gut 1999; 44(5):720–726.

37. Erickson RA, Sayage-Rabie L, Beissner RS. Factors predicting the number of EUS-guided fine-needle passes for diagnosis of pancreatic malignancies. Gastrointest Endosc 2000; 51(2):184–190.

38. Koito K, Namieno T, Nagakawa T, Shyonai T, Hirokawa N, Morita K. Solitary cystic tumor of the pancreas: EUS-pathologic correlation. Gastrointest Endosc 1997; 45(3):268–276.

39. Ahmad NA, Kochman ML, Lewis JD, Ginsberg GG. Can EUS alone differentiate between malignant and benign cystic lesions of the pancreas? Am J Gastroenterol 2001; 96(12):3295–3300.

40. Le Borgne J, de Calan L, Partensky C. Cystadenomas and cystadenocarcinomas of the pancreas: a multiinstitutional retrospective study of 398 cases. French Surgical Association. Ann Surg 1999; 230(2):152–161.

41. O'Toole D, Palazzo L, Arotcarena R, Dancour A, Aubert A, Hammel P, et al. Assessment of complications of EUS-guided fine-needle aspiration. Gastrointest Endosc 2001; 53(4):470–474.

42. Wiersema MJ, Sandusky D, Carr R, Wiersema LM, Erdel WC, Frederick PK. Endosonography-guided cholangiopancreatography. Gastrointest Endosc 1996; 43(2 Pt 1):102–106.

43. Brandwein SL, Farrell JJ, Centeno BA, Brugge WR. Detection and tumor staging of malignancy in cystic, intraductal, and solid tumors of the pancreas by EUS. Gastrointest Endosc 2001; 53(7):722–727.

44. Brugge WR. Role of endoscopic ultrasound in the diagnosis of cystic lesions of the pancreas. Pancreatology 2001; 1(6):637–640.

45. Sand JA, Hyoty MK, Mattila J, Dagorn JC, Nordback IH. Clinical assessment compared with cyst fluid analysis in the differential diagnosis of cystic lesions in the pancreas. Surgery 1996; 119(3):275–280.

46. Zimmer T, Stolzel U, Bader M, Koppenhagen K, Hamm B, Buhr H, et al. Endoscopic ultrasonography and somatostatin receptor scintigraphy in the preoperative localisation of insulinomas and gastrinomas. Gut 1996; 39(4):562–568.

47. Zimmer T, Scherubl H, Faiss S, Stolzel U, Riecken EO, Wiedenmann B. Endoscopic ultrasonography of neuroendocrine tumours. Digestion 2000; 62 Suppl 1:45–50.

48. Voss M, Hammel P, Molas G, Palazzo L, Dancour A, O'Toole D, et al. Value of endoscopic ultrasound guided fine needle aspiration biopsy in the diagnosis of solid pancreatic masses. Gut 2000; 46(2):244–249.

49. Dancygier H, Classen M. Endosonographic diagnosis of benign pancreatic and biliary lesions. Scand J Gastroenterol Suppl 1986; 123:119–122.

50. Amouyal P, Amouyal G, Levy P, Tuzet S, Palazzo L, Vilgrain V, et al. Diagnosis of choledocholithiasis by endoscopic ultrasonography. Gastroenterology 1994; 106(4):1062–1067.

51. Palazzo L, Girollet PP, Salmeron M, Silvain C, Roseau G, Canard JM, et al. Value of endoscopic ultrasonography in the diagnosis of common bile duct

stones: comparison with surgical exploration and ERCP. Gastrointest Endosc 1995; 42(3):225–231.

52. Scheiman JM, Carlos RC, Barnett JL, Elta GH, Nostrant TT, Chey WD, et al. Can endoscopic ultrasound or magnetic resonance cholangiopancreato-graphy replace ERCP in patients with suspected biliary disease? A prospective trial and cost analysis. Am J Gastroenterol 2001; 96(10):2900–2904.

53. Zidi SH, Prat F, Le Guen O, Rondeau Y, Rocher L, Fritsch J, et al. Use of magne-tic resonance cholangiography in the diagnosis of choledocholithiasis: prospec-tive comparison with a reference imaging method. Gut 1999; 44(1):118–122.

54. Liu CL, Lo CM, Chan JK, Poon RT, Fan ST. EUS for detection of occult cholelithiasis in patients with idiopathic pancreatitis. Gastrointest Endosc 2000; 51(1):28–32.

55. Norton SA, Alderson D. Endoscopic ultrasonography in the evaluation of idiopathic acute pancreatitis. Br J Surg 2000; 87(12):1650–1655.

56. Tandon M, Topazian M. Endoscopic ultrasound in idiopathic acute pancreatitis. Am J Gastroenterol 2001; 96(3):705–709.

57. Chak A, Hawes RH, Cooper GS, Hoffman B, Catalano MF, Wong RC, et al. Prospective assessment of the utility of EUS in the evaluation of gallstone pancreatitis. Gastrointest Endosc 1999; 49(5):599–604.

58. Prat F, Edery J, Meduri B, Chiche R, Ayoun C, Bodart M, et al. Early EUS of the bile duct before endoscopic sphincterotomy for acute biliary pancreatitis. Gastrointest Endosc 2001; 54(6):724–729.

59. Lees WR. Endoscopic ultrasonography of chronic pancreatitis and pancreatic pseudocysts. Scand J Gastroenterol Suppl 1986; 123:123–129.

60. Wallace MB, Hawes RH, Durkalski V, Chak A, Mallery S, Catalano MF, et al. The reliability of EUS for the diagnosis of chronic pancreatitis: interobserver agreement among experienced endosonographers. Gastrointest Endosc 2001; 53(3):294–299.

61. Nattermann C, Goldschmidt AJ, Dancygier H. Endosonography in chronic pancreatitis—a comparison between endoscopic retrograde pancreatography and endoscopic ultrasonography. Endoscopy 1993; 25(9):565–570.

62. Hollerbach S, Klamann A, Topalidis T, Schmiegel WH. Endoscopic ultra-sonography (EUS) and fine-needle aspiration (FNA) cytology for diagnosis of chronic pancreatitis. Endoscopy 2001; 33(10):824–831.

63. Kahl S, Glasbrenner B, Leodolter A, Pross M, Schulz HU, Malfertheiner P. EUS in the diagnosis of early chronic pancreatitis: a prospective follow-up study. Gastrointest Endosc 2002; 55(4):507–511.

64. Wiersema MJ, Wiersema LM. Endosonography-guided celiac plexus neuro-lysis. Gastrointest Endosc 1996; 44:656–662.

65. Gress F, Schmitt C, Sherman S, Ciaccia D, Ikenberry S, Lehman G. Endo-scopic ultrasound-guided celiac plexus block for managing abdominal pain associated with chronic pancreatitis: prospective single center experience. Am J Gatroenterol 2001; 96:409–416.

66. Gress F, Schmitt C, Sherman S, Ikenberry S, Lehman G. A prospective randomised comparison of endoscopic ultrasound-and computed

tomography-guided celiac plexus block for managing chronic pancreatitis pain. Am J Gastroenterol 1999; 94:900–905.

67. Gunaratman NT, Sarma AV, Norton ID, Wiersema MJ. A prospective study of EUS-guided celiac plexus neurolysis for pancreatic cancer pain. Gastrointest Endosc 2001; 54:316–324.

68. Fockens P, Johnson TG, van Dullemen HM, Huibregtse K, Tytgat GN. Endosonographic imaging of pancreatic pseudocysts before endoscopic transmural drainage. Gastrointest Endosc 1997; 46:412–416.

69. Norton ID, Clain JE, Wiersema MJ, DiMagno EP, Petersen BT, Gostout CJ. Utility of endoscopic ultrasonography in endoscopic drainage of pancreatic pseudocysts in selected patients. Mayo Clin Proc 2001; 76:794–798.

70. Giovaninni M, Pesenti C, Rolland AL, Moutardier V, Delpero JR. Endoscopic ultrasound-guided drainage of pancreatic pseudocysts or pancreatic abscesses using a therapeutic echo endoscope. Endoscopy 2001; 33:473–477.

71. Kobayashi H, Danbara T, Tamaki S, Kitamura S, Hata E, Fukushima K, Kira S. Detection of the mediastinal lymph nodes metastasis in lung cancer by endoscopic ultrasonography. Jpn J Med 1988; 27:17–22.

72. Hawes RH, Gress F, Kesler K.A, Cummings OW, Conces DJ Jr. Endoscopic ultrasound versus computed tomography in the evaluation of the mediastinum in patients with non-small-cell lung cancer. Endoscopy 1994; 26:784–787.

73. Laudanski J, Kozlowski M, Niklinski J, Chyczewski L. The preoperative study of mediastinal lymph nodes metastasis in lung cancer by endoscopic ultrasonography (EUS) and helical computed tomography (CT). Lung Cancer 2001; 34(suppl 2):S123–S126.

74. Gress FG, Savides TJ, Sandler A, et al. Endoscopic ultrasonography, fine-needle aspiration biopsy guided by endoscopic ultrasonography, and computed tomography in the preoperative staging of non-small cell lung scancer: a comparison study [see comments]. Ann Int Med 1997; 127:604–612.

75. Wallace MB, Silvestri GA, Sahai AV, Hawes RH, Hoffman BJ, Durkalski V, Hennesey WS, Reed CE. Endoscopic ultrasound-guided fine needle aspiration for staging patients with carcinoma of the lung. Ann Thorac Surg 2001; 72:1861–1867.

76. Serna DL, Aryan HE, Chang KJ, Brenner M, Tran LM, Chen JC. An early comparison between endoscopic ultrasound guided fine needle aspiration vs, mediastinoscopy for diagnosis of mediastinal malignancy. Am Surg 1998; 64:1014–1018.

77. Aabakken L, Silvestri GA, Hawes R, Reed CE, Marsi V, Hoffman B. Cost-cfficacy of endoscopic ultrasonography with fine-needle aspiration vs. mediastinotomy in patients with lung cancer and suspected mediastinal adenopathy. Endoscopy 1999; 31:707–711.

78. Fritscher-Ravens A, Soehendra N, Schirrow L, et al. Role of trans-esophageal endosonography-guided fine-needle aspiration in the diagnosis of lung cancer. Chest 2000; 117:339–345.

79. Fritscher-Ravens A, Sriram PVJ, Topalidis T, et al. Diagnosing sarcoidosis using endosonography-guided fine needle aspiration. Chest 2000; 118; 928–935.
80. Roberts SA, Davies G, Howell S, Banks J. Endoscopic ultrasound guided biopsy of subcarinal lymph nodes. Clin Radiol 2000; 55:832–836.
81. Nguyen P, Feng JC, Chang K. Endoscopic ultrasound (EUS) and EUS-guided fine needle aspiration (FNA) of liver lesions. Gastrointest Endosc 1999; 50:357–361.
82. Chang KJ, Erickson RA, Nguyen P. Endoscopic ultrasound (EUS) and EUS-guided fine-needle aspiration of the left adrenal gland. Gastrointest Endosc 1996; 44:568–572.
83. Chang KJ, Albers CG, Nguyen P. Endoscopic ultrasound-guided fine-needle aspiration of pleural and ascitic fluid. Am J Gastroenterol 1995; 90:148–150.
84. Nguyen PT, Chang KJ. EUS in the detection of ascites and EUS-guided paracentesis. Gastrointest Endosc 2001; 54:336–339.
85. Pasricha PJ, Ravich WJ, Hendrix TR, et al. Intrasphincteric botulinum injection for the treatment of achalasia. N Engl J Med 1995; 332:774–778.
86. Hoffman BJ, Knapple WL, Bhutani MS, et al. Treatment of achalasia by injection of botulinum toxin under endoscopic ultrasound guidance. Gastrointest Endosc 1997; 45:77–79.
87. Birk JW, Khan AM, Gress F. The use of endoscopic ultrasound to evaluate response to intrasphincteric botulinum toxin in the treatment of achalasia (abstr). Gastrointest Endosc 1998; 47:AB141.
88. Harada N, Kouza T, Arima M, et al. Endoscopic ultrasound-guided pancreatography: a case report. Endoscopy 1995; 27:612–615.
89. Wiersema MJ, Sandusky D, Carr R, et al. Endosonography-guided cholangiopancreatography. Gastrointest Endosc 1996;44:102–106.
90. Giovannini M, Moutardier V, Pesenti C, Bories E, Lelong B, Delpero JR. Endoscopic ultrasound-guided bilioduodenal anastomosis: a new technique for biliary drainage. Endoscopy 2001; 33:898–900.
91. Erickson RA, Garza AA. EUS with EUS-guided fine-needle aspiration as the first endoscopic test for the evaluation of obstructive jaundice. Gastrointest Endosc 2001; 53:475–484.
92. Van Dam J, Rice TW, Catalano MF, Kirby T, Sivak MV Jr. High-grade malignant stricture is predictive of esophageal tumor stage. Risks of endosonographic evaluation. Cancer 1993 May 15;71(10):2910–2917.

12

Imaging Rectal Cancer

Andrea Maier
University of Vienna, Vienna, Austria

Steve Halligan
St. Mark's Hospital, London, England

INTRODUCTION

In recent years it has become well established that prognosis for patients with rectal cancer is dependent upon both the stage of their cancer and the skill of their surgeon. Most importantly, new techniques for surgical resection require precise preoperative determination of local tumor stage so that patients who need preoperative radiotherapy/chemotherapy can be identified while avoiding over-treatment in those whose tumors are less advanced. Imaging assessment plays the pivotal role in answering these questions.

PREOPERATIVE STAGING OF RECTAL CANCER

Miles's (1) radical abdomino-perineal resection is no longer the standard surgical treatment for rectal cancer. A variety of alternative operations are currently possible, including low anterior resection combined with total mesorectal excision (TME), and abdomino-perineal resection is now reserved for only the lowest of tumors, where sphincter integrity cannot be preserved. Furthermore, locally extensive tumors may be downstaged or rendered nonviable ("sterilized") prior to surgery by using radiotherapy (55 or 25 Gy, respectively) with or without chemotherapy, and so become operable. The choice of operation and the decision whether to employ pre-operative therapy is based on the location of the tumor (for example, radiotherapy to proximal rectal tumors risks small-bowel enteritis) and preoperative staging. Preoperative staging aims to predict postoperative histopathological staging as accurately as possible.

Local staging of rectal cancer has focused on the relationship of the tumor to the rectal wall, namely the muscularis propria; i.e., the circular and longitudinal smooth muscle of the rectum. While Cuthbert Dukes's staging system has been used extensively, the more subtle TNM system (2) (Table 1) has now been adopted generally and is the system that should be used. Tumor penetration through the rectal wall, into the perirectal tissues, is associated with a poorer prognosis in terms of both metastatic disease and local recurrence (3–6). Whether local lymph nodes are involved or not is also a strong prognostic indicator. A patient whose tumor is confined to the mucosa or submucosa and who has no evidence of malignant lymph nodes has a recurrence risk of only 5%, which increases to 10% if the tumor invades the muscularis propria but does not reach the perirectal tissues (T2 tumor). However, once the rectal wall is penetrated (T3 tumor), the risk of recurrence rises to at least 25%, and it reaches 50% if neighboring structures are involved (T4 tumor).

While many studies have demonstrated increased recurrence for those tumors that have penetrated the rectal wall (7–9), it is now well appreciated that the degree to which the tumor has penetrated (i.e., the extent of extrarectal spread) also directly influences survival (10,11). The depth of tumor penetration through the muscularis propria is a measure of

TABLE 1   Comparison of Dukes Staging of Rectal Carcinoma and TNM Classification for Colorectal Cancer

Dukes stage		TNM classification	
A	Tumor confined to bowel wall	T1	Tumor involves submucosa
		T2	Tumor involves muscularis propria
B	Tumor penetrates bowel wall	T3	Tumor beyond muscularis propria
		N0	No involved nodes
C	Regional lymph nodes involved	N1	Up to 3 perirectal/colic nodes
		N2	4 or more perirectal/colic nodes
		N3	Apical node involved
		M0	No distant metastasis
D	Distant metastasis	M1	Distant metastasis

lateral tumor spread towards the pelvic side walls. Elegant work by Quirke et al. (12) has highlighted the importance of this measurement. Accurate preoperative assessment of lateral spread has become central to optimal management of rectal cancer because of the general adoption of TME for mid and low rectal tumors. In TME, the surgical specimen containing the tumor is excised by circumferential sharp dissection around the mesorectal fascia (which envelops the mesorectum), a plane that then becomes the postsurgical "circumferential resection margin" (CRM). If a T3 tumor has penetrated far enough through the rectal wall to breach the mesorectum (and thus the CRM), then it is highly likely that residual tumor will be left in the pelvis, greatly enhancing the risk of local recurrence (13). The margin between tumor and mesorectal fascia is therefore a vital piece of pre-operative information:

> Some surgeons believe that patients whose tumors have penetrated the rectal wall (i.e., T3) but which are well away from the meso-rectal fascia may be safely treated by surgery alone since the risk of incising tumor or leaving residual tumor in the pelvis is low for a competent surgeon. Administering radiotherapy to these patients increases side-effect morbidity and treatment cost for little incremental benefit.

> Patients whose tumors are near to, contact, or breach the mesorectal fascia will need preoperative radiotherapy with or without chemo-therapy in order to render tumor potentially in the surgical field nonviable and so minimize the chance of postoperative recurrence.

It should be borne in mind that there is still considerable controversy surrounding the most appropriate treatment for rectal cancer and the regime chosen will vary, especially from country to country. For example, many Europeans would choose to administer preoperative radiotherapy whatever the extent of a T3 tumor and also to those T2 tumors where positive mesorectal nodes are thought likely. In the United States, post-operative radiotherapy/chemotherapy is more prevalent. Nevertheless, this should not detract from the importance of accurate preoperative staging by imaging.

In addition to factors concerning the primary tumor itself, it is well established that dissemination of tumor cells to local lymph nodes greatly influences disease recurrence and prognosis. The number of involved nodes is an important prognostic factor, regardless of the depth of tumor invasion (14–16). Other tumor-related variables have also been shown to be independent prognostic factors. Mucin production, DNA content, tumor growth pattern, vascular invasion and lymphatic invasion (17–20) are all important variables that influence recurrence and survival. However, knowledge of the anatomical spread of the primary tumor remains the most powerful single predictor of patient survival (21).

It should also be borne in mind that accurate staging applies not only to advanced cancers but also to those that are very superficial. Tumors that have not invaded the muscularis propria are amenable to local resection. Local, transanal resection is a relatively noninvasive and well-tolerated procedure and is therefore especially suitable for elderly patients whose risk of operative morbidity and mortality is highest. However, embarking on a local resection only to find that the tumor has actually invaded the rectal wall defeats this objective.

In summary, the decision as to the best surgical approach for treatment of a patient with rectal cancer depends on several factors: tumor location, penetration of the rectal wall, the depth of penetration into peri-rectal tissues, lymph node involvement, and tumor grade. Most of these variables are described by tumor stage, which remains the most sensitive predictor of prognosis and which is central to clinical decision making in these patients (22). For many years digital palpation of the tumor by an experienced surgeon has been the mainstay of preoperative staging, an approach that is now known to be notoriously inaccurate. For this reason, imaging is central to modern preoperative determination of tumor stage. A number of imaging modalities may be applied to preoperative staging, each with their own merits, disadvantages, and advocates.

TRANSRECTAL ULTRASOUND

Transrectal ultrasound (TRUS) was introduced into clinical practice in 1983 (23,24). Initial studies using a relatively low frequency of 3.5 and 4.0 MHz were able to demonstrate the rectum as a two- or three-layer structure. With the introduction of 7.5 MHz transducers, five distinct rectal layers could be identified regularly (25,26) (Fig. 1,2): the first layer (hyperechoic) corresponds to the water-filled balloon and interface with the superficial mucosa, the second layer (hypoechoic) to the deep mucosa, the third layer (hyperechoic) to the submucosa, the fourth layer (hypoechoic) to muscularis propria, and the fifth layer (hyperechoic) to the interface between muscularis propria and perirectal tissues (Fig. 2). Because, in general, these layers broadly correspond to the different histological layers that are relevant to staging, Hildebrandt and Feifel (27) proposed that endosonographic staging should be based on the TNM classification. Thus, a T1 tumor is confined to the first three layers (Fig. 3), a T2 tumor penetrates the fourth layer (Fig. 4), a T3 tumor extends through the fifth layer (Fig. 5) into the perirectal fat, and a T4 tumor invades any adjacent organ that can be visualized during endosonographic examination.

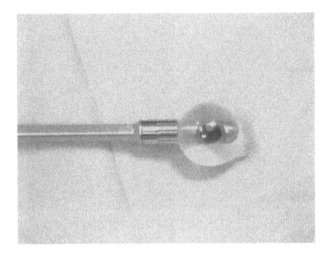

FIGURE 1   B and K 10 MHz transducer with rectal balloon filled with water for acoustic coupling.

The accuracy for rectal tumor staging using TRUS ranges from 64 to 95% overall, with an average of 84% (28–37). It is well established that T2 tumors are commonly overstaged as T3, an error that is due to peritumoral inflammation (38–40). Peritumoral inflammation appears hypoechoic on ultrasound and, because it surrounds the primary tumor, tends to merge with it and therefore artefactually increases its extent. Overstaging results in overtreatment, usually because the patient receives radiotherapy where none was actually warranted. Alternatively, understaging may be caused by failure to detect microscopic areas of tumor infiltration because they are below the limits of resolution of the equipment. Other variables that influence the accuracy of tumor staging include operator experience (31,33,41) and the level of the tumor; accuracy is reduced for low rectal tumors, especially those on the anterior and posterior aspect of the ampulla, presumably because the ultasound beam is no longer tangential to the tumor (36,42). On the other hand, anal sphincter infiltration can be assessed precisely (43). Higher tumors at the limit of the reach of the probe and stenotic tumors also pose a problem. Indeed, it may be impossible to traverse the tumor in up to 17% of cases (38). After chemotherapy and/or radiotherapy, the accuracy of TRUS in predicting local stage falls to 50% overall (44,45). Posttreatment evaluation is impaired because tumor margins become generally indistinct in addition to diffuse rectal wall thickening following radiation.

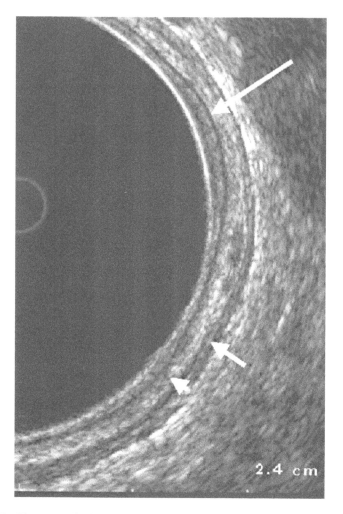

FIGURE 2 Transrectal ultrasound of normal rectal wall: The deep mucosa is visualized as the innermost hyporeflective band (long white arrow). The submucosa is visualized as a hyper reflective band (arrowhead), which is just medial to the muscularis propria (short white arrow). In this case, separation of the muscularis propria into circular and longitudinal components is visible in places.

Endorectal ultrasound is particularly suitable for those patients whose tumor is potentially curative by local excision (53), i.e., T1 tumors, because its near-field spatial resolution is excellent. Although distinguishing between T1 and T2 tumors may occasionally be a problem,

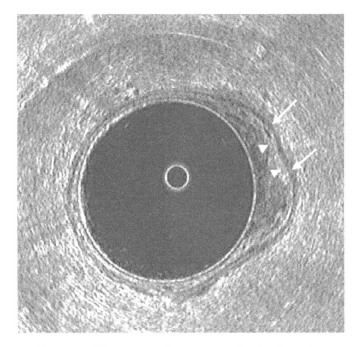

Figure 3   uT1 tumor: There is an intact layer of reflective submucosa (white arrowheads) medial to the muscularis propria (white arrows).

one study found that distinguishing between T1 and T2-3 tumors, and between T1-2 and T3 tumors, yielded positive predictive values of 93% and 100%, respectively, and negative predictive values of 94% and 93% (54).

As stated above, lymph node status is a strong prognostic variable. However, lymph node staging by TRUS is less accurate than primary tumor staging. Different echogenic patterns have been described (46–48). Two main groupings can be discerned: hypoechoic and hyperechoic. Lying intermeditate to these are nodes that are neither one type nor the other—a mixed pattern (Fig. 5). Hyperechoic nodes are believed to represent inflamed nodes, whereas those that are hypoechoic or mixed are believed to represent metastatic disease. Several investigators have applied these criteria for differentiation, with an accuracy of approximately 73–83%. As with most imaging techniques, however, a small focus of micrometastasis within the node is unlikely to be identified, raising the false-negative rate (49,50). Furthermore, lymph nodes located beyond the field of view of the transducer will remain undetected, irrespective of their size

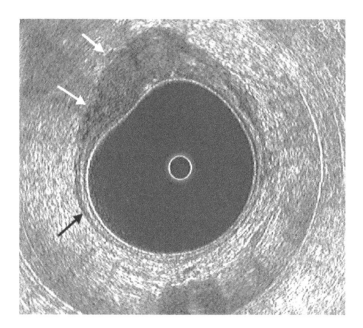

FIGURE 4 UT2 tumor: The tumor merges with the muscularis propria (black arrow), confirming that it is invaded. However, although the lateral aspect of the muscularis is expanded (white arrows), there is no evidence of any definite tumor beyond it. This was a T2 tumor on histopathology.

or echogenicity. This is especially the case for more proximal tumors (51). In general, morphological characteristics such as size, shape, or outer border have not been sufficiently discriminatory to recommend their adoption (52).

TRUS TECHNIQUE

Both rigid and flexible endoprobes may be used, but it should be borne in mind that a transducer capable of providing a radial 360-degree image of the rectal wall is necessary for optimal results (Fig. 1). Probably because this usually requires dedicated equipment, the examination generally remains confined to specialized units and has not disseminated to the same degree as prostatic ultrasound, for example. Rigid probes are able to examine the distal 12 cm of rectum. The transducer is surrounded by a distensible balloon that must be filled with degassed water for acoustic coupling, eliminating all retained air in the process. The entire assembly is then covered by a condom that has been lubricated on its inner and outer

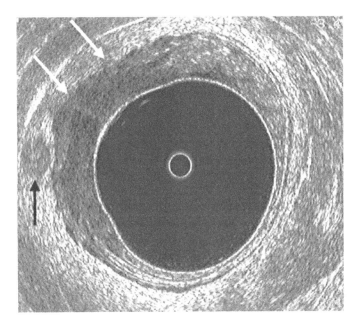

FIGURE 5 UT3 tumor: In contrast to Fig. 4, the outer aspect of the muscularis is nodular and irregular (white arrows), diagnosing tumor infiltration beyond the rectal wall, into perirectal tissues. There is also a large mesorectal lymph node (black arrow) of mixed reflectivity.

surfaces. It is practical to empty the rectum beforehand, for example, by administering two glycerine suppositories and asking the patient to void. Alternatively, the assembly may be used without the covering condom and sterilized between each patient.

Examination is generally performed with the patient lying in the left lateral position but may also be performed in the lithotomy position if specialized examination couches are available. The endoprobe may either be inserted through a rigid sigmoidoscope, which allows direct visualisation of the tumor, or alternatively passed directly into the rectum. If using the latter approach, digital examination beforehand will help identify the tumor quadrant and level in order to facilitate correct probe placement. Once in the rectum, the balloon is inflated to acoustically couple the transducer to the tumor. Examination should encompass the entire tumor, which is best achieved by inserting the transducer above the level of the tumor and then slowly withdrawing it. It is important to attempt to keep the transducer at 90 degrees to the tumor at all times, although this is often not possible.

COMPUTED TOMOGRAPHY

Initial reports of the use of computed tomography (CT) for local tumor staging of rectal cancer were encouraging. Early published results indicated agreement in the order of 90% between preoperative CT staging and ultimate histopathological assessment (55–58). However, in hindsight many of the patients recruited to these early studies had advanced disease, and this spectrum bias may have prejudiced results. While TRUS has remained relatively static over the last few years, significant technological advances in CT continue unabated, which makes meaningful comparative studies very difficult both to perform and report before the technology used in them is outdated.

In 1981 Thoeni et al. (55) proposed a classification system dividing rectal tumors into four stages based on the measured thickness of the rectal wall on CT. A somewhat similar system was suggested the same year by Dixon et al. (59). Lymph nodes where classified as either enlarged or not enlarged. Neither of these two systems corresponds directly with modern TNM staging, which limits their clinical application. More recent studies (60,61) are equivocal, with overall local staging accuracies ranging from 47 to 75%. A major limitation of CT is its low inherent contrast resolution, which means that it is unable to distinguish the various layers of the rectal wall, notably the muscularis propria. While rectal distension with air or water has been advocated as a means by which to improve local staging, this does not overcome this inherent limitation. The result is that reliable differentiation between T1 and T2 tumors is presently impossible. Furthermore, tumor infiltration into the anal sphincters and its extent cannot be detected. However, CT staging improves the further the tumor extends through the rectal wall, and several authors have found CT reliable in this regard. For example, Angelelli et al. (62) reported an accuracy of 83% when comparing CT with Dukes's classification determined from the resected specimen. However, spectrum bias may be partly responsible for these results since only 10% of recruited patients had Dukes' A tumors, with most suffering from more advanced disease.

The importance of the relationship between tumor and the mesorectal fascia has already been stated. Grabbe et al. (57) brought the perirectal fascia to the attention of radiologists but suggested that it normally cannot be identified due to limited spatial resolution. It should be borne in mind that the advent of modern helical multidetector machines will undoubtedly mean that this suggestion needs reevaluation. It should also be noted that the mesorectum becomes easily identified when it is thickened by adjacent pathological processes, such as tumor infiltration or inflammation. Under such circumstances tumor growth beyond the fascia may be detectable, indicating either unresectability or the need for pre-operative therapy. While some authors maintain that differentiation between inflammation and tumor infiltration is possible (63), most would agree that this distinction is often unreliable when using CT.

With the advent of multidetector machines, lymph nodes down to approximately 3 mm can be can be visualized on CT, but it remains generally impossible to reliably ascertain whether enlargement is due to malignant infiltration or reactive inflammation unless enlargement is gross. A common approach is to define nodal metatsasis on the basis of size (64,65). Many authors have applied different criteria and definitions, for example from 5 mm to 15 mm, and positive and negative predictive values vary accordingly. Clearly, as the size criteria for a positive node decrease, sensitivity increases but specificity decreases in tandem. Depending on the criteria used, sensitivities range from 22 to 88% while specificities range from 64 to 96%. Such findings inevitably reduce the clinical value of CT as an investigative tool for detection of lymph node metastases.

Studies that compare CT with TRUS for local tumor staging consistently show the latter to be more accurate for both tumor stage and lymph node status (66–71). The net result is that the role of CT for local staging of rectal cancer is currently disappointing and accurate assessment of local spread can only be achieved for advanced tumors. At the time of writing, however, the advent of multidetector CT and the promise of isotropic imaging indicate that these conclusions may well change in the near future. However, the inability of CT to resolve the various components of the rectal wall remains a major handicap, whatever collimation can be currently employed, suggesting that CT will never be useful when attempting to determine local resectability. Studies that investigate whether multidetector machines can reliably visualize the mesorectal fascia are eagerly anticipated.

MAGNETIC RESONANCE IMAGING

MR imaging for staging rectal cancer was first described in 1986 (72,73). It was hoped that improved contrast resolution when compared to CT would enhance staging while the pelvic location of these tumors would serve to combat motion artefact. However, using a conventional body coil, the rectal wall appeared as one layer and MR imaging was unable to evaluate the depth of tumor penetration. Furthermore, substantial problems were encountered in early in vivo studies as a result of extensive motion artifacts. However, as with CT, MR imaging has been subject to substantial technical advances over the last decade, and its role in preoperative staging of rectal cancer is now firmly established.

The development of endorectal receiver coils held great promise for accurate determination of local tumor stage. Structures near the coil surface are depicted with high spatial resolution, so it seems sensible to expect that tumors originating from the rectal epithelium will be well visualized. Such coils are able to resolve the individual layers of the rectum (74,75). Using T2-weighted sequences the following can be resolved: An inner layer of high signal intensity representing the mucosa and muscularis mucosae; a middle layer of high signal intensity representing the submucosa; and a second layer of low signal intensity representing the muscularis propria; and an outer layer of high signal intensity representing perirectal fat. Using these criteria, Schnall and coworkers (75) found that prospective staging using endorectal MR imaging agreed with the pathological stage in 29 of 36 patients (81%). The extent of invasion was overestimated in seven cases mostly because irregularity of the presumed extraluminal tumor border was used to indicate a T3 lesion. Lymph nodes were described as infiltrated if no fat could be identified within them. Using this definition 16 of 36 patients had N1 lesions, which resulted in a specificity of 78% for differentiating between N1 and N0 disease, with a sensitivity of 81%. Despite these initially promising results, it is now generally accepted that endorectal coils suffer many of the specific disadvantages that affect TRUS. In particular, the coils may be difficult to place across stenotic tumors, and they are also relatively uncomfortable for the patient, especially since examination times are much longer than for TRUS. It may also be difficult to image as far proximally as TRUS (76). Furthermore, flare artefact can significantly impair depiction of very superficial tumors, and field-of-view limitations mean that they may fail to adequately demonstrate more advanced tumors. Studies that directly compare endorectal MR imaging and endorectal ultrasound have found MR imaging inferior to ultrasound for T and N staging (77–80).

The use of phased-array coils (81) results in better spatial resolution, and, in particular, those that have used a high-resolution, thin-section technique have recently reported very promising results (82,83). Brown and coworkers (82) evaluated local tumor stage in 28 consecutive patients using such a technique and found that MR imaging correctly predicted the T stage in every case. The authors focused on the depth of transmural tumor penetration into the mesorectal fat and found close agreement between the MR estimate and ensuing pathological measurement. In a subsequent study of 76 patients that used a similar high-resolution technique, Beets-Tan and coworkers (83) found MR imaging prediction of T stage only moderately accurate, but preoperative prediction of involvement of the mesorectal fascia was much stronger: of 29 patients in whom pathology found a clear circumferential resection margin by at least

10 mm, MR imaging correctly predicted this in 28 and 27 cases, respectively, for two readers (83). MR imaging also correctly predicted an involved margin in all 12 who had such on subsequent histopathology. A regression analysis of the remaining cases suggested that a histological clearance of at least 1 mm could be confidently predicted with a measured MR imaging distance of 5 mm (83). Although a question mark remains regarding the accuracy of preoperative T staging using MR imaging, these studies suggest that high-resolution, phased-array techniques can accurately predict the depth of any extramural penetration and, more importantly, predict the relationship between this and the mesorectal fascia. If this accuracy is maintained in larger studies from multiple centers, then surgeons will be able to confidently direct individual patients towards appropriate treatment strategies on the basis of MR imaging alone.

MR IMAGING TECHNIQUE

The MR imaging technique employed for high-resolution imaging is relatively straightforward, but a pelvic phased-array coil is mandatory. A common approach is to obtain initially sagittal T2-weighted fast spin echo scans through the pelvis, which will image the configuration of the rectum and tumor. Common parameters would include a 4 mm slice thickness, small interslice gap, 24 cm FOV and 256 × 256 matrix. This is then used as the template from which to plan high-resolution T2-weighted scans that are obtained in the axial plane with respect to the tumor (i.e., perpendicular to its long axis) using a thinner collimation, smaller FOV, and higher matrix (3 mm, 16 cm, and 512 × 512, for example). These latter scans will be the most useful from which to determine the local tumor stage since they will image its relationship to the muscularis propria and mesorectal fascia in an anatomically relevant plane. It may also be necessary to perform coronal T2-weighted scans in order to best appreciate the relationship between the tumor and pelvic sidewalls/mesorectal fascia and also to the anal canal and pelvic floor if the tumor is low. It is also useful to obtain axial scans through the entire pelvis to search for more distant lymphadenopathy.

On T2-weighted imaging, tumor appears as epithelial-based thickening with a signal intensity slightly higher than the muscularis propria, which appears as a low signal circumferential band surrounding the rectal lumen (Fig. 6). The outermost aspect of the muscularis propria will remain intact with T2-tumors or less (Fig. 6). Differentiation between T2 and T3 tumors is critical but can be difficult. The crucial finding is tumor penetration into perirectal fat, but, as with ultrasound, this is complicated by desmoplastic extramural reaction, which is evidenced by low signal spiculated strands extending out into the perirectal tissues (Fig. 7). While

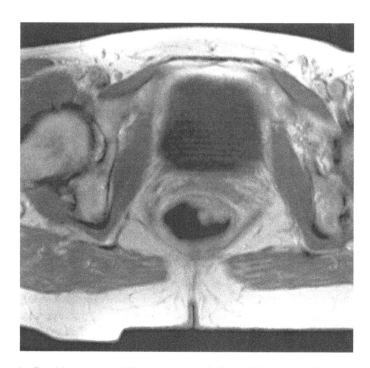

Figure 6   Double-contrast MR imaging technique: There is a T2 rectal cancer arising from the left anterior rectal quadrant. The underlying muscularis propria is visualized as a band of lower signal and there is no evidence of enhancing tumor beyond this.

some workers have suggested it is easy to distinguish this from tumor (82), others have found it more difficult, resulting in overstaging (83). It has been suggested that extramural broad-based tissue with the same signal characteristics as the bulk of the intramural tumor is necessary for confident diagnosis of a T3 stage (82) (Fig. 8,9). It should also be noted that small discontinuities in the muscularis can be due to penetrating vessels and should not in themselves suggest a T3 stage. T4 tumors are diagnosed by infiltration into an adjacent organ (Fig. 10) or muscle or by tumor that reaches the peritoneal surface.

The mesorectal fascia is generally easy to identify on MR imaging and is manifest as a thin low signal envelope surrounding the rectum, and, for the reasons already discussed, this will be the potential CRM in patients undergoing TME. T3 tumors that are well away from the potential CRM (Fig. 8) can be distinguished from those that are not (Fig. 9). However, there are problem areas that have not been fully addressed in the literature

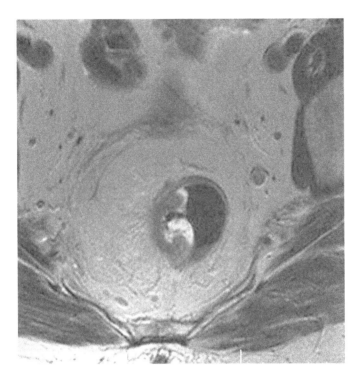

FIGURE 7 There are several strands extending from the tumor base into perirectal fat. At histopathological examination these proved to be due to a desmoplastic reaction rather than tumor cells.

to date. For example, the muscularis propria and mesorectal fascia converge anteriorly and also converge as they funnel towards the anal canal. In these locations a very early T3 lesion can still potentially involve the mesorectal fascia. Tumor deposits remote from the primary tumor can also involve the mesorectal fascia. These can be due to involved mesorectal nodes, isolated mesorectal metastatic deposits, or venous invasion, and are diagnosed by nodular masses with the same signal intensity as the primary tumor (Fig. 11). Attempts to determine nodal involvement have generally been based on size criteria and are consequently of limited clinical use. However, the application of lymph node–specific contrast agents to rectal cancer raises the possibility of imaging cancer in normal-sized nodes, and further work in this area is eagerly awaited.

There are many other MR imaging approaches to local staging of rectal cancer. In particular, many workers employ intravenous gadolinium in an attempt to discriminate enhancing tumor from adjacent reactive

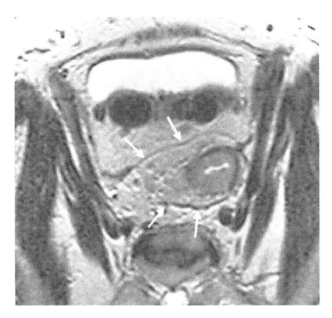

FIGURE 8   There is a T3 tumor evidenced by medial disruption of the muscularis propria. However, its margins are several mm away from the surrounding mesorectal fascia (arrows).

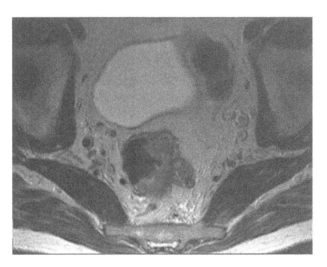

FIGURE 9   T3 tumor arising from the left lateral aspect of the rectum. In this case there is tumor penetration through the muscularis for several mm, and the tumor approaches the potential circumferential resection margin.

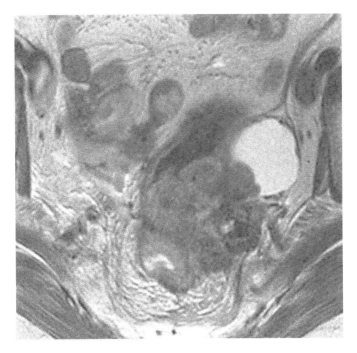

FIGURE 10   Advanced rectal cancer which is directly invading the left ovary.

tissue. Wallengren and coworkers (84) combined this with rectally administered SPIO contrast agents in order to produce a double-contrast technique, an approach that was followed by a randomized phase II dose-ranging trial (85). The double-contrast technique aims to image the rectal wall as a two-layer structure: a hyperintense mucosa/submucosa and a hypointense muscularis propria (Fig. 6). Using these criteria, accuracy for staging rectal cancer higher than T2 was 82%. In addition, this double-contrast technique is an elegant method with which to determine anal sphincter involvement in low tumors (86).

CONCLUSION

Treatment for rectal cancer has improved dramatically over the last decade, and low local recurrence rates are possible with modern surgical techniques. Imaging now plays the pivotal role in directing individual patients towards appropriate treatment strategies, most importantly identifying those in whom preoperative treatment is required in order

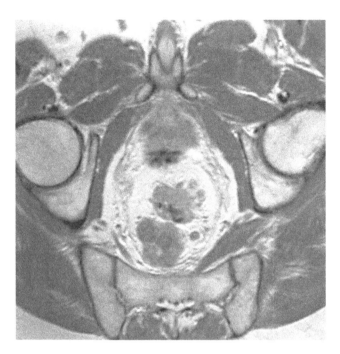

FIGURE 11 In this case the rectal tumor is remote from the potential circumferential resection margin, but there is a huge posterior nodal mass that contacts the mesorectal fascia, indicating that preoperative therapy will be needed if postoperative resection margins are to be negative.

to achieve the best chance of cure. TRUS and MR imaging have complementary roles to play in this selection process, and both should be available in all centers performing rectal cancer surgery.

REFERENCES

1. Miles WE. Cancer of the rectum. Trans Med Soc 1923; 46:27.
2. Sobin LH, Wittekind CH, eds. UICC: TNM Classification of Malignant Tumors. 5th ed. New York: Wiley, 1997.
3. Chapuis PH, Fisher R, Dent OF, Newland RC, Pheils MT. The relationship between different staging methods and survival in colorectal cancer. Dis Colon Rectum 1985; 28:158–161.
4. Fielding LP, Phillips RK, Hittinger R. Factors influencing mortality after curative resection for large bowel cancer in elderly patients. Lancet 1989; 1:595–597.

5. Hermanek P, Guggenmoos-Holzmann I, Gall FP. Prognostic factors in rectal carcinoma. A contribution to the further development of tumor classification. Dis Colon Rectum 1989; 32:593–599.
6. Ondera H, Maetani S, Nishikawa T, et al. The reappraisal of prognostic classification for colorectal cancer. Dis Colon Rectum 1989; 32: 609–614.
7. Lockhart-Mummery HE, Ritchie JK, Hawley PR. The results of surgical treatment for carcinoma of the rectum of St. Mark's Hospital from 1948 to 1972. Br J Surg 1976; 63:673–677.
8. Rao AR, Kagan AR, Chan PM, Glibert HA, Nussbaum H, Hintz BL. Patterns of recurrence following curative resection alone for adenocarcinoma of the rectum and sigmoid cancer. Cancer 1981; 48:1492–1495.
9. Pilipshen SJ, Heilweil M, Quan SH, Strenberg SS, Enker WE. Patterns of pelvic recurrence following definitive resections of rectal cancer. Cancer 1984; 53:1354–1362.
10. Nicholls RJ, Mason AY, Morson BC, Dixon AK, Fry IK. The clinical staging of rectal cancer. Br J Surg 1982; 69:404–409.
11. Nicholls RJ, Galloway DJ, Mason AY, Boyle P. Clinical local staging of rectal cancer. Br J Surg 1985; 72(suppl):551–552.
12. Quirke P, Durdey P, Dixon MF, Williams NS. Local recurrence of rectal adenocarcinoma due to inadequate surgical resection. Histopathological study of lateral tumor spread and surgical excision. Lancet 1986; 2: 996–999.
13. Cawthorn SJ, Parums DV, Gibbs NM, A'Hern RP, Caffarey SM, Broughton GI, et al. Extent of mesorectal spread and involvement of lateral resection margin as prognostic factors after surgery for rectal cancer. Lancet 1990; 335:1055–1059.
14. Dukes CE, Bussey HJR. The spread of rectal cancer and its effect on prognosis. Br J Cancer 1958; 12:309–320.
15. Wolmark N, Fisher B, Weiand HS. The prognostic value of the modification of the Dukes'C class of colorectal cancer. An analysis of the NSABP clinical trials. Ann Surg 1986; 203:115–122.
16. Jass JR, Atkin WS, Cuzick J, Bussey HJ, Morson BC, Northover JM, et al. The grading of rectal cancer: historical perspectives and a multivariate analysis of 447 cases. Histopathology 1986; 10:437–459.
17. Symonds D, Vickery A. Mucinous carcinoma of the colon and rectum. Cancer 1976; 37:1891–1900.
18. Jones DJ, Moore M, Schofield PF. Prognostic significance of DNA ploidy in colorectal carcinoma: a prospective flow cytometric study. Br J Surg 1988; 75:28–33.
19. Garlon CA, Fabris G, Arslan-Pagnini C, Pluchinotta AM, Chinelli E, Carniato S. Prognostic correlation of operable carcinoma of the rectum. Dis Colon Rectum 1985; 28:47–50.
20. Talbot IC, Ritchie S, Leighton MH, Hughes AO, Bussey HJ, Morson BC. The clinical significance of invasion of veins by rectal cancer. Br J Surg 1980; 67:439–442.

21. Fielding LP, Fenoglio-Preiser CM, Freedman LS. The future of prognostic factors in outcome prediction for patients with cancer. Cancer 1992; 70:2367–2377.

22. Williams NS, Durdey P, Quirke P, Robinson PJ, Dyson JE, Dixon MF, et al. Pre-operative staging of rectal neoplasm and its impact on clinical management. Br J Surg 1985;72:868–874.

23. Dragsted J, Gammelgaard J. Endoluminal ultrasonic scanning in the evaluation of rectal cancer. Gastrointest Radiol 1983; 8:367–369.

24. Hildebrandt U, Feifel G, Zimmermann FA, Goebbels R. Significant improvement in clinical staging of rectal carcinoma with intrarectal ultrasound scanner. J Exp Clin Cancer Res (suppl) 1983; 2:53.

25. Beynon J, Foy DM, Temple LN, Channer JL, Virjee J, Mortensen NJ. The endosonic appearance of normal colon and rectum. Dis Colon Rectum 1986; 29:810–813.

26. Kimmey MB, Martin RW, Hagitt RC, Wang KY, Franklin DW, Silverstein FE. Histologic correlates of gastrointestinal ultrasound images. Gastroenterology 1989; 96:433–441.

27. Hildebrandt U, Feifel G. Preoperative staging of rectal cancer by intrarectal ultrasound. Dis Colon Rectum 1985; 28:42–46.

28. Beynon J, Mortensen NJ, Rigby HS. Rectal endosonography, a new technique for the preoperative staging of rectal carcinoma. Eur J Surg Oncol 1988; 14:297–309.

29. Yamashita Y, Machi J, Shirouzu K, Morotomi T, Isomoto H, Kakegawa T. Evaluation of endorectal ultrasound for the assessment of wall invasion of rectal cancer. Dis Colon Rectum 1988; 31:617–623.

30. Glaser F, Schlag P, Herfarth C. Endorectal ultrasonoraphy for the assessment of invasion of rectal tumors and lymph node involvement. Br J Surg 1990; 77:883–887.

31. Orrom WJ, Wong WD, Rothenberger DA, Jensen LL, Goldberg SM. Endorectal ultrasound in the preoperative staging of rectal tumors. A learning experience . Dis Colon Rectum 1990; 33:654–659.

32. Konishi F, Ugajin H, Ito K, Kanazawak K. Endorectal ultrasonography with a 7.5 MHz linear array scanner for the assessment of invasion of rectal carcinoma. Int J Colorect Dis 1990; 5:15–20.

33. Tio TL, Coene PP, van Delden OM, Tytgat GN. Colorectal carcinoma: preoperative TNM classification with endosonography. Radiology 1991; 179:165–170.

34. Katsura Y, Yamada K, Ishizawa T, Yoshinaka H, Shimazu H. Endorectal ultrasonography of wall invasion and lymph node metastases in rectal cancer. Dis Colon Rectum 1992; 35:362–368.

35. Feifel G, Hildebrandt U. New diagnostic imaging in rectal cancer: endosonography and immunoscintigraphy. World J Surg 1992; 16:841–847.

36. Herzog U, von Flue M, Tondelli P, Schuppisser JP. How accurate is endorectal ultrasound in the preoperative staging of rectal cancer? Dis Colon Rectum 1993; 36:127–134.

37. Cho E, Nakijama M, Yasuda K, Ashihara T, Kawai K. Endoscopic ultrasono-
    graphy in the diagnosis of colorectal cancer invasion. Gastrointest Endosc
    1993; 39:521–527.
38. Hawes RH. New staging techniques. Endoscopic ultrasound. Cancer 1993;
    71(suppl 12):4207–4213.
39. Hulsmans FJ, Tio TL, Fockens P, Bosma A, Tytgat GN. Assessment of tumor
    infiltration depth in rectal cancer with transrectal sonography: caution is
    necessary. Radiology 1994; 190:715–720.
40. Maier AG, Barton PP, Neuhold NR, Herbst F, Teleky BK, Lechner GL. Peri-
    tumoral tissue reaction at transrectal US as a posibble cause of overstaging:
    histopathologic correlation. Radiology 1997; 203:785–789.
41. Solomon MJ, McLeod RS, Cohen EK, Simons ME, Wilson S. Reliability and
    validity studies of endoluminal ultrasound for anorectal disorders. Dis
    Colon Rectum 1994; 37:546–551.
42. Sailer M, Leppert R, Bussen D, Fuchs KH, Thiede A. Influence of tumor
    position on accuracy of endorectal ultrasound staging. Dis Colon Rectum
    1997; 40:1180–1186.
43. Maier AG, Kreuzer SH, Herbst F, Wrba F, Schima W, Funovics MA,
    Teleky BK, Lehner GL. Transrectal sonography of anal sphincter infiltration
    in lower rectal cancer. AJR 2000; 175:735–739.
44. Napoleon B, Pujol B, Berger F, Valette PJ, Gerard JP, Souquet JC. Accuracy
    of endosonography in the staging of rectal cancer treated by radiotherapy.
    Br J Surg 1991; 78:785–788.
45. Glaser F, Kuntz C, Schlag P, Herfarth C. Endorectal ultrasound for control
    of preoperative radiotherapy of rectal cancer. Ann Surg 1993; 217:64–71.
46. Hildebrandt U, Klein T, Feifel G, Schwarz HP, Koch B, Schmitt RM.
    Ensonography of pararectal lymph nodes. In vitro and in vivo evaluation.
    Dis Colon Rectum 1990; 33:863–868.
47. Nielsen MB, Qvitzau S, Pedersen JF. Detection of pericolonic lymph nodes in
    patients with colorectal cancer: an in vitro and in vivo study of the efficacy
    of endosonography. AJR 1993; 161:57–60.
48. Hulsmans FH, Bosma A, Mulder PJ, Reeders JW, Tytgat N. Perirectal lymph
    nodes in rectal cancer: in vitro correlation of sonoraphic parameters and
    histopathologic findings. Radiology 1992; 184:553–560.
49. Beynon J, Mortensen NJ, Foy DM, Channer JL, Righy H, Virjee J. Pre-
    operative assessment of mesorectal lymph node involvement in rectal cancer.
    Br J Sur 1989; 76:276–279.
50. Dworak O. Number and size of lymph node metastases in rectal carcinomas.
    Surg Endosc 1989; 3:96–99.
51. Rosch T, Lorenz R, Classen M. Endoscopic ultrasonography in the evaluation
    of colon and rectal disease. Gastrointest Endosc 1990; 36(suppl 2):33–39.
52. Hildebrandt U, Feifel G. Endosonoraphy in the diagnosis of lymph nodes.
    Endoscopy 1993; 25:243–245.
53. Banerjee AK, Jehle EC, Shorthouse AJ, Buess G. Local excision of rectal
    tumors. Br J Surg 1995; 82:1165–1173.

54. Detry R, Kartheuser A. Endorectal ultrasonoraphy in staging small rectal tumors. Br J Surg 1992; 79(suppl):30.
55. Thoeni RF, Moss AA, Schnyder P, Margulis AR. Detection and staging of primary rectal and rectosigmoid cancer by computed tomography. Radiology 1981; 141:135–138.
56. Zaunbauer W, Haertl M, Fuchs WA. Computed tomography in carcinoma of the rectum. Radiology 1981; 6:79–84.
57. Grabbe W, Lierse W, Winkler R. The perirectal fascia: morphology and use in staging of rectal carcinoma. Radiology 1983; 149:241–246.
58. Balthazar EJ, Megibow AJ, Hulnick D, Naidich DP. Carcinoma of the colon: detection and preoperative staging by CT. AJR 1988; 150:301–306.
59. Dixon AK, Kelsey Fry I, Morson BC, Nicholls RJ, York Mason A. Preoperative computed tomography of carcinoma of the rectum. Br J Radiol 1981; 54:655–659.
60. Freeny PC, Marks WM, Rayan JA, Bolen JW. Colorectal carcinoma evaluation with CT: preoperative staging and detection of postoperative recurrence. Radiology 1986; 158:347–353.
61. Bech-Shriver E, Bachmann-Nielsen M, Qvitzan S, Christiansen J. Comparison of precontrast, postcontrast and delay scanning for the staging of rectal carcinoma. Gastrointest Radiol 1992; 17:267–270.
62. Angelelli, Marcarini L, Lupo L, Caputi-Jambrenghi O, Pannarale O, Memeo V. Rectal carcinoma: CT staging with water as contrast medium. Radiology 1990; 177:511–514.
63. Williams NS, Durdey P, Quirke P, Robinson PJ, Dyson JED, Dixon MF, Bird CC. Pre-operative staging of rectal neoplasm and its impact on clinical management. Br J Surg 1985; 72:868–874.
64. Thoeni RF. Colorectal cancer. Radiologic staging. Radiol Clin North Am 1997; 35:457–485.
65. Thompson WM, Halvorsen RA, Foster WL Jr, Roberts L, Gibbons R. preoperative and postoperative CT staging of rectosigmoid carcinoma. AJR 1986; 146:703–710.
66. Rifkin MD, Ehrlich SM, Marks G. Staging of rectal carcinoma: prospective comparison of endorectal US and CT. Radiology 1989; 170:319–322.
67. Waizer A, Zitron S, Ben-Baruch D, Baniel J, Wolloch Y, Dintsman M. Comparative study for preoperative staging of rectal cancer. Dis Colon Rectum 1989; 32:53–56.
68. Holdsworth PJ, Johnston D, Chalmers AG, Chenells P, Dixon MF, Finan PJ, et al. Endoluminal ultrasound and computed tomography in the staging of retal cancer. Br J Surg 1988; 75:1019–1022.
69. Beynon J, Mortensen NJ, Foy DM, Channer JL, Virjee J, Golddard P. Pre-operative assessment of local invasion in rectal cancer: digital examination, endoluminal sonography or computed tomography? Br J Surg 1986; 73:1015–1017.
70. Goldman S, Arviddson H, Norming U, Lagerstedt U, Magnusson L, Frisell J. Transrectal ultrasound and computed tomography in preoperative of lower rectal adenocarcinoma. Gastrointest Radiol 1991; 16:259–263.

71. Akasu T, Sunouchi K, Sawadw T, Tsioulias GJ, Muto T, Morioka Y. Preoperative stging of rectal carcinoma: prospective comparison of transrectal ultrasonography and computed tomography (abstr). Gastroenterology 1990; 98:28.
72. Hodgman CG, MacCarty RL, Wolff BG, May GR, Berquist TH, Sheedy PF, et al. Preoperative staging rectal carcinoma by computed tomography and 0.5T magnetic resonance imaging. Preliminary report. Dis Colon Rectum 1986; 29:446–450.
73. Butch RJ, Stark DD, Wittenberg J, Tepper JE, Saini S, Simeone JF, et al. Staging rectal cancer by MR and CT. AJR 1986; 146:1155–1160.
74. Chan TW, Kressel HY, Milestone B, Tomachefski J, Schnall M, Rosato E, Daly J. Rectal carcinoma: staging at MR imaging with endorectal surface coil. Radiology 1991; 1181:461–467.
75. Schnall MD, Furth EE, Rosato EF, Kressel HY. Rectal tumor stage: correlation of endorectal MR imaging and pathologic findings. Radiology 1994; 190:709–714.
76. Okizuka H, Sugimura K, Ishida T. Preoperative local staging of rectal carcinoma with MR imaging and a rectal balloon. J Magn Reson Imaging 1993; 3:329–335.
77. Waizer A, Powsner E, Russo I, Hadar S, Cytron S, Lombrozo R, et al. Prospective comparative study of magnetic resonance imaging versus transrectal ultrasound roe preoperative staging and follow-up of rectal cancer. Preliminary report. Dis Colon Rectum 1991; 34:1068–1072.
78. Thaler W, Watzka S, Martin F, La Guardia G, Psenner K, Bonatti G. et al. Preoperative staging of rectal cancer by endoluminal ultrasound vs. magnetic resonance imaging. Preliminary results of a prospective comarative study. Dis Colon Rectum 1994; 37:1189–1193.
79. Joosten FB, Jansen JB, Rosenbusch G. Staging of rectal carcinoma using MR double surface coil, MR endorectal coil, and intrarectal ultrasound: correlation with histopathologic findings. J Comput Assisted Tomogr 1995; 19:752–758.
80. Zagoria RJ, Schlarb CA, Ott DJ, Bechtold RI, Wolfmann NT, Scharling ES, et al. Assessment of rectal tumor infiltration utilizing endorectal MR imaging and comparison with endoscopic rectal sonography. J Surg Oncol 1997; 64:312–317.
81. Hadfield MB, Nicholson AA, MacDonald AW, et al. Preoperative staging of rectal carcinoma by magnetic resonance imaging with a pelvic phased-array coil. Br J Surg 1997; 84:529–531.
82. Brown G, Richards CJ, Newcombe RG, Dallmore NS, Radcliff AG, Carey DP, Bourne MW, Williams GT. Rectal carcinoma: thin-section MR imaging for staging in 28 patients. Radiology 1999; 211:215–222.
83. Beets-Tan RG, Beets GL, Vliegen RF, Kessels AG, Van Boven H, De Bruine A, von Meyenfeldt MF, Beaten CG, van Engelshoven JM. Accuracy of magnetic resonance imaging in prediction of tumout-free resection margin in rectal cancer surgery. Lancet 2001; 357:497–504.

84. Wallengren NO, Holtas S, Andren-Sandberg A, Jonsson E, Kristoffersson DT, McGill S. Rectal carcinoma: double-contrast MR imaging for preoperative staging. Radiology 2000; 215:108–114.

85. Maier AG, Kersting-Sommerhoff B, Reeders JWAJ, et al. Staging of rectal cancer by double-contrast MR imaging using the rectally adminstered superparamagnetic iron oxide contrast agent ferristene and iv gadodiamide injection: results of a multicenter phase II trial. J Magn Reson Imaging 2000; 12:651–660.

86. Urban M, Rosen HR, Hölbling N, Feil W, Hochwarther G, Hruby W, Schiessel R. MR Imaging for the preoperative planning of sphincter-saving surgery for tumors of the lower third of the rectum: use of intravenous and endorectal contrast materials. Radiology 2000; 214:503–508.

13

Self-Expanding Metal Colonic Stents

Steve Halligan
St. Mark's Hospital, London, England

INTRODUCTION

Large bowel obstruction is a common surgical emergency. In the developed world the most common underlying cause is an occluding colorectal cancer. Unfortunately, emergency surgery for malignant large bowel obstruction is particularly badly tolerated by patients; mortality may be as high as 40%, a figure that drops to less than 5% in elective cases (1). A review of 272 patients presenting as an emergency with colorectal cancer found that this group were more likely to have a stoma fashioned, took longer to become fully ambulatory after their operation, and spent longer in hospital when compared to patients undergoing elective treatment (2). Furthermore, patients were more likely to die both during initial admission and over the subsequent 5 years (2). The reasons for these appalling statistics are seemingly obvious; tumors that present with obstruction tend to be of a higher stage, and only 50% are candidates for a cure. However, while this is true, it cannot represent the whole story because stage-for-stage survival is also reduced (3). Rather, morbidity and mortality is increased in this group because of the considerable systemic disturbance that accompanies malignant large bowel obstruction; the result is a very poor general condition by the time of hospital presentation. Emphasizing this point, patients presenting acutely have twice the frequency of wound infection, 11 times the frequency of renal failure, and 25 times the rate of respiratory complications compared to patients who are operated on electively (3). It is now well established that poor general condition is the major cause of mortality in patients presenting with malignant large bowel obstruction and far outweighs local factors related to the primary tumor.

The site of the primary tumor influences whether it is likely to cause obstruction or not, and obstruction is surprisingly a feature that is again relatively independent of stage (4). Seventy percent of obstructing cancers are left sided, which itself adds a degree of surgical uncertainty. While curative surgery for obstructing right-sided tumors is uncontroversial (right hemicolectomy and primary anastamosis) and these patients tend to do well as a group, surgery for left-sided obstruction is less clear-cut and a variety of approaches are possible. Some surgeons advocate a three-stage procedure, with initial relieving colostomy followed by resection and then finally by closure. However, 40% of these patients never have intestinal continuity restored. Others advocate a two-stage procedure with primary resection and either a Hartmann's (i.e., formation of a blind rectal stump) or mucous fistula. A more recent approach is a single-stage resection with on-table colonic lavage.

All of this is complicated by the underlying possibility that the disease is incurable and the surgery therefore merely palliative. Median survival for patients with disseminated colorectal cancer is only 7 months, and, if at all possible, surgery should be generally avoided in this group so that quality of remaining life is as best as it can be. However, adequate staging of the disease is frequently impossible when patients present as a surgical emergency, and, moreover, no patient should be allowed to die from large bowel obstruction. The result is that many patients who are incurable are unavoidably subjected to major surgery in what will prove to be the last few months of their life.

The Holy Grail of surgery for obstructing colorectal cancer would therefore be a relatively noninvasive procedure that could be applied to left-sided tumors. This would also allow time for the patient's general condition to be stabilized so that the risk of any subsequent curative surgery would equal that of elective procedures for similar stage tumors. Furthermore, such a procedure would also buy time for adequate staging of the disease in order to facilitate sensible management decisions. If the patient were found to have incurable disease in the interim, then the procedure could potentially offer definitive palliation while avoiding the need for a stoma. Self-expanding metal colorectal stents can potentially fulfill these requirements.

SELF-EXPANDING METAL COLORECTAL STENTS

Self-expanding metal stents are well established for palliation of esophageal malignancy, and the rationale for their use in the colon is clear from the previous discussion; the left colon is potentially accessible to metal stents, which can be placed to relieve obstruction with minimal intrusion, buying time to stabilize and improve the patient's general condition and allowing time for staging of the disease. If the patient is found not to be a candidate for cure, either because of disseminated disease or because of frailty and associated operative risk, the stent can be left in situ for definitive pallia-tion, thus avoiding the need for surgery and possibly also a stoma. It has also become evident that stent deployment is possibly beneficial in some patients suffering from malignant colonic obstruction due to causes other than primary colorectal carcinoma, and there may also be a further role in benign disease where surgery is not an easy option.

DEPLOYMENT TECHNIQUE

First it is important to establish both the diagnosis of obstruction and its underlying cause in any scenario where stent placement is being consid-ered. Furthermore, for stent deployment to be practicable, obstruction should be confined to a single, well-defined area of colon. Referrals will gen-erally fall into one of two groups: those presenting acutely as an emergency and those with more indolent disease, who are thought by their clinicians likely to obstruct in the very near future. The latter group will usually have a well-established diagnosis and may include those with a known colorectal cancer, perhaps on a waiting list for definitive surgery. Alternatively, patients may have other disseminated malignancies where colonic obstruc-tion is a complication of their underlying disease, for example, ovarian carcinoma. In this (or indeed any) scenario, it is important that the stenting radiologist directly inspects any preexisting imaging, rather than accept the clinician's story. In the author's experience, the clinical diagnosis of obstruction is frequently unconfirmed on contemporaneous imaging. Also, inspection by a competent radiologist may also reveal that obstruction is either at several separate locations or extends over several centimeters, which may mean deployment is impracticable (or may mean more than one stent is necessary for colonic decompression) (Fig. 1). Thorough assessment of the clinical situation will prevent the stenting team from being pointlessly assembled, often in the middle of the night! Colonic stenting does not suit everyone with large bowel obstruction, and careful patient selection is the key to both technical and clinical success.

Similarly, patients presenting as acute emergencies will also tend to fall into one of two groups; those with an established diagnosis of colorectal cancer (usually awaiting elective surgery scheduled for the near future) and those with no known prior diagnosis. In the latter case it is again especially important to establish the underlying diagnosis before contemplating

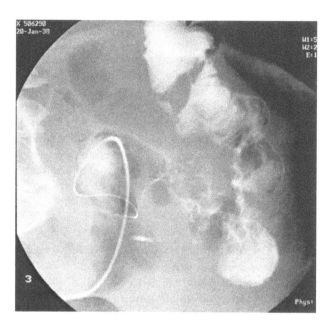

FIGURE 1   A sigmoid stricture has been reached by an aniographic catheter and guidewire. Contrast injection reveals extensive proximal extrinsic disease over a long segment in this patient with peritoneal metastases. There is no dominant stricture, and stenting is unlikely to be helpful.

a stent. This point cannot be stressed enough. At the very least, a diagnosis of acute large bowel obstruction should be made from abdominal radiographs that have been seen by the stenting radiologist; in the author's experience, junior surgeons and physicians are increasingly unable to diagnose obstruction from abdominal films, and it is courting disaster to rely on their assessment. If obstruction is present, a water-soluble enema is perhaps the easiest way to establish the underlying cause, although computed tomography (CT) is an increasingly useful alternative, especially when patients are frail or in extremis. Computed tomography also allows distant staging where the underlying cause is a carcinoma. Inevitably, in some cases it will be difficult to establish the cause using imaging alone, and in such instances there should be a low threshold to employ endoscopy.

Once the diagnosis of colonic obstruction and its cause have been established and a stent considered the best option, then the team can be assembled. There are essentially three philosophical approaches to colonic stenting: radiologist alone, endoscopist alone, or a combined procedure. The approach chosen will depend on local circumstances such as staff and room availability (e.g., endoscopy suite or fluoroscopy/interventional room), clinician enthusiasm to develop the procedure, and perceived turf battles. However, there can be no doubt that the skills possessed by radiologists and endoscopists are complementary, so the best approach would seem to be combined. For obvious reasons, tumor cannulation is usually easiest when attempted under direct vision using an endoscope. This is especially true when the tumor ostium is narrow or when the tumor has bulky, rolled margins. However, endoscopists tend to lack the catheter and guidewire manipulation skills possessed by trained radiologists. Furthermore, in some instances it is impossible to deploy the stent through the colonoscope (often because fixity due to adjacent disease prevents scope angulation). Alternatively, in other situations this may be the only option (especially relevant to very proximal tumors). The author prefers a combined approach, which undoubtedly accelerates the procedure (Fig. 2).

Once the patient has been consented for the procedure, light conscious sedation and analgesia is administered intravenously with appropriate monitoring facilities in place. With the patient in the left-lateral position on a fluoroscopy couch, the endoscope (colonoscope or sigmoidoscope) is introduced to the level of the known occlusion, which is then directly inspected. Occasionally, the endoscope can easily traverse the stricture, in which case the team should reconsider the rationale of placing a stent at that time. The author has found it very helpful to place a small metal mucosal clip at the distal tumor margin because this helps identify this site during subsequent stricture imaging and stent deployment and aids accurate placement. The tumor ostium can then be cannulated using a thin ERCP-type catheter passed through the scope channel and contrast injected to define the stricture length and general morphology. In most circumstances, the author has found stent deployment easiest when performed in isolation rather than through the endoscope. To achieve this when using endoscopic cannulation, the scope must be withdrawn while leaving the catheter across the stricture, a tricky procedure at the best of times! Ideally, the scope is carefully withdrawn while the catheter position is monitored using fluoroscopy. Once the tip of the scope is free of the anus, the catheter can be cut (allowing the endoscope to be completely removed) and a guidewire then inserted through the catheter to cross the stricture. In order to facilitate this maneuver, as much catheter as possible should be deployed above the stricture and a short scope (ie sigmoidoscope or pediatric colonoscope) used where possible. If catheter dislodgement is likely, then an ERCP guidewire or alternative can be passed through the catheter and is usually a little easier to maneuver proximal to the occlusion because it is stiffer.

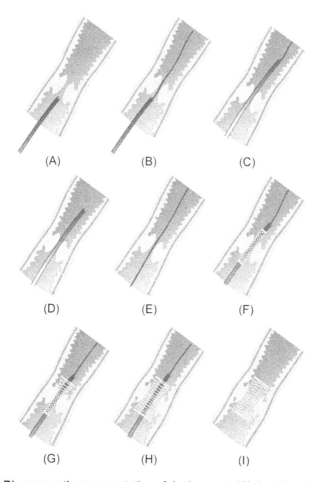

(A)   (B)   (C)

(D)   (E)   (F)

(G)   (H)   (I)

FIGURE 2   Diagrammatic representation of deployment. (A) A catheter is advanced
to the distal margin of the stricture using either an endoscope or guidewire. (B) The
stricture is cannulated by a soft hydrophilic guidewire. (C) The catheter is
advanced over the guidewire, through the stricture. (D) The guidewire is withdrawn. (E) A stiff guidewire is introduced through the catheter and the catheter
withdrawn. (F) The stent is advanced into position over the guidewire. (G) The
stent is deployed with a flange above the stricture, and then pulled down into the
stricture during further deployment. (H) The stent is fully deployed to cross
the stricture. (I) The guidewire and deployment mechanism are withdrawn, leaving
the stent in situ.

If the exchange cannot be performed, there are two options: either the stent is deployed through the endoscope or deployment is attempted solely using radiology. The approach used will depend on the site and morphology of the stricture, but the author would usually attempt radiological cannulation first. The stricture must be reached using a catheter; the author favors a 6.5 French biliary manipulation catheter for recto-sigmoid lesions or a longer angiographic catheter for more proximal occlusions. However, like angiographic practice, the site and type of stricture encountered will usually determine the final catheter configuration chosen. A combination of guidewire probing followed by catheter advance will usually be needed to reach the stricture if this is proximal to the rectosigmoid junction; more distal strictures are easily reached merely by inserting the catheter directly. Contrast should also be used liberally to outline the bowel lumen and disclose the required direction for probing. Gas insufflation is also vital to open out and distend the bowel lumen. Like endoscopic cannulation, changes in patient position may be necessary to achieve catheter advance. For more proximal strictures it is frequently necessary to continually alternate between a hydrophilic wire and a stiffer type since the characteristics of the latter help prevent catheter looping within mobile bowel. If hand movements do not seem to be effectively transmitted to the catheter or wire tip, then it is worth screening distally to look for catheter looping within the lumen or looping of the bowel itself (a frequent cause of failed colonoscopy). Catheter looping within the rectum is a particular problem, especially when trying to reach proximal strictures, and some sort of stiffening device may need to be employed; the author uses a 9 French peel-away sheath, which has the advantage that it can be easily removed when it is time to deploy the stent.

Once the stricture is encountered, water-soluble contrast injected down the catheter will help identify the general direction of the tumor ostium, which is cannulated using torque to direct the catheter tip in combination with probing using a hydrophilic guidewire. Again, patient positional change may be necessary to observe the direction of the ostium and facilitate cannulation. Tumors with shouldered margins and tight ostia may take a considerable time to cannulate, but this is usually possible if the catheter can reach the tumour. Once the guidewire has passed the stricture the catheter is advanced over it (Fig. 3A), the wire withdrawn, and contrast injected to define stricture length and morphology (Fig. 3B).

At this time, the type of stent used should be chosen. The author has experience of two types, the Memotherm (Bard) and the Wallstent (Boston Scientific), although the Ultraflex (Boston Scientific) knitted nitinol type is also available, which is polyurethane coated and has a proximal

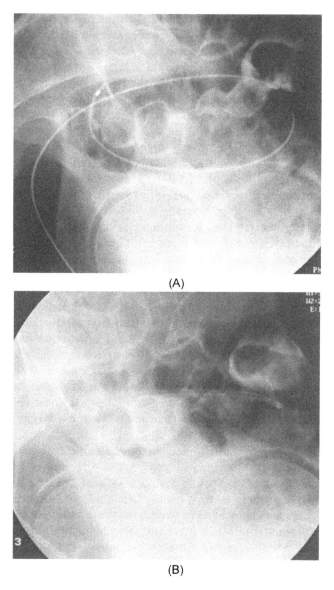

(A)

(B)

FIGURE 3 Deployment of a stent across a proximal rectal stricture. (A) The rectal stricture is crossed by the catheter and soft hydrophilic guidewire. (B) The guidewire is withdrawn and contrast injected in order to define the stricture so that an appropriate stent can be chosen. (C) A stiff guidewire is placed across the stricture, straightening the deployment path. (D) A Memotherm stent is delivered over the stiff guidewire. (E) Final position of the deployed stent.

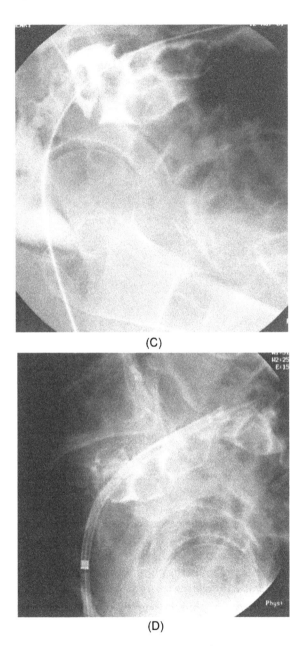

(C)

(D)

FIGURE 3 (*continued*)

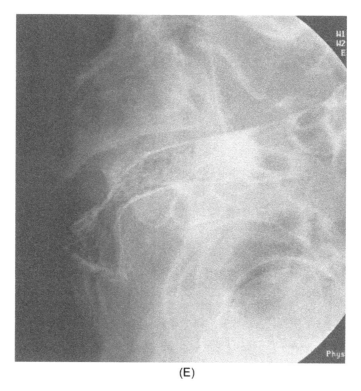

(E)

FIGURE 3   (continued)

flange (a type extensively used for esophageal stenting). A variety of stent lengths and diameters are available. Generally, the most useful is the largest, which is 10×3 cm at the time of writing. The stent is deployed over a stiff guidewire, and it may be necessary to preform a curve on the stent and delivery system to achieve passage around a tight fixed curve, even with the degree of straightening achieved using a stiff guidewire (Fig. 3C,3D). This is especially a problem with the relatively stiff and bulky Memotherm; the key to success is to straighten the colon as much as possible; it may even be necessary to use two guidewires in tandem to achieve this. Most importantly, a short delivery system facilitates tracking the stent over the guidewire because the guidewire can exit the distal end of the delivery system and be "fixed" by the radiologist or assistant. The major benefit of the Memotherm delivery system is its reasonable length. In contrast, although the Wallstent is more flexible and easier to track, its major disadvantage is its excessive length—225 cm. This stent was originally designed for endoscopic delivery with the result that it is far too long for the guidewires generally employed in radiology. With a system so long, it is impossible to pass the guidewire out of the distal end of the delivery system and thus very difficult to track the stent proximally. However, at the time of writing a shorter delivery system has been designed with radiologists in mind, which will overcome this major disadvantage. The author would generally choose the Memotherm excepting those circumstances where there are tracking difficulties (especially if the tumor is distal), in which case the relative flexibility of the Wallstent is very advantageous. The Wallstent must be used for any deployment through the endoscope.

Depending on the stricture morphology, the aim is to deploy the stent so that there is a good flange upstream of the tumor margin, the aim of which is to prevent subsequent migration due to peristalsis. Indeed, for localized strictures approximately two thirds of the stent should be upstream. If a mucosal clip has been placed, then this will facilitate accurate deployment of the distal stent margin relative to the stricture. Balloon dilatation prior to deployment is not recommended because it potentially risks tumor perforation and dissemination. Deployment should be slow and careful. In the author's experience, it is helpful to deploy approximately one third or more of the stent well upstream of the stricture and then to continue deployment with traction on the delivery system, with the effect that the stent is pulled into the stricture. This maneuver helps achieve both a stable position within the stricture and a good upstream flange. Because the aim is to deploy the distal aspect of the stent just beyond the tumor margin, deployment without some degree of traction can result in the stent springing above the stricture altogether. The Memotherm in particular has a tendency to leap upstream if deployment is too rapid, and this should be borne in mind. However, the Memotherm does not shorten during deployment, and its eventual position is thus probably easier to predict overall. Furthermore, the pistol-grip deployment mechanism is easy and comfortable to use. The Memotherm stent cannot be retracted once delivery has commenced, whereas it is possible to retract the Wallstent if no more than 50% of the stent has been released. However, the Wallstent delivery system is primitive and relatively difficult to use, and the stent also shortens during delivery with the result that its final position can occasionally be difficult to predict. When the stricture length approaches or exceeds the individual stent length, overlaying two stents together may be used to traverse long strictures. For rectal tumors it should also be borne in mind that care should be taken so that the distal stent does not impinge on the anus, which can cause very distressing tenesmus. Indeed, the distal stent margin should ideally be several centimeters clear of the anus (Fig. 3E). For this reason it is probably best to consider stenting only proximal ampullary tumors.

AFTERCARE AND COMPLICATIONS

Adequate postprocedural pain relief is vital, especially since expansion occurs during the first 24 hours following deployment. Just because a stent has been placed does not mean that clinical decompression definitely follows, and the symptoms and signs of obstruction must still be monitored carefully. Patency can be checked using a water-soluble contrast enema (Fig. 4). Stool softeners should be administered to prevent impaction within the stent. Perforation is a serious complication and is related to both excessive guidewire manipulation and balloon dilatation. It is sensible to perform a water-soluble enema if there is any suspicion of perforation. Indeed, the stricture should be kept well visualized with contrast throughout the procedure. Migration is the most common later complication and often occurs within the first 24 hours (Fig. 5). An abdominal film the day following deployment is useful to check for this, to document stent expansion, and to monitor signs of obstruction. Digital retrieval should be cautious since the stents have sharp prongs that can easily puncture a gloved finger. Stent fracture is a reported late complication (5) as is perforation into an adjacent viscus, the bladder, for example (6). Reobstruction due to tumor ingrowth can also occur and can be potentially treated by a second stent, if necessary.

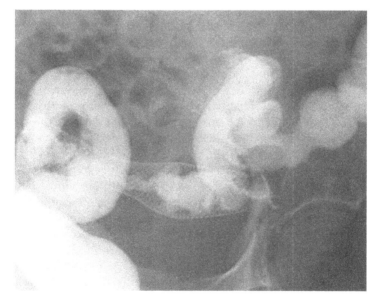

FIGURE 4   Water-soluble enema following stent insertion shows good patency.

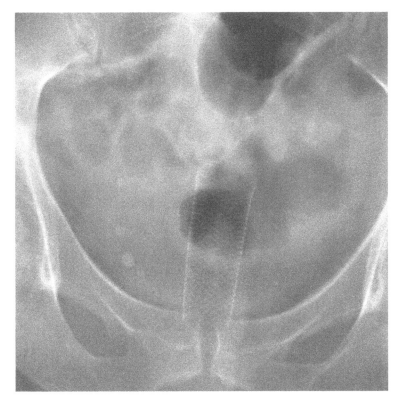

Figure 5   Abdominal films the day after stent deployment shows rectal migration.

LITERATURE REVIEW

The first description of deployment of a self-expanding metal stent to treat colonic carcinoma was a single case report in 1991 (7). By 2001 there were 40 reports of the procedure in the literature, indicating rapid and widespread acceptance (8). In addition to the treatment of colonic obstruction due to primary colorectal cancer, there are now articles that focus specifically on palliative series (9), patients with extrinsic malignant disease (10) (Fig. 6), and benign indications (11) (Fig. 7). The largest individual series to date comprises 80 patients (12), but the problems of addressing the literature have largely been resolved by a recent systematic review (13). Technical success was achieved in 551 (92%) of 598 patients (90% of palliative procedures and 85% where deployment was as a "bridge to surgery"). Predictably, the most common cause for technical failure was inability to cannulate the tumor ostium with a guidewire. Five percent

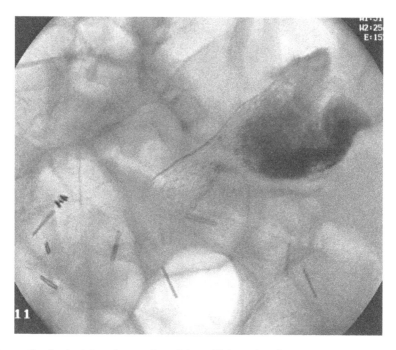

FIGURE 6   A stent has been placed to palliate extensive recurrent anastamotic carcinoma.

of patients in whom technical success was achieved failed to clinically decompress. Three of 598 patients died, giving a mortality of 1%, which compares excellently with even the most optimistic figures for operative mortality in this group of patients. Fatalities were due to laparotomy that was needed to treat perforation. Indeed, perforation occurred in 4% of cases (10% of those where a balloon was used to predilate the stricture vs. 2% where it was not). Migration occurred in 10% of deployments, half of these within 3 days. Interestingly, many of these patients required no further intervention.

SUMMARY

Deployment of colorectal self-expanding metal stents is technically feasible and well within the capabilities of many interventional radiologists, especially those familiar with esophageal procedures. For potentially curative cases it appears that morbidity and mortality compare extremely favorably with surgery, and there are also clear benefits to avoiding surgery in those patients who need palliation. Furthermore, there are likely to be

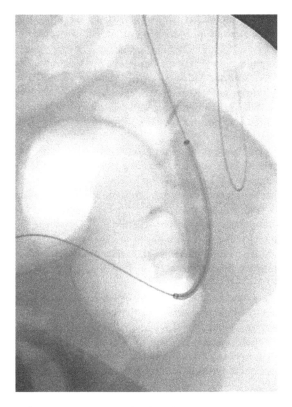

Figure 7 Stent placement to treat a benign descending colon stricture in a young woman with Crohn's disease who was too unfit for operation.

considerable financial savings, although no detailed economic analysis has been performed to date. The results of prospective randomized trials comparing stenting with surgery are awaited with great interest, although the results from case-control series are so promising that the opportunity for a randomized trial may actually have been lost.

REFERENCES

1. McIntyre R, Reinbach D, Cuschieri RJ. Emergency abdominal surgery in the elderly. J R Coll Edin 1997; 42:173–178.
2. Scott NA, Jeacock J, Kingston RD. Risk factors in patients presenting as an emergency with colorectal cancer. Br J Surg 1995; 82:321.
3. Runkel NS, Schlag P, Schwarz V, Herfarth C. Outcome after emergency surgery for cancer of the large intestine. Br J Surg 1991; 78:183–188.

4. Aldridge MC, Phillips RK, Hittinger R, Fry JS, Fielding LP. Influence of tumour site on presentation, management and subsequent outcome in large bowel cancer. Br J Surg 1986; 73:663–670.
5. Suzuki N, Saunders BP, Thomas-Gibson S, Marshall M, Halligan S, Northover JMA. Complications of colonic stenting: a case of stent migration and fracture. Endoscopy 2003; 35:1085.
6. Marshall M, Suzuki N, Halligan S, Ackle C, Saunders BP. Self-expandable metal stents for benign and malignant colonic obstruction. Eur Radiol 2001; 11:C14.
7. Dohmoto M. Endoscopic implantation of rectal stent for palliation of malignant stenosis. Endoscopica Digestiva 1991; 3:1507–1512.
8. Harris GJ, Senagore AJ, Lavery IC, Fazio VW. The management of neoplastic colorectal obstruction with colonic endoluminal stenting devices. Am J Surg 2001; 181:499–506.
9. Aviv RI, Shyamalan G, Watkinson A, Tibbals J, Ogunbaye G. Radiological palliation of malignant colonic obstruction. Clin Radiol 2002; 57:347–351.
10. Miyayama S, Matsui O, Kifune K, et al. Malignant colonic obstruction due to extrinsic tumour: palliative treatment with a self-expanding nitinol stent. AJR 2000; 175:1631–1637.
11. Paul L, Pinto I, Gomez H, Fernandez-Lobato R, Moyano E. Metallic stents in the treatment of benign diseases of the colon: preliminary experience in 10 cases. Radiology 2002; 223:715–722.
12. Camunez F, Echen Agusia A, Simo G, Turegano F, Vazquez J, Barreiro-Meiro I. Malignant colorectal obstruction treated by means of self-expanding metallic stents:effectiveness before surgery and in palliation. Radiology 2000; 216:492–497.
13. Khot UP, Wenk-Lang A, Murali K, Parker MC. Systematic review of the efficacy and safety of colorectal stents. Br J Surg 2002; 89:1096–1102.

14

Imaging the Anal Canal

Andrew B. Williams, Gordon Buchanan,
and Steve Halligan

St. Mark's Hospital, London, England

INTRODUCTION

Over the last decade, advances in anal imaging have had a significant impact on the management of patients with anal disorders, particularly in the investigation and treatment of peri-anal sepsis and anal incontinence. This chapter will detail the basic anatomy of the anal canal and describe the imaging appearances of the anal canal using two main techniques, endoanal ultrasound and magnetic resonance imaging, after which practical applications in both incontinence and sepsis will be considered.

ANATOMY

The anal canal in adults is approximately 4 cm long and begins as the rectum narrows and passes backwards between the levator ani muscles (1) and has an upper limit at the pelvic floor and a lower limit at the anal verge (2). The upper anal canal is lined by mucosa comprised of simple columnar epithelium, whereas the lower canal is lined by stratified squamous epithelium (3), with the transition zone known as the dentate line. Beneath the mucosa lies the subepithelial layer, a layer of connective tissue and smooth muscle (1). This layer increases in thickness throughout life and forms the basis of the vascular cushions thought to be important for maintenance of continence (4,5).

The caudal continuation of rectal circular smooth muscle condenses to form the internal anal sphincter, which lies lateral to the subepithelial layer (3), whereas the caudal continuation of rectal longitudinal smooth muscle forms the longitudinal muscle of the anus (Fig. 1). The longitudinal muscle thus lies between the internal and the external anal sphincters, within the intersphincteric space, and its smooth muscle fibers are augmented with striated muscle originating from the levator ani (6), puborectalis (7), and pubococcygeus (8). Fibers from the longitudinal muscle traverse the external anal sphincter and form septae that insert into the perianal skin as the corrugator cutis ani muscle, which is thought to prevent anal eversion during defecation (7,9).

The striated muscle of the external sphincter surrounds the longitudinal muscle and forms the outer border of the intersphincteric space. The external sphincter is conventionally described in three parts (7,10–12), with deep, superficial, and subcutaneous portions. While the deep and subcutaneous portions form rings of muscle around the anus, the elliptical fibers of the superficial external sphincter run between the perineal body anteriorly and coccyx posteriorly. The external sphincter has also been considered as a single muscle contiguous with the puborectalis muscle (3,13). Important structural differences have been shown between men and women using anal endosonography. Most importantly, the anterior external anal sphincter is shorter in women than in men (14–16).

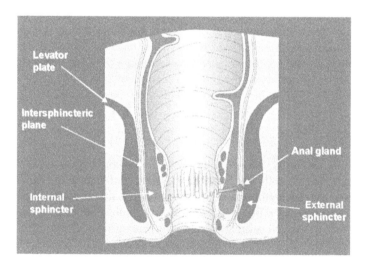

FIGURE 1 Coronal diagram of the anal canal showing the external and internal sphincters and the longitudinal muscle.

ANAL ENDOSONOGRAPHY

Anal endosonography (AES) was first described in 1989 by Law and Bartram (17) and was a consequence of minor modification to an ultrasound probe already in use to stage rectal tumors (18). Anal endosonography is quick to perform, relatively cheap, and increasingly available. While technically very simple, interpretation can be rather difficult, especially as this remains a developing and evolving field.

Endosonography overcomes many of the problems incurred when imaging deep structures using conventional transcutaneous ultrasound. By placing the transducer in a body cavity (endosonography), it is sited in close proximity to the structures of interest, allowing a higher frequency transducer to be employed. This improves spatial resolution while avoiding interference from intervening structures. The reduction in tissue penetration due to the increase in frequency is of no consequence due to the transducer proximity to the target (although increasingly important if areas of interest are relatively remote from the sphincter complex). Anal endosonography generally utilizes a transducer mounted on a rotating rod that is enclosed within a rectal tube and which produces 360° radial images. The transducer is surrounded by a sonolucent cone, which is filled with degassed water for acoustic coupling. The most commonly used system is the type 1850 Bruel and Kjaer rotating endoprobe (B & K Medical, Sandhoften, Denmark) (Fig. 2). Initially a 7 MHz crystal was used (17), but image resolution has been greatly improved with the advent of the 10 MHz probe, which has a focal length of 1–4 cm and a beam width of 0.8 mm (16). Sonolucent gel is applied to the cone of the assembled probe, which is then covered by a condom. After lubrication the unit is ready for insertion into the anus. Anal endosonography may be performed with the patient in the left lateral or prone position. It is preferable to examine in the prone position because this improves the symmetry of the images obtained (19).

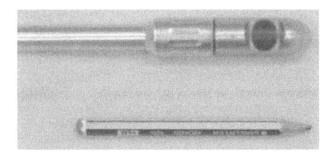

FIGURE 2   B and K Medical anal endosonography probe.

The probe is inserted through the anus into the lower rectum, where contact is lost between the probe surface and the bowel wall, which leads to characteristic reverberation echo distortion. As the probe is withdrawn further, the first anatomical landmark seen is the sling of the puborectalis muscle. The examination then begins in earnest and anal canal distal to this level is carefully examined. The probe is oriented such that the anterior part of the anal canal is uppermost on the image, mimicking conventional cross-sectional imaging orientation. Such orientation also facilitates division of the sphincter circumference into the hours of a clock face, i.e., 12 o'clock corresponds to directly anterior and 6 o'clock to directly posterior.

The endosonographic appearance of the anal canal has been well established (17,20,21) and is continually being refined, especially in the light of endoanal MR imaging (22). The anal canal mucosa is not seen because it is lost within the bright reflection from the outside of the probe cone. The subepithelial tissue is highly reflective and is surrounded by a low reflection produced by its interface with the internal anal sphincter. The width of the internal sphincter increases with age: normal width for a patient 55 years old or younger is 2.4–2.7 mm, but above this age the normal range increases to 2.8–3.4 mm. As the width of the sphincter increases, it becomes progressively more reflective and indistinct, which may be due to a relative increase in the fibroelastic content of this muscle as a consequence of aging (23). The external anal sphincter is of moderate reflectivity with the longitudinal muscle of a similar reflectivity situated between the two sphincters in the intersphincteric space (Fig. 3).

THREE-DIMENSIONAL ANAL ENDOSONOGRAPHY

It is now fairly simple to create three-dimensional (3D) ultrasound images from two-dimensional (2D) datasets. The basic component of an image is the pixel, with a height and width that depends on the size of the matrix of the ultrasound scanner. Each pixel may be assigned a brightness value ranging from 0 to 255, which is directly proportional to the intensity of the echo received by the transducer in that part of the matrix. Depth is added to the 2D pixel to create a voxel (volume and element; voXel). Each voxel may also be assigned a brightness value. The height and width of the voxel are likewise governed by the matrix configuration, but the depth is created in a 3D program and depends on the gap between the images. Interpolation may be used to create intervening images to form symmetrical voxels that avoid image degradation when the image is viewed in different planes.

Algorithms within the program calculate the difference in brightness between adjacent voxels and adjust the change in each interpolated image to give a smooth transition in brightness. If too many interpolated images

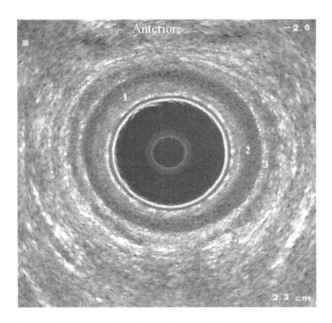

FIGURE 3 Normal AES in a female, mid canal level. 1 = subepithelial tissues; 2 = internal anal sphincter; 3 = external anal sphincter; 4 = external anal sphincter.

are introduced, the image may become unrepresentative. There are a variety of approaches to correct registration for the position of each image. The transducer may be tilted, mechanical, or electromagnetic positioning devices or complex software algorithms used to link multiple images. Precise registration is required for accurate 3D measurement, which is simplest to achieve using a mechanical device. Endosonography of the anal canal requires the probe to be slowly drawn down through the canal in a straight line, so that a mechanical linear translation rig is suitable for this examination. A manual system has been decribed (16,24,25), although an automated motorized system has subsequently been developed (26). This automatic system does not rely upon interpolation; all data displayed is "real," although the voxel depth is assumed by the rate of acquisition of the system (26).

The great advantage of 3D imaging is that once a dataset has been obtained, the volume contains all of the data for that examination. Standard 2D AES, as with most ultrasound examinations, is a dynamic process that is observer dependent. The patient is assessed in real time and any diagnosis made as the scan progresses. "Hard copy" generally poorly represents the total examination, and a complete recording is usually impossible without videotape. In contrast, 3D systems acquire a volume of digital data that can be archived for subsequent review. This separates diagnosis from the time of examination and enables sonographers unskilled in AES diagnosis to perform examinations for subsequent radiologist review. Another advantage of a data volume is that it may be imaged, and structures measured, in any plane. The anal sphincters are circular structures. Their thickness is easily measured axially and the size of any defect recorded in hours, but the cranio-caudal extent of any tear or abnormality may only be referred to in general terms by dividing the canal into high, mid, and low levels. These are not constant, making the longitudinal appreciation of any lesion imprecise, a disadvantage immediately overcome by multiplanar imaging.

Unfortunately, differences in tissue contrast between layers on AES are not marked and the reflectivity of some layers is not constant, so that techniques assigning transparency, opacity, maximum intensity projection, or surface rendering algorithms have not proved clinically useful. Three-dimensional reconstruction of anal endosonography is now increasingly available (16,24,25) and while its clinical role is uncertain it does permit multiplanar assessment of sphincter injury using ultrasound for the first time (Fig. 4).

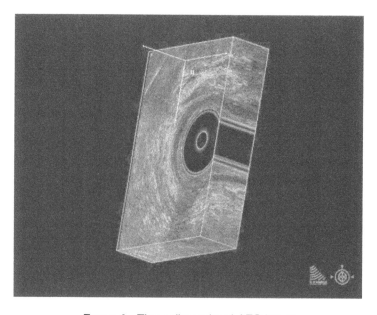

FIGURE 4 Three-dimensional AES image.

MAGNETIC RESONANCE IMAGING

Magnetic resonance imaging is now well established for imaging assessment of the anal canal and pelvis. Tissue differentiation using MR imaging is excellent, and T2-weighted sequences are especially suited to imaging both pathology and anatomical structures simultaneously in great detail. However, spatial resolution is generally insufficient to image the anal sphincter complex well enough to characterize the individual morphological abnormalities encountered in patients with anal incontinence, although improved when using a pelvic phased array coil. In contrast, the spatial resolution in the immediate vicinity of the coil is greatly enhanced when using an endoanal receiver coil, while maintaining excellent tissue differentiation. Much has been learned regarding anal anatomy via endoanal MR imaging. Demonstration of sphincter anatomy using MR imaging has been validated and confirmed using MR scans of cadavers with subsequent histological sectioning (27–30). Furthermore, intra-individual comparisons using both AES and endoanal MR imaging have refined our understanding of the structures seen on both modalities (22); structures that are distinct using MR imaging (e.g., the lateral border of the external sphincter) can be detailed on the ultrasound and vice versa (e.g., the internal sphincter).

On T2-weighted images the external sphincter and longitudinal muscle return a relatively low signal, whereas the internal sphincter returns a relatively high signal and enhances further with gadolinium (Fig. 5). The subepithelial tissue has a signal intensity value between that of the internal and external sphincters. The lateral border of the external anal sphincter is well defined on endocoil MR imaging, especially when compared with the rather indistinct images of AES (31). It should be noted that endoanal imaging, both ultrasound and MR, suffers from field-of-view limitations.

ANAL INCONTINENCE

Anal imaging is now generally considered mandatory for patients complaining of anal incontinence, a common condition that affects 2% of the general population older than 45 years, a figure that rises to 7% over the age of 65 years. A clinical distinction should be made between anal incontinence, which includes involuntary loss of gas and/or stool, and fecal incontinence, which specifically describes stool loss. Incontinence will be underestimated if only stool loss is considered. Various clinical symptom-grading systems are used, but there is no doubt that the more sophisticated the questionnaire employed, the higher the prevalence of incontinence. Population-based studies of anal incontinence have shown

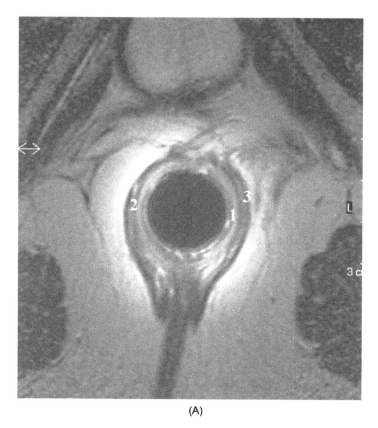

(A)

FIGURE 5 Endocoil MR images in an asymptomatic volunteer. (A) Axial image.
1 = internal sphincter; 2 = longitudinal muscle; 3 = external anal sphincter.
(B) Coronal image. 1 = external sphincter; 2 = puborectalis; 3 = levator plate.

a small but significant prevalence in uncomplaining, young individuals.
A relationship with childbirth has long been recognized, and variables such
as forceps delivery are known to increase the likelihood of anal incontinence following vaginal delivery. Postal questionnaire studies of postpartum women have revealed that frank fecal incontinence reaches
a prevalence of nearly 10%. Similar estimates of anal incontinence
have approached 25%. Clinically, much of this misery is invisible
because symptoms are underreported, probably due to embarrassment,
preoccupation with the newborn baby, and perceptions of inevitability.

Pelvic neuropathy had been considered the most likely cause of incontinence ever since physiological tests demonstrated impaired pudendal
nerve conduction following vaginal delivery, presumably due to soft tissue

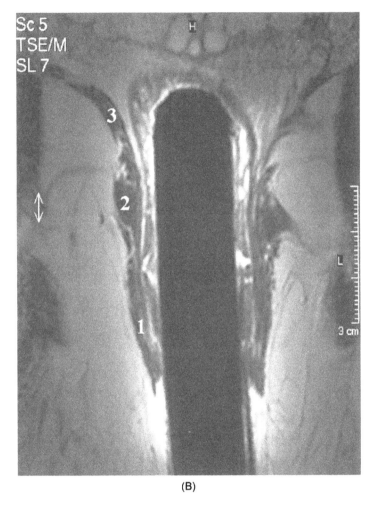

(B)

FIGURE 5   (continued)

stretching during birth, a finding that led directly to the concept of "neuro-pathic fecal incontinence." At that time, detailed imaging of the various components of the anal sphincter was unavailable. However, with the development of anal endosonography at St. Mark's Hospital, London, high-resolution imaging of the anal sphincter complex became possible (17). For the first time, detailed images of the external and internal sphinc-ters surrounding the anus could be easily and rapidly acquired. It quickly became clear that not only could childbirth damage pelvic nerves, but the anal sphincter complex was frequently disrupted as well. Tears in the sphincter were easily diagnosed as a discontinuity in the normally circumferential sphincter ring (Fig. 6). While adequate clinical history and anal physiological testing may assess severity and suggest sphincter trauma, anal ultrasound is now the gold standard for the diagnosis and assessment of surgically remediable sphincter disruption.

Indeed, the endosonographic localisation of sphincter tears has been confirmed by histological examination of biopsies taken during sphincter repair (32). Sonographic sphincter trauma is seen as either a localized area of low reflectivity in an otherwise highly reflective external sphincter or as an amorphous area of mixed reflectivity (26,32,33) (Fig. 6). The internal sphincter is practically always also disrupted during obstetric injury. The diagnosis of postobstetric anterior sphincter defects may be enhanced by the reduction in the length of the perineal body (34), and normal postpartum changes in sphincter morphology are now well recognized (35). Three-dimensional reconstruction of AES may also demonstrate the full extent of a sphincter injury (36), and a direct correlation exists between

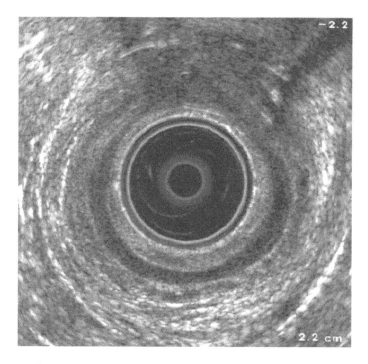

FIGURE 6 Extensive anterior external and internal sphincter defect following obstetric injury in a young women.

the length of a defect and the arc of displacement of the two ends of the sphincter (24).

Diagnosis of obstetric sphincter tears is important because these women may be helped by surgery that aims to restore integrity to the sphincter ring. This usually takes the form of an overlapping sphincter repair, where the external sphincter is mobilized, the scar excised, and the free ends of the sphincter overlapped and sutured. Symptomatic improvement is of the order of 85%, dropping to approximately 50% on long-term follow-up. The prime role of anal imaging, whether sonography or MR, is therefore to detect those patients who have an underlying tear and direct them to surgery. Just as important, imaging can confidently exclude those patients who have no laceration, sparing them an operation likely to be unhelpful and instead directing them to more appropriate treatments such as biofeedback behavioral therapy, sacral nerve stimulation, or sphincter reconstruction, using either muscular flaps or implantable devices.

Many clinically unsuspected sphincter injuries have been diagnosed using AES. In a group of 11 patients with a clinical diagnosis of idiopathic fecal incontinence thought to be unrelated to sphincter trauma, four were actually shown to have a sphincter defect on AES that was later confirmed by EMG studies (37). AES is superior in the differentiation between those patients with idiopathic fecal incontinence and those with a sphincter defect when compared with either simple manometric assessment or vector volume studies (38,39).

The anal sphincter complex in the female may also be examined via the trans-vaginal route. The results of trans-vaginal scanning using the same probe as that used for endoanal work were disappointing, although they have provided images of the anal sphincters in a nondistended state (40). The endoanal probe is difficult to control when used in the vagina due to the divergent axes of the anal canal and the vagina, and the distal canal is often difficult to image (41). The use of a shorter, side-firing scanner probe has greatly improved the images acquired (42), such that trans-vaginal scanning may now be a useful method of assessing women for sphincter trauma.

In a landmark publication that employed anal endosonography in women before and after vaginal delivery, the incidence of anal sphincter tears was estimated at approximately one third of all births (43), a staggeringly high figure subsequently confirmed by several other workers (44). Symptoms of anal incontinence and markers of physiological deterioration were strongly associated with sonographic sphincter tears (43). These findings eventually led to a complete change in obstetric emphasis; anal incontinence following childbirth is now thought to be predominantly due to sphincter tears. It is also clear that approximately 50% of women with sphincter tears can initially be asymptomatic for a variable time, often many years. Only subsequently, with the cumulative effects of aging and menopause, do symptoms of anal incontinence manifest themselves. Unsurprisingly, the temporal separation between delivery and symptoms means that sphincter tears are not usually considered when the patient presents. It is interesting to note that the vast majority of anal sphincter tears go unrecognized at the time of delivery; one prospective study of 2883 deliveries found 95 tears, an incidence of 3.3% (45), yet when these same authors used anal endosonography in a consecutive group of unselected vaginal deliveries, the incidence was 35% in primiparous women (43).

More recently, endocoil MR imaging has also been used to diagnose and assess anal sphincter trauma (46,47) (Fig. 7). Endocoil MR is considered by some to be superior to AES for the detection and assessment of external sphincter defects, largely because of superior external anal sphincter definition (48). Alternatively, others have found that AES remains equally effective for diagnosis of sphincter disruption (49). In reality, differences may actually reflect individual familiarity with the techniques used rather than any inherent technical deficiency (50). However, following the surge of interest in structural sphincter damage precipitated by the development of AES, it is increasingly well recognized that anal incontinence is not always a result of disruption and attention is again returning to the concept of neuropathic sphincter damage. Much of this change in attitude has been brought about by endocoil MR imaging, which has revealed that intact sphincters may be ineffective because they have been largely replaced by fat and fibrous tissue, a phenomenon known as external sphincter atrophy (51–53) (Fig. 8). This finding is important because patients who have both an atrophic external sphincter and a coexisting sphincter defect have been found to fare poorly after surgical repair of the defect, presumably because residual muscle is functionally inadequate (51,54). The degree of fat replacement may be precisely quantified using MR (53), but the appearances of atrophic muscle are equally well appreciated by simple inspection once the investigator has sufficient experience to recognize the morphology of normal muscle; an atrophic external sphincter has reduced bulk when compared to a normal sphincter and the quality of that muscle which is present is patchy and indistinct (Fig. 8).

Sphincter atrophy may also affect the internal sphincter, a phenomenon known as idiopathic internal anal sphincter degeneration (55). The internal sphincter normally thickens with age (56), but patients with idiopathic degeneration show progressive thinning, a finding that is probably best assessed using AES since this technique visualises the internal sphincter with greatest precision (49) (Fig. 9). Generally, a diagnosis of idiopathic degeneration should be considered in any adult

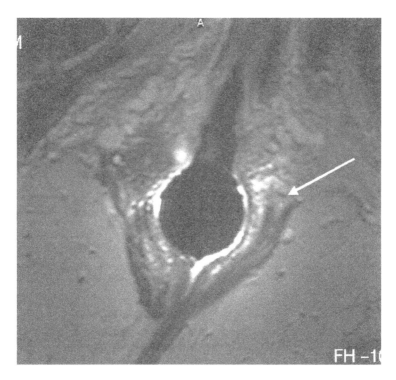

FIGURE 7   Axial endoanal MR image demonstrating an anterior sphincter tear (arrow) following obstetric injury.

patient with passive incontinence in combination with a thin but intact internal sphincter. The internal sphincter may also be damaged as an innocent bystander during trans-anal surgical procedures, and it is now well recognized that anal dilatation (57) or hemorrhoidectomy (58) may unintentionally damage the internal sphincter and cause passive incontinence (Fig. 10). Furthermore, sphincterotomy, which is used to treat anal fissures, is frequently overextensive in female patients and may also precipitate incontinence (59).

In summary, anal imaging for incontinence aims to characterize morphological sphincter abnormalities so that treatment is directed appropriately (60). The common combinations encountered, and their likely cause, are shown in Table 1.

FISTULA-IN-ANO

Fistula-in-ano is a relatively common condition and one in which, like incontinence, anal imaging has had tremendous impact over the last

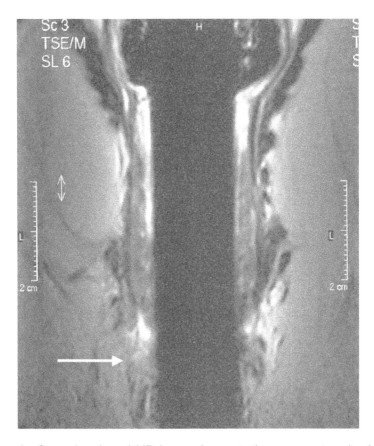

FIGURE 8 Coronal endoanal MR image demonstrating gross external sphincter atropy (arrow).

decade. By definition, a fistula describes an abnormal track that connects two epithelial surfaces. For fistula-in-ano, the external opening is usually perianal and the internal opening most often in the anal canal. The disease therefore manifests as chronic perianal suppuration and discomfort. Treatment is surgical, and while most anal fistulas are easily treated, some have a tendency to recur, by as much as 25% in some series (61). Recurrence is almost always due to occult sepsis that has initially escaped surgical detection and has thus gone untreated. Recurrent fistulas pose a notoriously difficult surgical challenge, and multiple failed operations are the rule rather than the exception in these patients. Such a state of affairs further complicates matters because the perianal scarring and distortion that inevitably accompanies multiple surgical attempts at cure impairs accurate

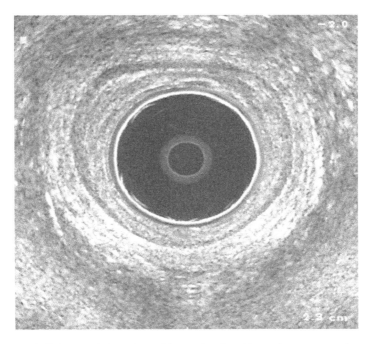

FIGURE 9 AES in an adult patient with passive fecal incontinence reveals an intact but thinned internal sphincter typical of idiopathic degeneration. The external sphincter boundaries are well preserved, suggesting that atrophy is confined to the internal sphincter.

preoperative assessment: digital palpation cannot easily distinguish sepsis from scarring. The inevitable result is that these individuals are progressively more difficult to treat, with both patient and surgeon becoming ever more exasperated.

The key to breaking this loop is accurate preoperative assessment, the main aim of which is to identify unsuspected areas of sepsis so that they can be targeted for subsequent treatment. Secondary aims are to define the relationship of the fistula to the anal sphincter complex, which serves to help predict the likelihood of postoperative anal incontinence. The surgeon therefore needs to answer two questions:

What is the relationship between fistula and anal sphincter? Will surgery risk incontinence and will sphincter-saving procedures be necessary?

Are there secondary extensions from the primary track that might cause relapse, and, if so, where are they?

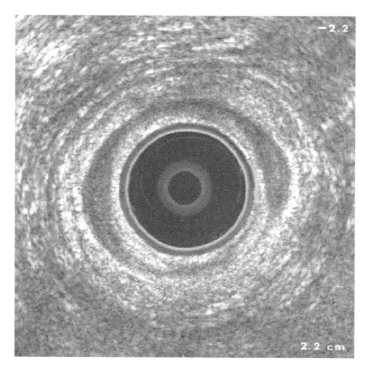

FIGURE 10   AES in a patient incontinent following hemorrhoidectomy reveals an extensive posterior internal sphincter defect.

TABLE 1   Common Morphological Sphincter Abnormalities in Anal Incontinence

Sphincter abnormality	Likely cause for incontinence
Combined anterior external and internal sphincter defects	Obstetric trauma
Isolated anterior external sphincter defect	Obstetric trauma
Isolated internal sphincter defect	Iatrogenic trauma, e.g., hemorrhoidectomy, anal dilatation
Thinned internal sphincter	Idiopathic internal anal sphincter degeneration
Thinned external sphincter	External sphincter atrophy
Thinned internal and external sphincter	Combined atrophy and degeneration
Sphincter defects combined with generalized sphincter thinning	Obstetric injury combined with long-standing underlying neuropathy

Anal fistulas are believed to be a consequence of sepsis that originates from anal glands that are located in the intersphincteric plane, between the internal and external sphincter (Fig. 11). These glands originate at the level of the dentate line, which is the where squamous epithelium meets columnar in the mid-anal canal and which is therefore where the internal opening of most anal fistulas can be found. The path that the fistula takes between the internal and external opening will define the type of fistula and will predict the degree of surgical difficulty. Parks exhaustively reviewed 400 consecutive patients with fistula-in-ano and concluded that all could be basically classified into four groups, defined by the relationship of the primary fistula track to the anal sphincter complex (62) (Fig. 11). Intersphincteric fistulas are the most common and do not cross the external sphincter. They are therefore usually easy to treat, and laying them open surgically does not involve division of the external sphincter. In contrast, all of the other fistula types penetrate the external sphincter or striated muscle of the pelvic floor (Fig. 11). It is important to note that a focus of infection in the intersphincteric space with communication to the anal canal is common to all intersphincteric, transsphincteric, and suprasphincteric fistulas, but extrasphincteric fistulas do not demonstrate this. Rather, they are usually due to primary rectal or perirectal disease, and the possibility of conditions such as carcinoma, Crohn's disease, and diverticular disease should be considered when this type is encountered. Correct determination of the height of the internal opening is also important. While most fistulas have an internal opening at dentate line level, some are higher, and generally the higher the internal opening, the more extensive sphincter division will be when the track is laid open.

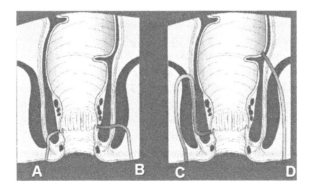

FIGURE 11   Diagram of Park's classification of fistula-in-ano. (A) Intersphincteric fistula; (B) transsphincteric fistula; (C) suprasphincteric fistula; (D) extrasphincteric fistula.

All fistulas may be complicated by "secondary tracks" or "extensions," which are areas of sepsis remote from the primary track. Extensions require specific treatment if the fistula is not to recur and will inevitably necessitate more extensive surgery for them to be adequately drained. Indeed, failure to detect and deal with extensions is the single most common cause of treatment failure. Extensions from the primary track may be intersphincteric, ischioanal, and supralevator (pararectal). Relapse is particularly common with supralevator sepsis because this is a difficult site to examine during examination under anesthetic (EUA) and, furthermore, the levator plate forms a relative barrier to free drainage even when an extension has been identified. The ischioanal (ischiorectal) fossa is the most common site to find an extension. Fistulas can also spread circumferentially in three planes: in the intrasphincteric space, in the ischioanal fossa, and in the supralevator space. Circumferential ramifications are termed "horseshoes" if they extend on either side of the internal opening and are important because extensive surgery is needed to drain them adequately.

CLINICAL VALUE OF IMAGING

Traditionally, EUA has been the method by which surgeons have explored the fistula and determined its relationship to the sphincter complex and identified the presence of any extensions. However, EUA is frequently misleading, especially in complex fistulas. This has driven the development of preoperative imaging. Unfortunately, fistulography is generally thought to be inadequate, mainly because the muscles of the pelvic floor are not visualized (63). AES held great promise, but while some authors have found it useful, others have found it no better than digital assessment in the clinic for assessment of complex fistulas (64). This is primarily because complex fistulas are frequently associated with extensions from the primary track, which are often beyond the field of view of the anal endoprobe and thus remain unrecognized. CT is of little use for fistula classification because its intrinsic contrast is relatively poor. On the other hand, MRI has excellent tissue contrast that renders it highly suitable both for the demonstration of sepsis and adjacent anatomical structures. Furthermore, the ability of MRI to easily image in any orientation means that the anal sphincter complex can be resolved in surgically relevant planes.

The first study to indicate the potential accuracy of MRI for preoperative classification of cryptogenic fistula-in-ano came from St. Mark's Hospital, where Lunniss and coworkers examined 16 patients with MRI and found that imaging classification agreed with subsequent surgical EUA (blind to MRI) in 14 (88%) (65). Interestingly, the two patients in whom there was disagreement (MRI had suggested sepsis, whereas EUA was normal) later presented with disease at the site initially predicted by MRI, a finding that led the authors to conclude that MRI was now the gold standard for fistula classification (65). Other authors have subsequently validated this work; Beckingham et al. found that MRI had a sensitivity of 97% and specificity of 100% for detection and classification of fistula in 42 subjects, 4 of whom were misdiagnosed during EUA (66). An interesting study from the same group separately classified patients on the basis of findings at preoperative MRI and subsequent EUA and discovered that MRI was the better predictor of postoperative relapse (67). That study clearly suggested that MRI was adept at identifying features likely to lead to postoperative recurrence, and Beets-Tan and colleagues extended this concept to determine the peri-operative impact of MRI, finding that imaging provided important additional information in 21% of cases (68). In the largest study of consecutive patients with recurrent disease to date, Buchanan and coworkers examined 71 patients with MRI and revealed the findings to the surgeon peri-operatively (69). The surgeon was then free to act on the imaging findings at their own discretion. The authors found a postoperative relapse rate of only 16% for those surgeons who always reexplored when MRI suggested they had missed disease, whereas the relapse rate was 57% for those surgeons who always ignored MRI, believing their own assessment to be superior. The authors concluded that preoperative MRI in patients with complex recurrent disease could reduce the incidence of postoperative relapse by approximately 75% (69), a dramatic effect of imaging in a clinical setting.

MR TECHNIQUE

A variety of MR imaging approaches may be taken to visualize fistulas, and T2-weighted sequences, STIR sequences, and T1-weighted sequences following gadolinium enhancement all have their advocates (70). It is now generally accepted that either a body coil or, preferably, a pelvic surface coil should be used. Whatever technique is adopted, it must be able to highlight both sepsis and adjacent structures. Most importantly, some form of fat suppression should be employed if using fast spin echo sequences since the high signal normally returned from fat can easily hide an active track or abscess. While endocoil MR exquisitely demonstrates the extent of the primary track, it may also miss distant extensions because of field of view problems, rather like AES, and should probably not be used in isolation unless there is good reason to believe that the fistula is definitely simple (71). The authors favor a simple approach: a sagittal T2-weighted scan through the midline is initially obtained, which reveals the extent and axis of the anal canal. Subsequent axial and coronal STIR sequences are planned from this and should encompass the full extent of the anal canal musculature and also extend into those areas that might hide distant extensions—the supralevator and presacral spaces, for example. Failure to align studies with respect to the anal canal axis is a major source of error, especially with respect to identification of the level of the track and its internal opening. Examination is rapid, well tolerated, relatively inexpensive, and no special patient preparation is necessary. Other sequences, imaging planes, or coils are used for problem solving after radiologist review.

Axial scans best relate the primary track to the sphincter complex and are the basis for fistula classification, whereas coronal scans best visualize the levator plate and facilitate diagnosis of both supralevator sepsis and the level of the internal opening. The external sphincter, puborectalis, and levator plate are of a signal similar to striated muscle elsewhere in the body, standing out against low signal ischiorectal and ischioanal fat on STIR sequences. In contrast, the internal sphincter returns high signal intensity on both STIR and T2-weighted scans, enabling it to be distinguished from the intersphincteric plane and external sphincter. It follows that an intersphincteric fistula is recognized as a high signal track that remains confined throughout its course by the external sphincter (Fig. 12). In contrast to

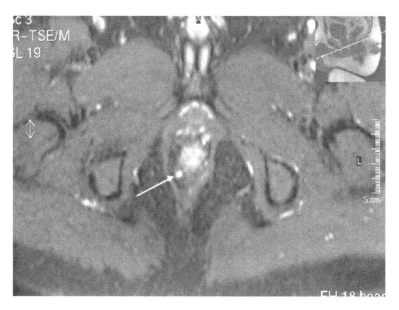

FIGURE 12   Axial STIR MR image shows a fistula track (arrow) that is medial to the external sphincter. Diagnosis: intersphincteric fistula.

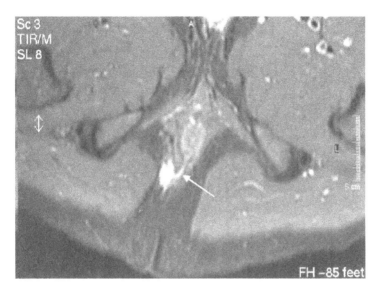

FIGURE 13 Axial STIR MR image shows a fistula track that is lateral to the external sphincter, in the ischioanal fossa. A portion of the track (arrow) crosses the external sphincter to reach a posterior internal opening at dentate line level. Diagnosis: transsphincteric fistula.

intersphincteric fistulas, transsphincteric fistulas penetrate the external sphincter in order to reach the ischioanal/ischiorectal fossa. Thus, a track in the ischioanal fossa generally indicates a transsphincteric fistula (Fig. 13). The level at which the external sphincter complex is breached is variable, but is most often at mid anal canal level, and the internal opening is usually posterior at dentate line level. Suprasphincteric fistulas do not traverse the external sphincter but arch over it instead. There will still be a primary track in the ischioanal fossa, but the track will cross the pubo-rectalis or levator plate instead of the external sphincter. The internal opening is usually at the dentate line. This type of fistula is best appreciated in the coronal plane, and in the authors' experience is both very uncommon and very difficult to differentiate from a high transsphincteric fistula. In any event, there is little practical difference because surgical management is similar; both types are likely to need sphincter conservation and should not be treated by simple fistulotomy since excessive sphincter division is inevitable. Extrasphincteric fistulas are recognized by the absence of any MR signal suggesting sepsis within the intersphincteric space. Again, there will be a primary track in the ischioanal fossa, but the internal opening will be rectal, a feature well appreciated on coronal views (Fig. 14).

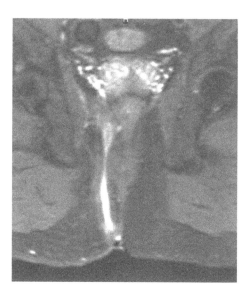

FIGURE 14   Coronal STIR MR image showing a right-sided extrasphincteric fistula. Note that the fistula enters the anorectal junction directly and there is no sepsis in the intersphincteric plane.

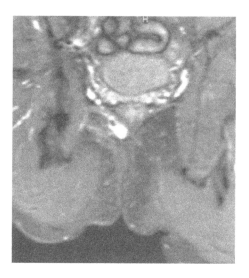

FIGURE 15   Coronal STIR MR image showing an anscess in the roof of the right ischioanal fossa. This finding was ignored during subsequent surgery because the abscess could not be palpated by the surgeon. The patient represented several months later with sepsis at the site initially predicted by MR.

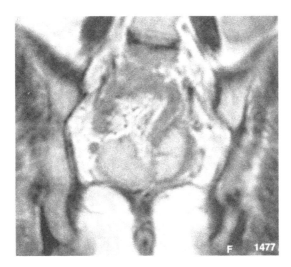

FIGURE 16 Coronal T2-weighted MR image showing bilateral supralevator abscesses.

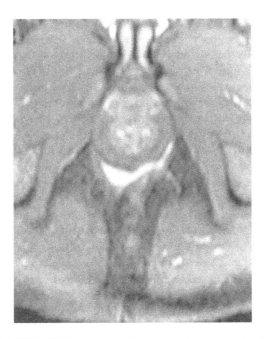

FIGURE 17 Axial STIR MR image reveals a horseshoe extension in the roof of the ischioanal fossa.

The location of external openings is of little relevance, as these can usually be seen on clinical inspection. However, occasionally the exit site may intermittently heal, and thus the presence of significant underlying disease may go unrecognized. This has recently become especially relevant since treatment of perianal Crohn's disease with anti-TNF-α agents is contraindicated in the presence of an underlying abscess (72). The level of the internal opening is more important since this will determine the extent of sphincter division during fistulotomy. Unfortunately, the dentate line cannot be identified on MRI as a discrete anatomical structure, and so its position must be inferred. Indeed, it is now recognized that an inability to precisely identify the level of the internal opening with respect to the dentate line is a relative deficiency of MRI (or indeed any imaging technique) and a common cause of misclassification (69); an insert showing the scan plane and level may help to precisely locate the midpoint of the anal canal. Furthermore, as with AES, a visible track extending right to the anal mucosal surface is frequently absent, and so the location of an internal opening must be inferred from the location of sepsis within the intersphincteric plane. Given this, if no enteric communication can be demonstrated, then a sinus should be diagnosed instead of a fistula.

In any event, the major role of MRI is to identify tracks and extensions that would otherwise have gone unrecognized. Secondary tracks and extensions are easily visualized as high signal collections in either the infralevator (Fig. 15) or supralevator compartments (Fig. 16) and are described with reference to their anatomical location and relationship to the primary track. It is important to recognize that sepsis medial to the puborectalis or levator on axial scans will be supralevator in location, whereas sepsis lateral to these muscles is infralevator. When a large track becomes an "abscess" is a matter of semantics, and a variety of definitions have been used, some of which rely on morphology, while others use diameter (e.g., > 1 cm). Horseshoe extensions are defined by sepsis that extends on both sides of the internal opening in the horizontal plane. Horseshoes may be intersphincteric, ischioanal, or supralevator (Fig. 17) and are important because they demand extensive incision in order to be drained adequately.

Fistula-in-ano is one area in which recent radiological developments, notably MRI, have made real and tangible differences to patients. It could easily be argued that failure to employ MRI is negligent in patients with recurrent disease. Furthermore, MRI is now generally available, and high-quality examination does not require special equipment. It suffers from none of the drawbacks associated with other imaging modalities, and for these reasons it could be argued there is little reason to request anything else when assessment of a complex fistula is required.

REFERENCES

1. Walls EW. Anatomy of the anal canal. Ann Roy Coll Surg England 1983:1–3.
2. Lawson JON. Pelvic anatomy, II. Anal canal and associated sphincters. Ann Roy Coll Surg England 1974; 54:287–300.
3. Goligher JC, Leacock AG, Brossy JJ. The surgical anatomy of the anal canal. Br J Surg 1955; 43:51–61.
4. Parks AG. The surgical treatment of haemorrhoids. Br J Surg 1956; 43: 337–351.
5. Haas PA, Fox TA. Age-related changes and scar formations of perianal connective tissue. Dis Colon Rectum 1990; 23(3):160–169.
6. Courtney H. Anatomy of the pelvic diaphragm and anorectal musculature as related to sphincter preservation in anorectal surgery. Am J Surg 1950; 79:155–173.
7. Milligan ETC, Morgan CN. Surgical anatomy of the anal canal with special reference to anorectal fistulae. Lancet ii 1934; 1213–1217.
8. Shafik A. A concept of the anatomy of the anal sphincter mechanism and the physiology of defecation. Dis Colon Rectum 1987; 30(12):970–982.
9. Lunniss PJ, Phillips RKS. Anatomy and function of the anal longitudinal muscle. Br J Surg 1992; 79:882–884.
10. Thompson P. The myology of the pelvic floor. London: McCorquodale & Co., 1899.
11. Holl K. Bardeleben's Handbuch der Anatomie des Menschen. Stuttgart: Fischer, 1897.
12. Gorsch RV. Proctologic Anatomy. 2ed. Baltimore: Williams & Wilkins, 1955.
13. Beersiek F, Parks AG, Swash M. Pathogenesis of anorectal incontinence. J Neurol Sci 1979; 42:111–127.
14. Nielsen MB, Pedersen JF, Hauge C, Rasmussen OO, Christiansen J. Endosonography of the anal sphincter: findings in healthy volunteers. AJR Am J Roentgenol 1991; 157(6):1199–1202.
15. Sultan AH, Kamm MA, Hudson CN, Nicholls JR, Bartram CI. Endosonography of the anal sphincters: normal anatomy and comparison with manometry. Clin Radiol 1994; 49(6):368–374.
16. Williams AB, Cheetham MJ, Bartram CI, Halligan S, Kmiot WA, Nicholls RJ. Gender differences in the longitudinal pressure profile of the anal canal related to anatomical structure as demonstrated on three-dimensional anal endosonography. Br J Surg 2000; 87:1674–1679.
17. Law PJ, Bartram CI. Anal endosonography: technique and normal anatomy. Gastrointest Radiol 1989; 14:349–353.
18. Hildebrandt U, Feifel G. Preoperative staging of rectal cancer by intrarectal ultrasound. Dis Colon Rectum 1985; 28:42–46.
19. Frudinger A, Bartram CI, Halligan S, Kamm M. Examination techniques for endosonography of the anal canal. Abdom Imaging 1998; 23(3):301–303.
20. Sultan AH, Nicholls RJ, Kamm MA, Hudson CN, Beynon J, Bartram CI. Anal endosonography and correlation with in vitro and in vivo anatomy. Br J Surg 1993; 80(4):508–511.

21. Tjandra JJ, Milsom JW, Stolfi VM, Lavery I, Oakley J, Church J, et al. Endoluminal ultrasound defines anatomy of the anal canal and pelvic floor. Dis Colon Rectum 1992; 35(5):465–470.

22. Williams AB, Bartram CI, Halligan S, Marshall MM, Nicholls RJ, Kmiot WA. Endosonographic anatomy of the normal anal canal compared to endocoil magnetic resonance imaging. Dis Colon Rectum 2000; 45: 176–183.

23. Burnett SJ, Bartram CI. Endosonographic variations in the normal internal anal sphincter. Int J Colorectal Dis 1991; 6(1):2–4.

24. Gold DM, Bartram CI, Halligan S, Humphries KN, Kamm MA, Kmiot WA. Three-dimensional endoanal sonography in assessing anal canal injury. Br J Surg 1999; 86:365–370.

25. Williams AB, Bartram CI, Halligan S. Review of three-dimensional anal endo-sonography. RAD 1999; 25(289):47–48.

26. Williams AB, Bartram CI, Halligan S, Spencer JA, Nicholls RJ, Kmiot WA. Sphincter damage after vaginal delivery—a prospective study. Obstet Gynaecol 2000; 97:770–775.

27. Hussain SM, Stoker J, Lameris JS. Anal sphincter complex: endoanal MR imaging of normal anatomy. Radiology 1995; 197:671–677.

28. deSouza NM, Puni R, Zbar A, Gilderdale DJ, Coutts GA, Krausz T. MR imaging of the anal sphincter in multiparous women using an endoanal coil: correlation with in vitro anatomy and appearances in fecal incontinence. AJR Am J Roentgenol 1996; 167(6):1465–1471.

29. Tan IL, Stoker J, Zwamborn AW, Entius CA, Calame J, Lameris JS. Female pelvic floor: endovaginal MR imaging of normal anatomy. Radiology 1998; 206(3):777–783.

30. Gerdes B, Kohler HH, Zielke A, Kisker O, Barth PJ, Stinner B. The anatomical basis of anal endosonography. A study in postmortem specimens. Surg Endosc 1997; 11(10):986–990.

31. Stoker J, Rociu E, Zwamborn AW, Schouten WR, Lameris JS. Endoluminal MR imaging of the rectum and anus: technique, applications and pitfalls. Radiographics 1999; 19(383):398.

32. Sultan AH, Kamm MA, Talbot IC, Nicholls RJ, Bartram CI. Anal endosono-graphy for identifying external sphincter defects confirmed histologically. Br J Surg 1994; 81(3):463–465.

33. Deen KI, Kumar D, Williams JG, Olliff J, Keighley MR. Anal sphincter defects. Correlation between endoanal ultrasound and surgery. Ann Surg 1993; 218(2):201–205.

34. Zetterstrom JP, Mellgren A, Madoff RD, Kim DG, Wong WD. Perineal body measurement improves evaluation of anterior sphincter lesions during endoanal ultrasonography. Dis Colon Rectum 1998; 41(6): 705–713.

35. Williams AB, Spencer JA, Bartram CI. Alteration of anal sphincter morphology following vaginal delivery revealed by three-dimensional anal endosonography. Br J Obstet Gynaecol 2002; 109:833–835.

36. Williams AB, Bartram CI, Halligan S, Spencer JA, Nicholls RJ, Kmiot WA. Anal sphincter damage after vaginal delivery using three-dimensional endosonography. Obstet Gynecol 2001; 97(5 pt 1):770–775.

37. Law PJ, Kamm MA, Bartram CI. Anal endosonography in the investigation of faecal incontinence. Br J Surg 1991; 78(3):312–314.

38. Sentovich SM, Blatchford GJ, Rivela LJ, Lin K, Thorson AG, Christensen MA. Diagnosing anal sphincter injury with transanal ultrasound and manometry. Dis Colon Rectum 1997; 40(12):1430–1434.

39. Felt-Bersma RJF, Cuesta MA, Koorevaar M, Strijers RL, Meuwissen SG, Dercksen EJ, et al. Anal endosonography; relationship with anal manometry and neurophysiologic tests. Dis Colon Rectum 1992; 35:944–949.

40. Sultan AH, Loder PB, Bartram CI, Kamm MA, Hudson CN. Vaginal endosonography. New approach to image the undisturbed anal sphincter. Dis Colon Rectum 1994; 37(12):1296–1299.

41. Frudinger A, Bartram CI, Kamm MA. Transvaginal versus anal endosonography for detecting damage to the anal sphincter. AJR Am J Roentgenol 1997; 168(6):1435–1438.

42. Stewart LK, Wilson SR. Transvaginal sonography of the anal sphincter: reliable, of not?Am J Roentgenol 1998; 173:179–185.

43. Sultan AH, Kamm MA, Hudson CN, Thomas J, Bartram CI. Anal sphincter disruption during vaginal delivery. N Engl J Med 1993; 329:1905–1911.

44. Fines M, Donnelly V, Behan M, O'Connell PR, O'Herlihy C. Effect of second vaginal delivery on anorectal physiology and faecal continence: a prospective study. Lancet 1999; 354:983–986.

45. Sultan AH, Kamm MA, Hudson CN, Bartram CI. Third degree obstetric anal sphincter tears: risk factors and outcome of primary repair. BMJ 1994; 308:887–891.

46. deSouza NM, Kmiot WA, Puni R, Hall AS, Burl M, Bartram CI, et al. High resolution magnetic resonance imaging of the anal sphincter using an internal coil. Gut 1995; 37(2)284–287.

47. Stoker J, Hussain SM, Lameris JS. Endoanal magnetic resonance imaging versus endosonography. Radiol Med (Torino) 1996; 92(6):738–741.

48. Rociu E, Stoker J, Eijkemans MJC, Schouten WR, Lameris JS. Fecal incontinence: endoanal US versus endoanal MR imaging. Radiology 1999; 212:453–458.

49. Malouf AJ, Halligan S, Williams AB, Bartram CI, Dhillon S, Kamm MA. Prospective assessment of accuracy of endoanal MR imaging and endosonography in patients with fecal incontinence. Am J Roentgenol 2000; 175:741–745.

50. Malouf AJ, Williams AB, Halligan S, Bartram CI, Dhillon S, Kamm MA. Prospective assessment of interobserver error for endoanal MRI in fecal incontinence. Abdom Imag 2001; 26:76–78.

51. Briel JW, Stoker J, Rociu E, Lameris JS, Hop WC, Schouten WR. External anal sphincter atrophy on endoanal magnetic resonance imaging adversely affects continence after sphincteroplasty. Br J Surg 1999; 86:1322–1327.

52. Williams AB, Bartram CI, Modhwadia D, Nicholls T, Halligan S, Kamm MA, et al. Endocoil magnetic resonance imaging quantification of external anal sphincter atrophy. Br J Surg 2001; 88:853–859.

53. Williams AB, Malouf AJ, Bartram CI, Halligan S, Kamm MA, Kmiot WA. Assessment of external anal sphincter morphology in idiopathic faecal incontinence with endo-coil magnetic resonance imaging. Digest Dis Sci 2001; 46:1466–1471.

54. Williams AB, Bartram CI, Chelvanayagam S, Norton C, Kamm MA, Halligan S, et al. Imaging predicts the results from anterior external anal sphincter repair following obstetric trauma. Colorectal Dis 2001; 3:82.

55. Vaizey CJ, Kamm MA, Bartram CI. Primary degeneration of the internal anal sphincter as a cause of passive faecal incontinence. Lancet 1997; 349:612–615.

56. Frudinger A, Halligan S, Bartram CI, Price AB, Kamm MA, Winter R. Female anal sphincter: age-related differences in asymptomatic volunteers with high-frequency endoanal US. Radiology 2002; 224:417–423.

57. Gattuso JM, Kamm MA, Halligan S, Bartram CI. The anal sphincter in idiopathic megarectum: effects of manual disimpaction under general anesthetic. Dis Colon Rectum 1996; 39:435–439.

58. Abbasakoor F, Nelson M, Beynon J, Patel B, Carr ND. Anal endosonography in patients with anorectal symptoms after haemorrhoidectomy. Br J Surg 1998; 85:1522–1524.

59. Felt-Bersma RF, van Baren R, Koorevaar M, Strijers RL, Cuesta MA. Unsuspected sphincter defects shown by anal endosonography afre anorectal surgery. Dis Colon Rectum 1995; 38:249–253.

60. Stoker J, Halligan S, Bartram CI. State-of-the-art: pelvic floor imaging. Radiology 2001; 218:621–641.

61. Lilius HG. Investigation of human foetal anal ducts and intramuscular glands and a clinical study of 150 patients. Acta Chir Scand 1968; suppl 383.

62. Parks AG, Gordon PH, Hardcastle JD. A classification of fistula-in-ano. Br J Surg 1976; 63:1–12.

63. Kuijpers HC, Schulpen T. Fistulography for fistula-in-ano: Is it useful? Dis Colon Rectum 1985; 28:103–104; 78:539–541.

64. Choen S, Burnett S, Bartram CI, et al. Comparison between anal endosonography and digital examination in the evaluation of anal fistulae. Br J Surg 1991; 78:445–447.

65. Lunniss PJ, Armstrong P, Barker PG, et al. Magnetic resonance imaging of anal fistulae. Lancet 1992; 340:394–396.

66. Beckingham IJ, Spencer JA, Ward J, et al. Prospective evaluation of dynamic contrast enhanced magnetic resonance imaging in the evaluation of fistula-in-ano. Br J Surg 1996; 83:1396–1398.

67. Chapple KS, Spencer JA, Windsor AC, Wilson D, Ward J, Ambrose NS. Prognostic value of magnetic resonance imaging in the management of fistula-in-ano. Dis Colon Rectum 2000; 43:511–516.

68. Beets-Tan RG, Beets GL, Der Hoop AG, Kessels AG, Vliegen RF, Baeten CG, van Engelshoven JM. Preoperative MR Imaging of anal fistulas: Does it really help the surgeon? Radiology 2001; 218:75–84.
69. Buchanan G, Halligan S, Williams A, Cohen CR, Tarroni D, Phillips RK, Bartram CI. Effect of MRI on clinical outcome of recurrent fistula-in-ano. Lancet 2002; 360:1661–1662.
70. Halligan S. Imaging fistula-in-ano. Clin Radiol 1998; 53:85–95.
71. Halligan S, Bartram CI. Magnetic resonance of fistula-in-ano: Are endo-anal coils necessary? Br J Radiol 1997; 70:125.
72. Bell SJ, Halligan S, Windsor AC, Williams AB, Wiesel P, Kamm MA. Response of fistulating Crohn's disease to infliximab treatment assessed by magnetic resonance imaging. Aliment Pharmacol Ther 2003; 17:387–393.

15

Dynamic Imaging of the Pelvic Floor

Harpreet K. Pannu
Johns Hopkins Medical Institutions, Baltimore, Maryland, U.S.A.

Frederick M. Kelvin
Methodist Hospital of Indiana and Indiana University School of
    Medicine, Indianapolis, Indiana, U.S.A.

INTRODUCTION

In patients with pelvic organ prolapse, imaging can be used as an adjunct to the physical examination, especially when pelvic examination is equivocal. Pelvic physical examination is the traditional and established method to evaluate patients with pelvic organ prolapse, and imaging is usually performed to answer specific questions such as the presence or absence of enteroceles, rectoceles, sigmoidoceles, rectal intussusception, and pelvic floor abnormalities. Imaging may also be performed in patients with severe or recurrent prolapse to delineate the pelvic compartments that are abnormal prior to repeat surgery or other therapy.

Pelvic organ prolapse is characterized by abnormal descent and protrusion of the pelvic organs into the vagina. The pelvis is divided into compartments relative to the vagina: the bladder and urethra are in the anterior compartment, the cervix in the middle compartment, and the cul-de-sac and rectum in the posterior compartment. Normally, these organs are supported by the endopelvic fascia and the muscles of the pelvic floor. The anterior portion of the endopelvic fascia between the bladder and vagina is called the pubocervical fascia, and the posterior portion between the rectum and vagina is called the rectovaginal fascia. Tears in the pubocervical fascia result in prolapse of the bladder (cystocele), tears in the superior portion of the rectovaginal septum result in enteroceles, and tears in the rectovaginal fascia result in anterior protrusion of the rectum (rectocele). The stress on the endopelvic fascia is relieved by the continuous tone of the levator ani muscle of the pelvic floor. Neuromuscular damage to this muscle can result in diminished tone and bulging, increasing the size of the pelvic hiatus.

Pelvic organ prolapse is common. The annual incidence of hospitalization for prolapse is reported as 0.20% and the rate of surgery as 1.58% per year for women who have had hysterectomy for prolapse (1). A survey of healthy perimenopausal women found that 16% had organ prolapse on physical examination (2). Prolapse almost invariably involves multiple organs; in one report, 95% of patients investigated radiologically for prolapse had abnormalities in all three pelvic compartments. It is advisable to identify all the areas of prolapse preoperatively because they may all require surgical correction, and ideally this is done at one operative setting (3).

CLINICAL UTILITY OF IMAGING

Imaging helps to confirm abnormalities detected on physical examination as well as to detect defects that may have been missed (4,5). Early experience with evacuation proctography suggested that this radiological technique detected enteroceles and sigmoidoceles not otherwise identifiable by physical examination (6). Subsequent comparative studies have confirmed the relative insensitivity of physical examination. The latter approach identifies only approximately 50% of enteroceles, but fares better for recognition of rectoceles and cystoceles (7–9).

Insensitivity of physical examination is almost certainly related in part to the patient's inability to strain maximally while being examined. Complete relaxation of pelvic floor muscles occurs only during or following defecation (and micturition), thereby allowing pelvic organ prolapse to manifest itself to the fullest extent. The degree of straining achieved by the patient while encumbered by an examining digit (with or without a vaginal speculum) is clearly likely to be less than that achieved during defecation.

A more fundamental benefit of imaging is that it directly visualizes the organs at the site of prolapse, whereas the position of these organs can only be inferred on physical examination. In patients with severe prolapse, the nature of the prolapsing viscera is also easier to determine on imaging than physical examination (4,10). It must be emphasized, however, that these two diagnostic approaches are based upon entirely different reference points: the hymeneal ring and the pubococcygeal line. A common reference system would be enormously beneficial (11). It appears likely that the limitations of physical examination have contributed to the frequent need for reoperation. One study found that the diagnosis of rectocele, enterocele, and cystocele was changed in 75% of patients in whom fluoroscopic cystoproctography was performed (12). Incomplete recognition of prolapse may be reduced by performing preoperative pelvic floor imaging, whether by fluroscopy or magnetic resonance imaging (MRI).

Similar to fluoroscopy, more defects are detected during MRI than on physical examination (5). In one study, additional diagnoses such as uterovaginal prolapse and enterocele were made on MRI in 34% of patients when compared with the physical examination (13). Incidental pelvic pathology is also demonstrated on MRI (14,15). In a study of imaging with both fluoroscopy and MRI, the operative plan was modified in 41% of cases due to additional diagnoses of sigmoidoceles, rectal intussusception, and levator ani abnormalities (16). Since the post-operative recurrence rate for pelvic floor disorders is approximately 30% and these disorders are often complex, imaging can be used to aid in patient management (16,17).

Imaging has been suggested as an objective method with which to assess pelvic floor defects. It can be used to quantify organ descent before surgery and to demonstrate improvement afterwards (3,5). Imaging, especially with MRI, provides a global evaluation of the entire pelvic floor. Additionally, the effects of prolapse in one compartment on adjacent compartments can be shown.

FLUOROSCOPIC CYSTOPROCTOGRAPHY

Introduction

Evacuation proctography (defecography) was initially utilized for the evaluation of anorectal dysfunction. In women, the role of this technique may be expanded by opacifying the small bowel and vagina in addition to the rectum, as this facilitates detection of an enterocele (6). The incorporation of a cystogram into the technique of proctography provides a more comprehensive radiological method of assessing the pelvic organs; this requires catheterization and opacification of the bladder in addition to opacifying the rectum, vagina, and small bowel. Sites of weakness involving these organs are then imaged at rest, during straining, during and after evacuation, and in the posttoilet state. The term dynamic cystoproctography (DCP) or, more completely, dynamic cystocolpoproctography has been attached to this procedure, as well as other terms such as colpocystodefecography and four-contrast defecography (7,18). This radiographic approach was developed to serve as a complement to the physical examination for the evaluation of pelvic organ prolapse. The varied sites of weakness may lead to protrusions of specific organs resulting in rectocele, cystocele, enterocele, and sigmoidocele, as well as symptoms of stress urinary incontinence and fecal incontinence. A global approach to pelvic floor imaging is preferable, as weakness of the pelvic floor in women usually involves multiple organ systems.

Technique

Several items of specialized equipment are required for the examination. These include a radiolucent commode, video-recording with slow motion play-back capability, and a thick barium paste that approximates the consistency of feces. The techniques of proctography are by no means standardized; although contrast filling of the vagina and rectum are almost universal, the small bowel is not routinely opacified and most investigators do not perform the cystographic phase. Because proctography depends upon opacification of multiple pelvic organs, it is unquestionably an intrusive procedure.

Irrespective of the form of proctography employed, it is crucial to explain the procedure thoroughly to the patient beforehand and to provide maximal privacy and reassurance for the patient during the procedure. Respect for the dignity of the patient in an unfamiliar environment is of paramount importance (19).

In most centers, DCP is performed in one phase after all the constituent pelvic organs have been opacified. There is, however, only a limited amount of space within the confines of the bony pelvis. As a result, unemptied organs may prevent recognition of other prolapsed organs which are competing for available space. This is particularly true of the bladder; an insufficiently drained cystocele often prevents descent of small bowel and may minimize a rectocele (20). Similarly, an incompletely emptied rectocele or rectum may hide an enterocele. In view of these common problems, a triphasic approach that is based upon sequential organ emptying is usually employed at our institution (19). The following account is a brief summary of this technique:

Initially, the pelvic small bowel is opacified with oral barium. The bladder is then catheterized, and approximately 50 mL of cystographic contrast material are introduced. Fifty milliliters is sufficient to fill the dependent part of the bladder and reduces the amount of drainage subsequently required; the depth of a cystocele is not affected by the amount of instilled cystographic contrast material. Lateral films of the bladder at rest and on maximal strain are obtained (cystographic phase) and the bladder then emptied as much as possible via the catheter before the latter is removed.

After further voiding in the bathroom, the vagina is then opacified with 20 mL of a barium suspension, and a folded gauze square is sometimes inserted in the urogenital introitus to limit loss of contrast from the vagina and thereby improve vaginal opacification (21). The rectum is then filled with approximately 200 mL of a high-viscosity barium paste, which is introduced via a caulking gun, and lateral films of the pelvis at rest and on voluntary contraction of the pelvic floor muscles ("squeezing") are obtained. The patient is then asked to evacuate as rapidly and completely as possible, and lateral films are taken during and following evacuation. The postevacuation film is obtained with the patient straining maximally.

The patient then goes to the bathroom again to attempt further evacuation and voiding before returning for the posttoilet phase, which consists of a final lateral film on the commode with the patient again straining maximally. The entire examination is recorded on videotape for subsequent review.

A more invasive variation of proctography is to combine it with simultaneous peritoneography to directly visualize herniation of the posterior peritoneal cul-de-sac (peritoneography) (22,23).

Radiological Definitions and Grading of Prolapse

Two basic considerations are relevant to the radiological assessment of pelvic organ prolapse. The first of these is to determine whether prolapse of a specific organ is indeed present. If so, then the degree of prolapse requires quantification. Grading is particularly important because minor degrees of prolapse are often asymptomatic. Unfortunately, radiologists have not yet developed universally accepted radiological criteria for defining prolapse of pelvic organs (11). Furthermore, little attention has been devoted to devising a system for the grading of organ prolapse.

Prolapse of pelvic organs is most often defined radiologically by reference to the pubococcygeal line, which extends from the inferior margin of the pubic symphysis to the sacrococcygeal junction (Fig. 1); this is considered to represent the approximate line of attachment of the pelvic floor muscles. A cystocele, enterocele or sigmoidocele (Fig. 1) and vaginal vault prolapse are defined by extension of the bladder base, small bowel or sigmoid colon, and vaginal apex, respectively, below this reference line. An enterocele has frequently been defined by the extension of small bowel

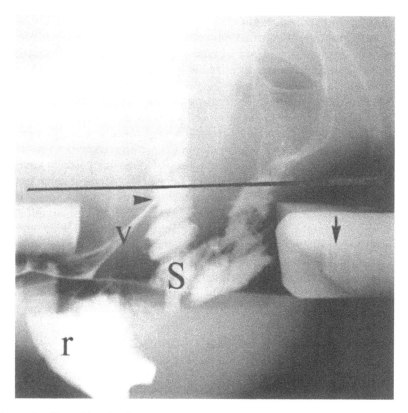

FIGURE 1   Sigmoidocele. Postevacuation image shows a loop of sigmoid colon (S) that extends below the pubococcygeal line (black line), indicating a sigmoidocele in the cul-de-sac. Note the radioopaque centimeter ruler (black arrow) within the commode. The sigmoidocele is of moderate size, extending 4.5 cm below the pubococcygeal line. v = vagina; arrowhead indicates vaginal apex. Note barium trapping within rectocele (r).

below the vaginal apex, but the vagina is both too mobile a structure and too high a reference point to be reliable. A radiological grading system for prolapse of the above organs has been described; prolapse of any of these organs is graded as small if there is organ descent up to 3 cm below the pubococcygeal line, moderate if this extension measures between 3 and 6 cm, and large if descent is greater than 6 cm (19). These measurements are all made on the images which show maximal organ descent. The radiological definition and grading of a rectocele is based on different criteria (see below). Correction for magnification is made possible by the incorporation of a midline radio-opaque centimeter ruler within the commode (Fig. 1).

Specific Sites of Organ Prolapse

The relative prevalence of prolapsed organs found at DCP in a large group of patients referred by urogynecology clinicians has been documented; a cystocele or a rectocele is present in more than 90% of such patients, and an enterocele is identified in approximately 30% (8). Sigmoidoceles are demonstrated in 4–5% of DCPs, but are more frequently identified by MRI. This is likely a consequence of limited retrograde filling of the sigmoid colon during DCP.

Rectocele

A rectocele is often defined radiologically as any anterior rectal bulge (6,7,24,25). When this definition is used, the size of a rectocele can be measured based upon its maximal depth measured at right angles to a line extended upward through the anterior wall of the anal canal (Fig. 2). With this measurement system, a rectocele has been considered small if less than 2 cm in depth, moderate if 2–4 cm in depth, and large if more than 4 cm in depth. Based on these criteria, the majority of asymptomatic women harbor a rectocele (26,27). Accordingly, this definition is flawed and has led others to restrict the diagnosis of rectocele to those anterior rectal bulges that are greater than 3 cm (28).

Proctography also determines whether barium is retained within the rectocele after evacuation (barium trapping) (Fig. 1; see also Fig. 5B). The likelihood of barium trapping is directly related to rectocele size (6). Trapping of contents is generally thought to explain the evacuation disturbance associated with a rectocele (29). Recent experience has shown that barium trapping diminishes considerably if a posttoilet image is obtained; this is presumably related to more effective evacuation in the privacy of the bathroom (30). Trapping is an important radiographic observation, because many surgeons are reluctant to operate on a rectocele unless it retains contrast.

If symptomatic, rectoceles usually are associated with straining and a sensation of incomplete evacuation. Patients may learn to obtain relief from the uncomfortable feeling associated with retained material by applying digital pressure to the vagina or perineum. The retained material within the rectocele may also cause dyspareunia due to pressure on the posterior vaginal wall. In some patients, impaired evacuation is probably associated with anismus rather than with the rectocele itself (31). Proctography may

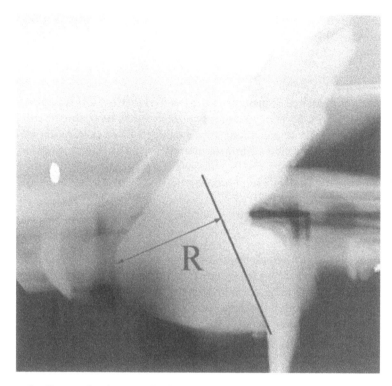

Figure 2 Rectocele. Image obtained during evacuation demonstrates a very prominent rectocele (R). The rectocele is large; it extends 5 cm (arrowed line) anterior to a line extended upwards from the anterior margin of the anal canal (black line).

suggest the presence of anismus and, therefore, the need for biofeedback therapy instead of surgery (32).

Historically, a variety of surgical techniques have been used for rectocele repair, including posterior colporrhaphy, transanal repair, and reinforcement of the rectovaginal septum with a graft (33). Discrete breaks in the rectovaginal fascia may account for many rectoceles; these fascial tears are amenable to direct surgical repair (34). The number of available surgical approaches reflects the variable results achieved by surgical correction. Postoperative assessment by DCP often shows that the rectocele persists despite symptomatic improvement, which is not accompanied by a corresponding reduction in rectocele size (35).

There is also an entity, sometimes referred to as a "posterior rectocele," in which an outpouching of the posterior rectal wall occurs. This outpouching is due to rectal herniation through a defect in the levator ani and is therefore more appropriately referred to as "perineal herniation." Unlike anterior rectoceles, these defects are usually lateralized to one side of the pelvic floor; they are therefore well visualized by either CT or MRI.

Enterocele

An enterocele is a herniation of small bowel either into the posterior peritoneal cul-de-sac in the rectovaginal space (Fig. 3) or into the vagina itself (see Fig. 5B). Definitive diagnosis therefore requires opacification of both the pelvic small bowel and the vagina. The incidence of enterocele has markedly increased as a result of widespread performance of both hysterectomy and cystourethropexy, both of which open up the posterior cul-de-sac. In one study, DCP revealed an enterocele in 64% of patients who had undergone a hysterectomy and in 27% of patients who had undergone cystopexy (18). Physicians performing surgery for stress

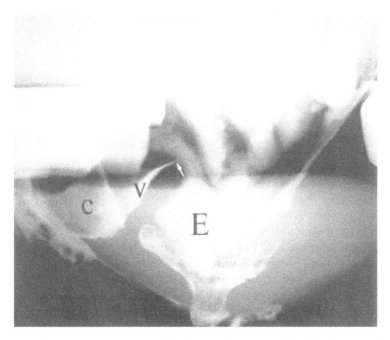

FIGURE 3   Enterocele. Postevacuation image shows considerable descent of loops of small bowel into the rectovaginal space, indicating an enterocele (E). Note downward displacement of anterior wall of vagina (v) by unopacified cystocele (c). Vaginal apex indicated by small arrow.

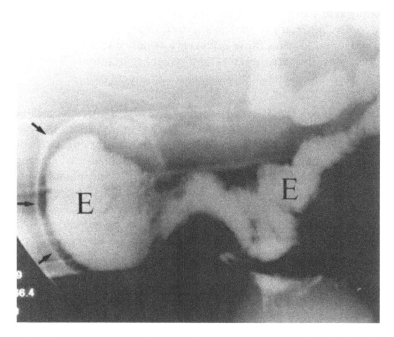

FIGURE 4   Massive enterocele following bladder neck suspension. Patient in whom cystourethropexy was performed 8 months previously for stress urinary incontinence now has a very large enterocele (E) demonstrated on posttoilet image. Arrows indicate contrast within anteriorly displaced vagina.

incontinence need to consider global evaluation of pelvic organs before undertaking such surgery (Fig. 4).

Unlike rectoceles, which are usually maximal during evacuation, enteroceles often become evident only at the end of evacuation. Repeated straining after evacuation may be essential for recognition of enteroceles. In one study, almost half (43%) of the enteroceles were only seen on postevacuation or posttoilet radiographs with the patient straining maximally, thus emphasizing the importance of this maneuver (8). Evacuation should be as complete as possible because the unemptied rectum or rectocele may prevent descent of an enterocele (Fig. 5) (20). Obtaining a posttoilet image after the patient has been to the bathroom to carry out further rectal evacuation therefore offers the best proctographic opportunity to detect an enterocele. Similar to the problem caused by an unemptied rectum, an insufficiently drained cystocele may result in a coexistent enterocele being overlooked or minimized.

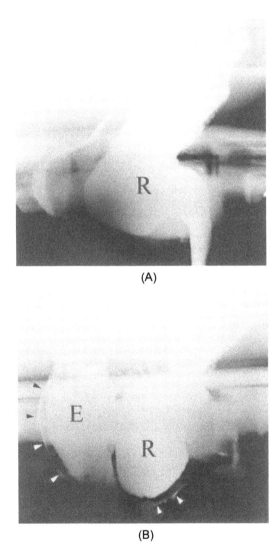

(A)

(B)

FIGURE 5   Competition for space between enterocele and rectocele. (A) Large rectocele (R) is demonstrated during evacuation (same image as in Fig. 2). (B) Postevacuation image shows that the rectocele (R) is now smaller, although it has retained considerable contrast (barium trapping). As a result of evacuation and straining, the anterior half of the grossly prolapsed vagina (arrowheads) is now occupied by an enterocele (E). (C) Preliminary image obtained after opacification of pelvic small bowel but before contrast filling of rectum demonstrates that the enterocele (E) is very large. Its full extent is only evident because the rectum is relatively collapsed.

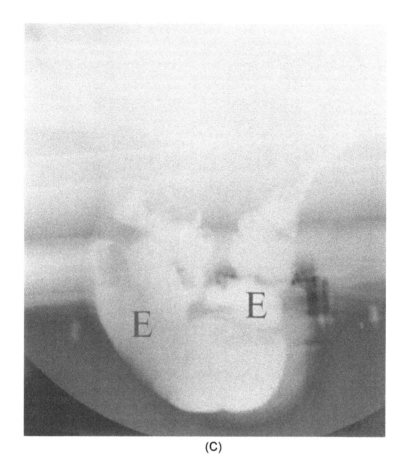

(C)

FIGURE 5   (continued)

Both enteroceles and rectoceles are well demonstrated by either DCP or MRI. Recently, detection of enteroceles by the technique of dynamic anorectal endosonography has also been described; in a small series, all enteroceles found in the pouch of Douglas by this endoluminal technique were confirmed by subsequent proctography (36). Anorectal endosonography is easier to perform and less cumbersome for the patient than proctography and deserves further evaluation.

The symptoms typically associated with an enterocele are a pelvic pressure or dragging sensation, especially when standing or bearing down. Symptoms of vaginal prolapse, pelvic fullness, and lower abdominal pain have been shown to disappear after enterocele repair (37). Enteroceles have long been held responsible for causing pressure on the rectum and thereby obstructing rectal evacuation, so-called defecation block (38). A more recent proctographic study showed that enteroceles do not impair rectal evacuation (39). Our impression, based on extensive proctographic studies, is that enteroceles descend only when the rectum starts to empty, and that it is the distended rectum that prevents enterocele descent rather than the rectum itself being obstructed by the enterocele. Not uncommonly, an enterocele accompanies a deep rectal intussusception or rectal prolapse.

Surgical repair of an enterocele requires obliteration of the herniated, bowel-containing cul-de-sac as well as resuspension of the unsupported vaginal axis and repair of other associated defects. Large enteroceles usually require a transabdominal approach so that concomitant abdominal sacrocolpopexy or a similar vaginal suspension procedure can be performed. Proctography is important in this respect, for the radiographic detection of a large, previously undiagnosed enterocele may change the surgical approach from a transvaginal to a transabdominal route of entry.

Peritoneocele

The combination of proctography and simultaneous peritoneography demonstrates the location and extent of the posterior peritoneal cul-de-sac. The term "peritoneocele" has been applied to herniation of the cul-de-sac. Bremmer et al. defined a peritoneocele as an extension of the rectouterine excavation below the upper third of the vagina (23).

When peritoneography is performed, only approximately 50% of peritoneoceles are found to contain bowel (22,23). In our MRI experience, however, either small or large bowel is usually present within a peritoneocele; this probably reflects our routine use of the posttoilet phase (19). Peritoneoceles have been classified as rectal, septal, or vaginal, depending on their location; rectal peritoneoceles are located within an associated rectal intussusception; septal peritoneoceles descend within the rectovaginal space; and vaginal peritoneoceles bulge into the vagina itself (23). Recognition of a peritoneocele, whether by peritoneography or MRI, is important because it predisposes to enterocele (or sigmoidocele) and suggests the need for operative closure of the cul-de-sac if pelvic floor reconstructive surgery is undertaken (19). The presence of a peritoneocele should be suspected at routine DCP if there is unexplained widening of the rectovaginal space; in our experience, this is found in 9% of DCPs (8).

Sigmoidocele

A sigmoidocele is a redundancy of the sigmoid colon that extends caudally into the cul-de-sac (Fig. 1) (40). They are less common than enteroceles on DCP, being found in approximately 5% of proctograms (8,40,41). As with other organ prolapses, there is no unanimity of definition. Fenner (41) defined a sigmoidocele as sigmoid colon extending more than 4 cm below the pubococcygeal line; according to our definition (see above), such a finding would constitute a moderate-sized sigmoid herniation (19,41).

Large sigmoidoceles are often associated with constipation (40,41). The redundant colon may compress the rectum and obstruct defecation; this is more likely to occur with a sigmoidocele than an enterocele because colonic content is more solid (41). Stasis of material within the redundant sigmoid colon may also be contributory by causing further discomfort and straining (40).

Sigmoidoceles, even when large, are usually not detected on physical examination (19,41). Sigmoid resection and/or sigmoidopexy have been shown to provide striking relief of associated constipation. Because bowel surgery is generally performed by a colorectal surgeon rather than a pelvic floor reconstructive surgeon, preoperative recognition by proctography is important (41). Obliteration of the cul-de-sac and repair of associated pelvic floor defects are usually accomplished at the same operative setting.

Vaginal Vault Prolapse

Vaginal vault prolapse involves prolapse of the apex of the vagina toward, through, or beyond the introitus, regardless as to whether a hysterectomy has been previously performed (42). External vaginal prolapse or vaginal prolapse to the introitus is usually clinically obvious. Vaginal vault prolapse is almost always associated with prolapse of other pelvic organs, the most common of which is an enterocele. This latter association usually reflects loss of support at the level of the vaginal apex, due to damage to the utero-sacral-cardinal complex at the time of hysterectomy.

Provided adequate vaginal opacification is maintained throughout the study, the location of the vaginal apex can usually be determined on the postevacuation and posttoilet images (Figs. 1 and 3). The degree of vaginal vault prolapse can then be assessed based on the grading system already described. However, when there is marked descent or eversion of the vagina, it is generally impossible to determine the location of the vaginal apex (Fig. 5B). With such gross vaginal prolapse, clinical inspection usually is self-declarative.

The degree of vaginal vault prolapse is important because it may influence both the route and type of surgical repair to be undertaken. For example, the less severe degrees of vault prolapse may be corrected transvaginally by a sacrospinous ligament suspension, whereas a trans-abdominal sacral colpopexy involving attachment of the vault to the sacral periosteum with a suspensory sling of synthetic material is often necessary for more severe vaginal descent. Obliteration of the cul-de-sac and repair of concomitant pelvic floor defects is carried out at the same time.

The direction of vaginal displacement is a valuable diagnostic adjunct. Anterior vaginal displacement indicates posterior vaginal wall failure, which traditionally is considered to be due to pressure from a rectocele. Proctography, however, reveals that approximately one third of patients with anterior displacement of the vagina have an enterocele or sigmoidocele (Fig. 4) (8). Inferior displacement of the vagina, on the other hand, is typically due to pressure from a cystocele (Fig. 3), although in

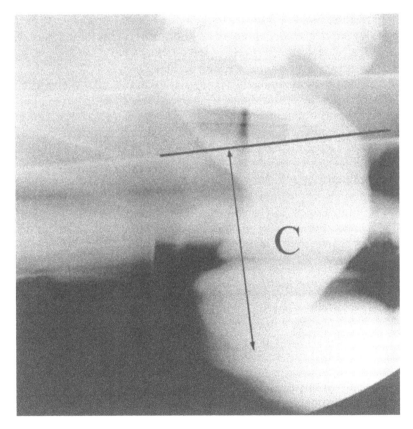

Figure 6 Cystocele. Cystogram image obtained on maximum strain shows a large cystocele (C). The base of the cystocele extends 7 cm (arrowed line) below the pubococcygeal line (straight line).

a small minority of patients this finding may be due to an intravaginal enterocele (8).

Cystocele

Cystoceles are the result of defects in the pubocervical fascia. Symptoms caused by a cystocele may be minimal until it reaches the introitus; the most common symptoms are a heaviness or "feeling of something bulging." Large cystoceles may also lead to voiding dysfunction.

Cystoceles are defined radiologically by descent of the bladder base below the pubococcygeal line (Fig. 6). Contrast opacification is not essential for the recognition of cystoceles, as they can be inferred by downward displacement of the vagina provided that the vagina is well opacified (see Fig. 3). If cystography is not performed, it is often nevertheless necessary to catheterize the bladder in order to facilitate bladder drainage. If this is not done, the large area occupied by an undrained cystocele may prevent detection of a coexistent enterocele or rectocele.

Retention of the catheter within the bladder may be useful during filming as it can indicate the axis of the urethra and identify the region of the bladder neck. The urethral axis is normally less than 35° to the vertical; a horizontally inclined urethra indicates a urethrocele. Funneling (beaking) of the bladder neck at rest may indicate intrinsic sphincter deficiency but is a nonspecific sign and may also be seen in continent women (43).

Symptomatic cystoceles are generally treated surgically; in recent years, abdominal or vaginal paravaginal repair has tended to replace anterior colporrhaphy. An anti-incontinence procedure is frequently included because elevation of the bladder often unkinks the bladder neck and unmasks urinary incontinence.

MAGNETIC RESONANCE IMAGING

Introduction

Reasons for using MRI to image pelvic organ prolapse include superior visualization of the soft tissues compared with fluoroscopy, decreased invasiveness of the study, lack of ionizing radiation, and flexibility to display pelvic anatomy in multiple planes (44). The limitations of MRI are imaging patients in the supine position and potential to underestimate rectal abnormalities, especially if rectal contrast is not used. Interest in this modality for pelvic floor imaging has been relatively recent, and validation of the accuracy of MRI and optimal technique for the study is still in the process of being determined.

MRI Compared with DCP

When MRI has been compared to fluoroscopic cystoproctography, the results have been variable. For the diagnosis of rectoceles, Delemarre et al. (45) found that the rectoceles were smaller on MRI, while Gufler et al. (46) found that equivalent information was obtained from both studies. However, both studies were performed without rectal contrast, and the former study was done with the patient in the prone position.

In contrast, Lienemann et al. (28), Vanbeckevoort et al. (9), and Kelvin et al. (19) compared MRI with fluoroscopy using rectal contrast. In the first study, 44 patients had MRI with rectal and vaginal contrast as well as fluoroscopy (28). Uterine prolapse and enteroceles were detected in greater numbers on MR than fluoroscopy. The superior soft tissue contrast on MRI allowed visualization of the cervix and defects involving the rectovaginal septum. However, Vanbeckevoort et al. found that more abnormal compartments were seen on fluoroscopy than on MRI in 35 patients (9). In another approach, Kelvin et al. studied 10 patients and specifically asked them to defecate rectal contrast during the MRI study (19). In this study, a similar number of rectoceles and cystoceles were detected on MRI and fluoroscopy, but the size of the abnormality was greater on fluoroscopy likely due to the seated position.

Studies in larger numbers of patients will help to clarify the sensitivity and accuracy of MRI as compared with DCP, which is the traditional test. When comparing MRI defecography in a vertical configuration magnet with fluoroscopy, both tests were found to be comparable for the detection of anorectal pathology, and soft tissue abnormalities in the pelvis were also diagnosed on MRI (47).

MRI Technique

On MRI, sagittal images of the pelvis are obtained as patients increase their intra-abdominal pressure. On these images, the bulging of the bladder, cervix, and rectum into the vagina can be appreciated as on physical examination and DCP. These abnormalities are also visible on axial images at the appropriate level, and inferior displacement of the viscera is seen on coronal images. Single shot fast spin echo T2-weighted images are usually obtained as bladder urine, pelvic fat, and rectal gel are high in signal, but gradient echo images have also been obtained (48).

The technique for MRI is not standardized, and different approaches have been reported in the literature. Midline sagittal straining images, sagittal images during patient defecation, and cystographic and proctographic phases have been reported (15,19,28). If rectal contrast is not given, patients are asked to strain maximally as the images are acquired. If rectal contrast is administered, patients are asked to defecate onto an absorbent pad placed on the MRI table. Rectal contrast agents include sterile lubricating jelly, ultrasound gel, and mashed potatoes mixed with gadolinium. Kelvin et al. have shown that contamination of the magnet is not a problem since the material used for rectal contrast is semi-solid (19).

The use of rectal contrast addresses concerns in the gynecological literature that pelvic floor defects may be inapparent due to suboptimal straining in the supine position during MRI (4,49). Another pitfall of asking patients to strain but not defecate during the MRI study is that they may inadvertently contract their muscles and actually raise the pelvic floor (50). Kelvin et al. found that 9 of 10 patients given rectal contrast were able to subsequently defecate in the supine position in the MRI magnet (19). An additional benefit of using rectal contrast is that abnormalities of rectal evacuation, such as rectal intussusception and anismus, that currently are evaluated by fluoroscopy can also be detected on MRI (51,52). Sample protocols for MRI are described in the following paragraphs.

Prior to starting the study, the examination is described to the patient, including the importance of bearing down maximally and defecating on request. Initially, the patient is asked to void to reduce bladder distention since, as described above, it has been shown to mask abnormalities on fluoroscopic studies (6). If a pessary is present in the vagina, the patient is asked to remove it since it hinders organ prolapse (53). The patient is positioned supine on a waterproof pad with a pelvic coil in place. The knees are flexed over a pillow to help the patient strain while supine (53). Approximately 120 mL of sterile lubricating jelly is inserted via a catheter tip syringe into the rectum and 15–20 mL of the same jelly is placed into the vagina.

After the scout images, a sagittal single shot fast spin echo T2-weighted scan of the pelvis is obtained. The midsagittal slice where the urethra, vagina, and anus are best seen is selected for performing the single location defecatory images. The patient is asked to defecate, and multiple images are obtained at this level as the degree of pelvic floor descent and organ prolapse are monitored until no further prolapse is seen. Following this sequence, additional images can be acquired in the sagittal plane to include the parasagittal tissues and in the axial and coronal planes to demonstrate organ descent and bulging of the pelvic floor. Both rest and strain images are obtained. Specific parameters are single shot fast spin echo sequence with time to echo of 60 ms, field of view of 28–32 cm, slice thickness of 6 mm with a 2 mm gap, matrix size of 256 x 256, bandwidth of 32 kHz, and an echo train length of 16. Another technique that can be used for pelvic floor MRI involves placing sonography gel in the rectum and vagina and a fixed volume of saline in the bladder (54). Rest, squeeze, strain, and defecation sagittal images are obtained with TR 5.8 ms, TE 2.5 ms, flip angle 70 degrees, slice thickness 7 mm, matrix 224 x 256, and the body coil.

Kelvin et al. described a triphasic method for the MRI examination similar to fluoroscopy (19). Initially, the bladder is catheterized and 50 mL of saline infused followed by mid-sagittal rest and strain images to evaluate bladder descent. Next the bladder is drained and ultrasound gel placed in the vagina and rectum for evacuation images in the midsagittal plane. The patient completes rectal evacuation in a restroom and is then rescanned to evaluate for enteroceles that may have been inapparent when the bladder and rectum were distended (4,6). Kelvin et al. no longer opacify the bladder during MRI; this was only done in their study population to exactly mimic the fluoroscopic examination.

An MRI technique without contrast involves initially obtaining sagittal images through the pelvis (53). Multiple midsagittal 5 mm thick single shot fast spin echo images are then obtained during patient straining.

Although MRI studies are generally performed with the patient supine, a few studies have been done on vertical configuration magnets (52,55,56). Both rest and strain images and defecatory images have been obtained (52,55,56). For defecation, a mixture of mashed potatoes and gadolinium has been placed in the rectum and gradient echo images obtained during evacuation (57).

Interpretation of the MRI Study

There is some variability in the criteria for diagnosing organ prolapse on MRI. The most commonly used reference is the pubococcygeal line, which itself is not defined consistently in the literature. It has been drawn on the midsagittal image from the inferior pubic symphysis to the last coccygeal joint, the sacrococcygeal joint, or the junction of the first and second coccygeal segments (Fig. 7) (2,17,50,53). Using this line, pelvic organ prolapse is diagnosed if the bladder base, uterine cervix, and vaginal apex descend below it (2,28,50). Widening of the rectovaginal space below the upper one third of the vagina by peritoneal fat, small bowel, or sigmoid colon is called peritoneocele, enterocele, or sigmoidocele (50). An anterior bulge in the rectal contour greater than 2 cm relative to the anal canal is called a rectocele (50). Goh et al. found that using these criteria, prolapse was only infrequently seen in normal volunteers and therefore these guidelines can be used to evaluate symptomatic patients (50).

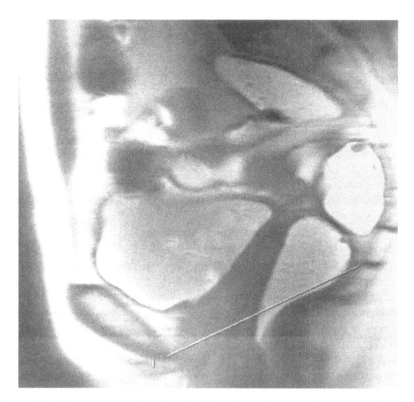

FIGURE 7   Pubococcygeal line. Sagittal T2-weighted image of the pelvis with rectal contrast. The pubococcygeal line is drawn from the inferior pubis to the last coccygeal joint.

Another measurement method is the "HMO" classification (15,53). The "H" line is the antero-posterior width of the pelvic hiatus. On a sagittal image, this line is drawn from the inferior pubic symphysis to the pubo-rectalis (Fig. 8). The normal length of this line is less than 6 cm. Organ prolapse is diagnosed when the organs have descended below the "H" line. Organ descent 0–2 cm below the "H" line is graded as small, 2–4 cm is moderate, and > 4 cm is large. The "M" line measures the descent of the levator plate relative to the pubococcygeal line and is normally less than 2 cm.

The most common method of using bony landmarks (pubococcygeal line) on MRI as opposed to using soft tissue landmarks on physical examination has resulted in difficulty comparing the two techniques (58).

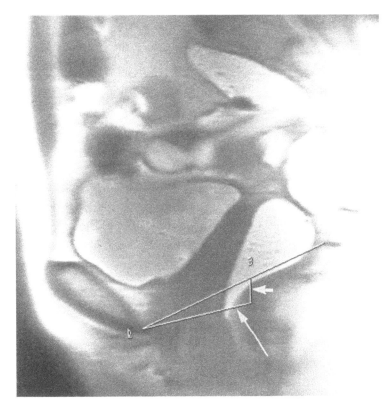

FIGURE 8   H and M lines. Sagittal T2-weighted image of the pelvis with rectal contrast. The "H" line (long arrow) is drawn from the inferior pubis to the puborectalis. The "M" line (short arrow) is drawn from the pubococcygeal line to the "H" line.

On physical examination, the hymenal ring is used for grading prolapse (58). A midpubic line on MRI has been proposed to approximate the hymenal ring for grading prolapse in a fashion similar to physical examination (59). The line is drawn on a sagittal image through the long axis of the pubic bone, and organ position is determined relative to this (Fig. 9).

Additional measurements that can be performed on MRI are the width and area of the pelvic hiatus on axial images and the angulation of the levator plate on sagittal images. The transverse diameter of the levator hiatus on axial images measures the extent of ballooning of the levator muscle from rest to strain.

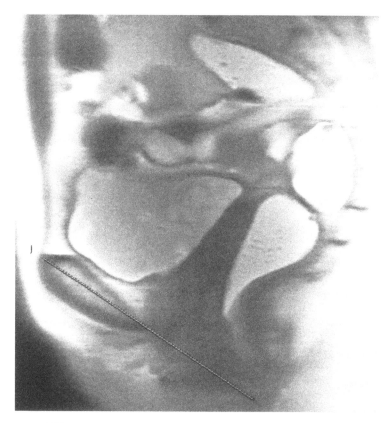

Figure 9 Midpubic line. Sagittal T2-weighted image of the pelvis with rectal contrast. The midpubic line is drawn through the long axis of the pubis.

Specific Sites of Organ Prolapse

Rectum

Abnormalities of the rectum seen on MRI include anterior rectoceles, perineal hernias, and intussusception. They are easily identified with the use of rectal contrast and during defecation. The rectal wall is outlined by the contrast and bulging of the contour or infolding can then be appreciated (Fig. 10; see also Fig. 13). Tears in the rectovaginal fascia result in anterior rectoceles and weakness or defects in the levator ani muscle result in perineal hernias (60). These areas of thinning and bulging of the levator muscle are inferred on DCP but directly visualized on MRI. In addition,

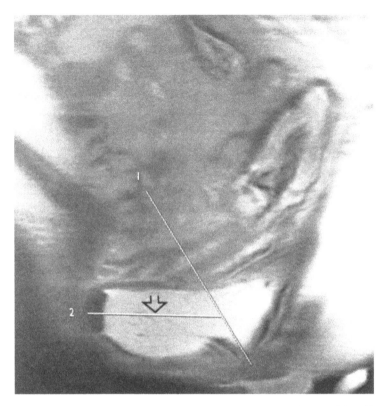

FIGURE 10 Anterior rectocele. Sagittal T2-weighted image of the pelvis with rectal contrast during patient defecation. There is a large anterior rectocele. The size is measured as the length (open arrow) anterior to the anal canal.

the multiplanar imaging capability allows for assessment of lateral rectal bulges.

Using fluoroscopic criteria, an anterior bulge of the rectal contour smaller than 2–3 cm is considered normal (27,61,62). As stated earlier, there is overlap in the size of rectoceles between asymptomatic and symptomatic women, and treatment is not based on size alone (61, 63–65). Symptoms such as discomfort from vaginal prolapse of a large rectocele or a sensation of incomplete emptying with defecation guide the need for surgical repair (61,62). Therefore, MRI findings must be correlated with the patient's symptoms. The sensitivity of supine MRI for detection of rectoceles is reported to be 76–100% and specificity as 50% (14,17).

MRI defecography performed on a vertical configuration magnet, if available, can also be used to assess patients with rectal symptoms. It has the potential to be the ideal test since the advantages of DCP and MRI are combined. Defecatory images are obtained with the patient in a seated position, and the soft tissues of the pelvis are visible. Similar to supine MRI defecography studies, rectoceles, anorectal junction descent and intussusception are seen on upright scans (51,52). With intussusception, prolapsing rectal folds are identified in the rectum or anus. In a study comparing supine MRI with patient straining and sitting MRI defecography, intussusceptions seen on the seated study were missed on the supine study (57). Whether the supine position or lack of defecation accounted for the lower detection of intussusception on the supine images is not known. However, the detection rate of other symptomatic abnormalities was similar on both tests. Lamb et al. also assessed defecatory studies in a vertical configuration magnet in 40 patients with defecatory dysfunction and found both the anterior and posterior compartments were satisfactorily evaluated (52).

An additional role of MRI is in evaluating the integrity of the anal sphincter (25). The internal and external anal sphincters can be assessed both for their thickness and for the presence of tears.

Cul-de-Sac

The prevalence of an enterocele type defect in the posterior/superior rectovaginal septum is 18–37% in patients with pelvic floor abnormalities (54). This defect allows herniation of peritoneal contents into the rectovaginal space. In normal individuals, no space between the rectum and vagina is identified at rest or with straining on MRI (54). In patients with pelvic floor dysfunction, a small space may be seen at rest that widens during straining (Fig. 11) (54). The contents of the space are easily identified on MRI without the need for oral or peritoneal contrast (14). These include mesenteric fat or fluid, small bowel, or large bowel (Fig. 12). Colon is the least common, being present in 5 of 49 cases in one MRI series (54). The sensitivity of MRI for detection of these defects is 87% and specificity is 80% (14).

Urethra, Vagina, and Bladder

In patients with deficient urethral support, there is excessive change in the urethral axis with increased abdominal pressure that is known as urethral hypermobility. As a result, when abdominal pressure increases with coughing or sneezing, it is transmitted preferentially to the bladder rather than the urethra and there is urine leakage. This gives rise to the symptom of genuine stress incontinence.

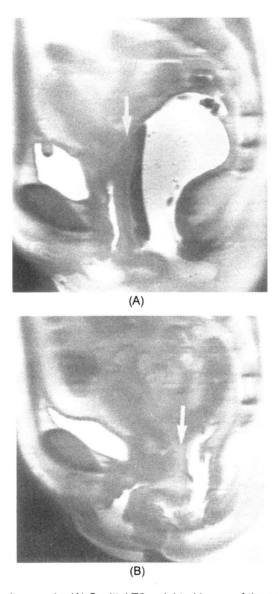

(A)

(B)

FIGURE 11   Peritoneocele. (A) Sagittal T2-weighted image of the pelvis with rectal and vaginal contrast. The patient is at rest and the vagina and rectum are closely apposed (arrow). (B) During defecation, there is widening of the rectovaginal space (arrow) with fat descent of the cervix also seen. (C) Parasagittal image during continued defecation shows increasing fat (arrow) in the rectovaginal space compatible with peritoneocele. C = cervix; R = rectum.

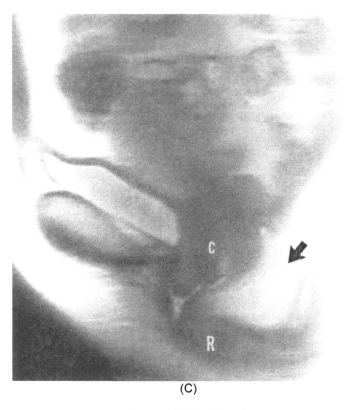

(C)

FIGURE 11   (continued)

On MRI, as on physical examination, a change in the urethral axis is seen with patient straining. On sagittal images, the urethra changes from a normal vertical position to an oblique or horizontal orientation (Fig. 13). A urethral angle greater than 30 degrees from the vertical is considered abnormal (15). Other findings described in women with incontinence include a dorsal oblique orientation of the ligaments suspending the urethra and increased volume of the retropubic space (66,67). Funneling or dilatation of the proximal urethral lumen can also occur with increased mobility of the posterior urethral wall (68). Patients with deficiency of the intrinsic urethral sphincter may be injected with collagen deep to the mucosa below the bladder neck. This injected collagen can be visualized on MRI (69).

The layers of the urethral wall are demonstrated on T2-weighted images obtained with a surface or endovaginal coil (70). The mucosa and

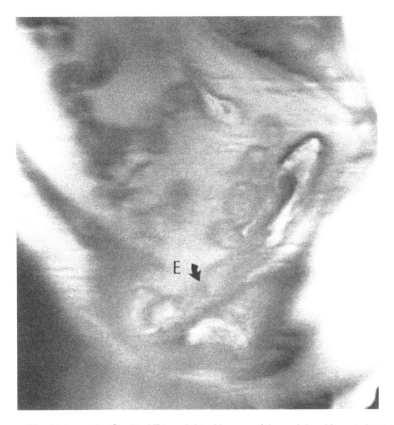

FIGURE 12   Enterocele. Sagittal T2-weighted image of the pelvis with rectal contrast shows small bowel loops (arrow) low in the pelvis compatible with enterocele (E).

submucosa are hypointense, the smooth muscle layer is hyperintense, and the outer striated muscle layer is hypointense on axial images (Fig. 14) (71). High-resolution images with an endourethral coil have been attempted to better delineate urethral anatomy (72). However, the correlation between muscle bulk on MRI and incontinence is not known at the present time.

On axial images, attempts have been made to identify the support ligaments of the urethra. The urethra is believed to be fixed either directly or indirectly to the pubic bone. It is not clear if ligaments directly attach the urethra to the pelvic sidewall or whether this lateral support is through the perivaginal fascia (70,73). Lateral ligaments extending from the urethra to the arcus tendineus fascia pelvis have been described in healthy volunteers and shown to have a dorsal oblique angulation in patients with

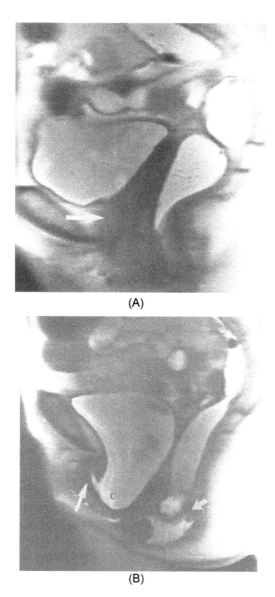

(A)

(B)

FIGURE 13 Urethral hypermobility and cystocele. (A) Sagittal T2-weighted image of the pelvis with rectal contrast. The patient is at rest and the urethra (arrow) is normal in orientation. (B) During patient defecation, the urethral axis changes from vertical to horizontal, the urethra lies under the pubis, and there is funneling (long arrow). A cystocele (c) also develops, and there is infolding of the rectal wall (short arrow) compatible with intussusception.

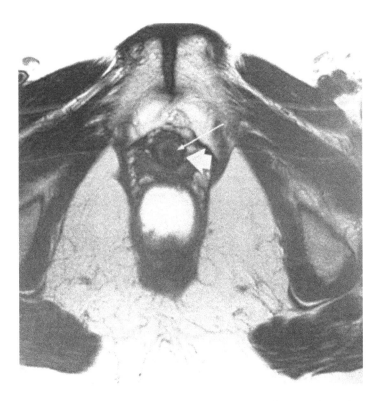

FIGURE 14   Urethral anatomy. Axial T2-weighted image of the urethra shows central hypointense submucosa (long arrow), middle hyperintense smooth muscle layer, and outer hypointense striated muscle layer (short arrow).

incontinence (67,74). Attenuation or absence of the ligaments from the posterior pubic symphysis to the anterior vaginal wall was also noted in a small study of incontinent women (66).

In addition to supporting ligaments, the mid and distal urethra is embedded in the anterior wall of the vagina. Lateral tears in the endopelvic fascia can also result in diminished urethral and vaginal support. Alteration in the morphology of the vagina is an indirect sign suggestive of this tear. On MRI performed in patients prior to and following surgery for lateral vaginal support defects, there was loss of the normal "H" shape of the vagina initially that was restored after surgery (75). The "H" shape is described on axial images where the lateral edges of the vagina are directed anteriorly towards the pubis while the center is posterior to the urethra (Fig. 15). This shape is felt to be due to the lateral insertions of the

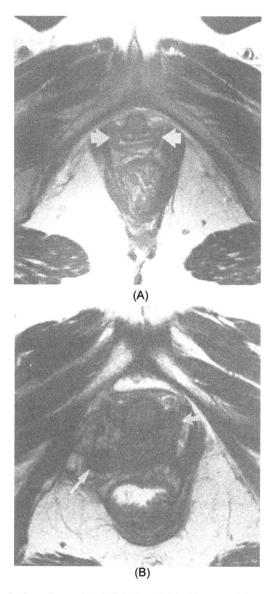

(A)

(B)

FIGURE 15   Vaginal anatomy. (A) Axial T2-weighted image of the pelvis shows normal "H" shape of the vagina with the lateral walls (arrows) extending anteriorly. (B)
Axial T2-weighted image of the pelvis in a patient with pelvic floor dysfunction
shows loss of the "H" shape with the right wall (long arrow) being posterior.
Normal left vaginal wall (short arrow). Findings possibly due to right paravaginal
fascial tear.

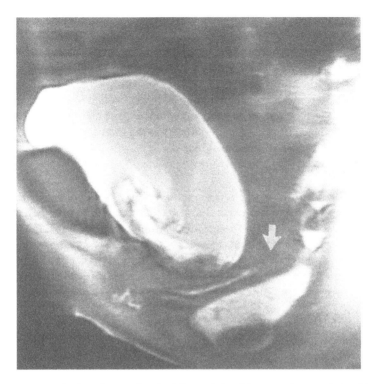

FIGURE 16 Vaginal prolapse. Sagittal T2-weighted image of the pelvis with rectal and vaginal contrast during patient defecation. The vagina (arrow) is low in the pelvis compatible with vaginal prolapse. A cystocele is also present.

endopelvic fascia overlying the anterior vaginal wall (66). Although loss of the normal "H" shape of the vagina is suggestive of deficient vaginal support, it has also been seen in normal nulliparous volunteers (67,74). Another sign of a lateral vaginal fascial tear described is lateral deviation of the anterior portion of the levator muscle (76).

On sagittal images, the proximal vagina has a backward angulation over the levator muscle (59). The attachment of the uterosacral ligaments from the cervix and upper vagina to the presacral fascia pulls the vagina over the levator plate. The vagina and vaginal apex are displaced inferiorly with straining in patients with prolapse (Fig. 16). The bladder may bulge into and deform the anterior wall and the rectum may deform the posterior wall. With complete prolapse beyond the hymen, there is a bulging mass out of the vagina and the vaginal mucosa is everted and exposed. In patients who have had a sacral colpopexy patch placed, a hypointense band can be seen extending from the vagina to the sacrum on T2-weighted images (77).

With cystoceles, there is descent of the bladder base that is readily evident on MRI (Fig. 13). A sensitivity of 100% and specificity of 83% is reported using the pubosacral line as a reference (14). The bladder base and cervical junction have been shown to be lower both at rest and straining in multiparous women when compared to nulliparous women (55). Also in patients with constipation, descent of the bladder and cervix is greater than in patients with fecal incontinence (78).

Pelvic Floor

The levator ani muscle with its three components, the iliococcygeus, the pubococcygeus, and the puborectalis, is part of the floor of the pelvis and is easily identified on MRI (79). The normal volume of the muscle is approximately 32–46 mL, and the normal thickness is approximately 3 mm for the iliococcygeus and 5–6 mm for the puborectalis (74,80,81). The right side of the puborectalis has been reported to be thinner than the left in normals; this difference may partly be due to technical reasons (82,74,81,82).

The iliococcygeus is posterior and superior and is normally convex cranially on coronal images of the posterior pelvis (80,81,83). In women without prolapse, the levator plate is nearly parallel to the pubococcygeal line on sagittal images and a line drawn from the levator plate crosses the pubis (74,84). However, in patients with prolapse, a line drawn from the levator plate is caudal to the pubis on sagittal images (84). With straining, the muscle bulges caudally and laterally and the pelvic hiatus enlarges (Fig. 17).

The pelvic hiatus is enclosed by the puborectalis muscle (81). The normal width of the hiatus on an axial image is approximately 31–42 mm (74,74). The size of the hiatus increases with straining in asymptomatic as well as symptomatic women, but the increase is greater in the latter group (Fig. 18). The mean area of the hiatus measured 2006 mm^2 at rest and 2783 mm^2 with straining in a study of 25 asymptomatic women (50). In another study of constipated women, the hiatus area increased by 159% in patients compared with an increase of 55% in normal controls (78). Both the size of the hiatus and caudal angulation of the levator may not change after surgery for prolapse (5).

Occasionally, focal bulges and thinning of the muscle with protrusion of pelvic fat and/or viscera may be seen on MRI (85). The signal intensity of the muscle may also appear increased on proton density images possibly due to fatty infiltration (82). Muscle movement with contraction and straining can also be dynamically monitored (86).

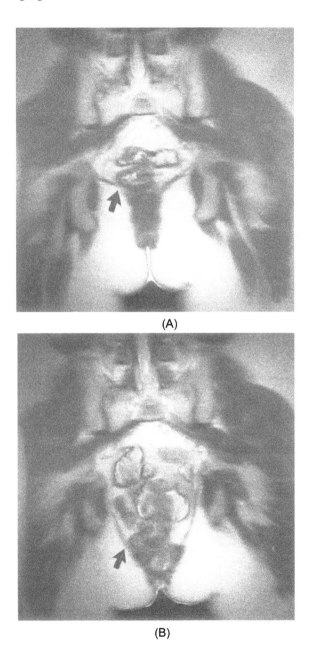

(A)

(B)

FIGURE 17 Bulging of the levator ani. (A) Coronal T2-weighted image of the posterior pelvis shows normal configuration of the levator ani (arrow). (B) During patient straining, there is caudal angulation and bulging of the muscle (arrow).

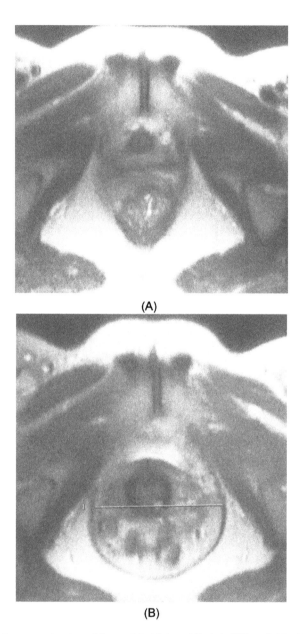

(A)

(B)

FIGURE 18   Increase in size of the pelvic hiatus. (A) Axial T2-weighted image of the pelvis with the patient at rest shows normal size of the pelvic hiatus enclosed by the levator ani muscle. (B) During patient straining, the width of the hiatus (line) increases abnormally, and there is descent of the cervix and bladder.

TREATMENT CONSIDERATIONS

A variety of nonsurgical approaches may be utilized in the management of pelvic organ prolapse if symptoms are not severe or if the patient refuses or is unfit for surgery. Nonsurgical options include pessaries, pelvic floor muscle exercises (Kegel exercises), and biofeedback therapy.

Goals of surgical therapy include symptomatic relief, restoration of anatomical relationships, and preservation of organ function. Many pelvic floor surgeons believe correction of all pelvic support defects should be attempted, whether symptomatic or not. If comprehensive repair is not done, coexisting asymptomatic support defects are likely to become symptomatic within a relatively short period of time (Fig. 4) (34).

More accurate preoperative assessment by DCP or MRI should hopefully reduce the incidence of operative failure. These techniques help the surgeon plan the different components of pelvic reconstructive surgery and, importantly, determine whether a transvaginal or transabdominal approach will be required. The current trend is toward the transabdominal route. Available evidence suggests that the reoperation rate is halved when the abdominal approach is employed (87). Large enteroceles and marked vaginal vault prolapse, in particular, are much more amenable to correction by transabdominal surgery. It should be recognized that enteroceles and sigmoidoceles often escape preoperative detection unless radiological evaluation is performed. Global assessment of pelvic organ prolapse is optimized by ensuring that competing organs are effectively emptied by virtue of a triphasic approach. As expressed succinctly by Halligan, "the global pelvic floor specialist has arrived, and his closest ally is the radiologist" (88).

REFERENCES

1. Bump RC, Norton PA. Epidemiology and natural history of pelvic floor dsyfunction. Obstet Gynecol Clin NA 1998; 25:723–746.
2. Yang A, Mostwin JL, Rosenshein NB, Zerhouni EA. Pelvic floor descent in women: dynamic evaluation with fast MR imaging and cinematic display. Radiology 1991; 179:25–33.
3. Maglinte DDT, Kelvin FM, Hale DS, Benson JT. Dynamic cystoproctography: a unifying diagnostic approach to pelvic floor and anorectal dysfunction. Am J Roentgenol 1997; 169:759–767.
4. Weidner AC, Low VHS. Imaging studies of the pelvic floor. Obstet Gynecol Clin 1998; 25:826–848.
5. Goodrich MA, Webb MJ, King BF, Bampton AEH, Campeau NG, Riederer SJ. Magnetic resonance imaging of pelvic floor relaxation: dynamic analysis and evaluation of patients before and after surgical repair. Obstet Gynecol 1993; 82:883–891.

6. Kelvin FM, Maglinte DDT, Hornback JA, Benson JT. Pelvic prolapse: assessment with evacuation proctography (defecography). Radiology 1992; 184:547–551.

7. Altringer WE, Saclarides TJ, Dominguez JM, Brubaker LT, Smith CS. Four-contrast defecography: pelvic "floor-oscopy.". Dis Colon Rectum 1995; 38:695–699.

8. Kelvin FM, Hale DS, Maglinte DDT, Patten BJ, Benson JT. Female pelvic organ prolapse: diagnostic contribution of dynamic cystoproctography and comparison with physical examination. Am J Roentgenol 1999; 173:31–37.

9. Vanbeckevoort D, Van Hoe L, Oyen R, Ponette E, Deprest J. Pelvic floor descent in females: comparative study of colpocystodefecography and dynamic fast MR imaging. J Magn Reson Imaging 1999; 9:373–377.

10. Brubaker L, Retzky S, Smith C, Saclarides T. Pelvic floor evacuation with dynamic fluoroscopy. Obstet Gynecol 1993; 82:863–868.

11. Kelvin FM, Maglinte DDT. Radiologic investigation of prolapse. J Pelv Surg 2000; 6:218–220.

12. Maglinte DDT, Kelvin FM, Fitzgerald K, Hale DS, Benson JT. Association of compartment defects in pelvic floor dysfunction. Am J Roentgenol 1999; 172:439–444.

13. Rentsch M, Paetzel C, Lenhart M, Feuerbach S, Jauch KW, Furst A. Dynamic magnetic resonance imaging defecography. Dis Colon Rectum 2001; 44: 999–1007.

14. Gousse AE, Barbaric ZL, Safir MH, Madjar S, Marumoto AK, Raz S. Dynamic half Fourier acquisition, single shot turbo spin-echo magnetic resonance imaging for evaluating the female pelvis. J Urol 2000; 164: 1606–1613.

15. Comiter CV, Vasavada SP, Barbaric ZL, Gousse AE, Raz S. Grading pelvic prolapse and pelvic floor relaxation using dynamic magnetic resonance imaging. Urol 1999; 54:454–457.

16. Kaufman HS, Buller JL, Thompson JR, Pannu HK, DeMeester SL, Genadry RR, Bluemke DA, Jones B, Rychcik JL, Cundiff GW. Dynamic pelvic magnetic resonance imaging and cystocolpoproctography alter surgical management of pelvic floor disorders. Dis Colon Rectum 2001; 44: 1575–1584.

17. Tunn R, Paris S, Taupitz M, Hamm B, Fischer W. MR imaging in posthysterectomy vaginal prolapse. Int Urogynecol J Pelvic Floor Dysfunct 2000; 11:87–92.

18. Hock D, Lombard R, Jehaes C, Markiewicz S, Penders L, Fontaine F, Cusumano G, Nelissen G. Colpocystodefecography. Dis Colon Rectum 1993; 36:1015–1021.

19. Kelvin FM, Maglinte DDT, Hale DS, Benson JT. Female pelvic organ prolapse: a comparison of triphasic dynamic MR imaging and triphasic fluoroscopic cystocolpoproctography. Am J Roentgenol 2000; 174:81–88.

20. Kelvin FM, Maglinte DDT. Dynamic cystoproctography of female pelvic floor defects and their interrelationships. Am J Roentgenol 1997; 169:769–774.

21. Ho LM, Low VHS, Freed KS. Vaginal opacification during defecography: utility of placing a folded gauze square at the introitus. Abdom Imaging 1999; 24:562–564.
22. Halligan S, Bartram CI. Evacuation proctography combined with positive contrast peritoneography to demonstrate pelvic floor hernias. Abdom Imaging 1995; 20:442–445.
23. Bremmer S, Mellgren A, Holmstrom B, Lopez A, Uden R. Peritoneocele: visualization with defecography and peritoneography performed simultaneously. Radiology 1997; 202:373–377.
24. Halligan S, Spence-Jones C, Kamm MA, Bartram CI. Dynamic cystoproctography and physiological testing in women with urinary stress incontinence and urogenital prolapse. Clin Radiol 1996; 51:785–790.
25. Stoker J, Halligan S, Bartram CI. Pelvic floor imaging. Radiology 2001; 218:621–641.
26. Bartram CI, Turnbull GK, Lennard-Jones JE. Evacuation proctography: an investigation of rectal expulsion in 20 subjects without defecatory disturbance. Gastrointest Radiol 1988; 13:72–80.
27. Shorvon PJ, McHugh S, Diamant NE, Somers S, Stevenson GW. Defecography in normal volunteers: results and implications. Gut 1989; 30:1737–1749.
28. Lienemann A, Anthuber C, Baron A, Kohz P, Reiser M. Dynamic MR colpocystorectography assessing pelvic-floor descent. Eur Radiol 1997; 7:1309–1317.
29. Van Dam JH, Ginai AZ, Gosselink MJ, Huisman WM, Bonjer HJ, Hop WC, Schouten WR. Role of defecography in predicting clinical outcome of rectocele repair. Dis Colon Rectum 1997; 40:201–207.
30. Greenberg T, Kelvin FM, Maglinte DDT. Barium trapping in rectoceles: Are we trapped by the wrong definition?. Abdom Imaging 2001; 26:587–590.
31. Johansson CD, Nilsson BY, Holmstram B, Dolk A, Mellgren A. Association between rectocele and paradoxical sphincter response. Dis Colon Rectum 1992; 35:503–509.
32. Halligan S, Bartram CI, Park HJ, Kamm MA. Proctographic features of anismus. Radiology 1995; 197:679–682.
33. Kahn MA, Stanton SL. Techniques of rectocele repair and their effects on bowel function. Int Urogynecol J Pelvic Floor Dysfunct 1998; 9:37–47.
34. Gill EJ, Hurt WG. Pathophysiology of pelvic organ prolapse. Obstet and Gynecol Clin North Am 1998; 25:757–769.
35. Van Laarhoven CJHM, Kamm MA, Bartram CI, Halligan S, Hawley PR, Phillips RKS. Relationship between anatomic and symptomatic long-term results after rectocele repair for impaired defecation. Dis Colon Rectum 1999; 42:204–210.
36. Karaus M, Neuhaus P, Wiedenmann B. Diagnosis of enteroceles by dynamic anorectal endosonography. Dis Colon Rectum 2000; 43:1683–1688.
37. Driebeek-van Dam JH, Schouten WR, Gosselink MJ, Huismann WM, Ginai AZ. Anorectal symptoms in recto–enterocele (abstr). Int Urogynecol J Pelvic Floor Dysfunct 1997; 8(suppl):55.

38. Wallden L. Defecation block in cases of deep rectogenital pouch. Acta Chir Scand 1952; 165(suppl):1–121.

39. Halligan S, Bartram C, Hall C, Wingate J. Enterocele revealed by simultaneous evacuation proctography and peritoneography: does "defecation block" exist?. Am J Roentgenol 1996; 167:461–466.

40. Jorge JMN, Yang Y-K, Wexner SD. Incidence and clinical significance of sigmoidoceles as determined by a new classification system. Dis Colon Rectum 1994; 37:1112–1117.

41. Fenner DE. Diagnosis and assessment of sigmoidoceles. Am J Obstet Gynecol 1996; 175:1438–1442.

42. Timmons MC, Addison WA. Vaginal vault prolapse. In: Brubaker LT, Saclarides TJ, eds. The Female Pelvic Floor: Disorders of Function and Support. Philadelphia: Davis, 1996:262–268.

43. Pannu HK, Kaufman HS, Cundiff GW, Genadry R, Bluemke DA, Fishman EK. Dynamic MR imaging of pelvic organ prolapse: spectrum of abnormalities. RadioGraphics 2000; 20:1567–1582.

44. Rodriguez LV, Raz S. Diagnostic imaging of pelvic floor dysfunction. Curr Opin Urol 2001; 11:423–428.

45. Delemarre JBVM, Kruyt RH, Doornbos J, Buyze–Westerweel M, Trimbos JB, Hermans J, Gooszen HG. Anterior rectocele: assessment with radiographic defecography, dynamic magnetic resonance imaging, and physical examination. Dis Colon Rectum 1994; 37:249–259.

46. Gufler H, Laubenberger J, DeGregorio G, Dohnicht S, Langer M. Pelvic floor descent: dynamic MR imaging using a half-Fourier RARE sequence. J Mag Resonan Imaging 1999; 9:378–383.

47. Schoenenberger AW, Debatin JF, Guldenschuh I, Hany TF, Steiner P, Krestin GP. Dynamic MR defecography with a superconducting, open-configuration MR system. Radiology 1998; 206:641–646.

48. Unterweger M, Marincek B, Gottstein-Aalame N, Debatin JF, Seifert B, Ochsenbein-Imhof N, Perucchini D, Kubik-Huch RA. Ultrafast MR imaging of the pelvic floor. Am J Roentgenol 2001; 176:959–963.

49. Brubaker L, Heit MH. Radiology of the pelvic floor. Clin Obstet Gynecol 1993; 36:952–959.

50. Goh V, Halligan S, Kaplan G Healy JC, Bartram CI. Dynamic MR imaging of the pelvic floor in asymptomatic subjects. Am J Roentgenol 2000; 174:661–666.

51. Hilfiker PR, Debatin JF, Schwizer W, Schoenenberger AW, Fried M, Marincek B. MR defecography: Depiction of anorectal anatomy and pathology. J Comput Assist Tomogr 1998; 22:749–755.

52. Lamb GM, De Jode MG, Gould SW, Spouse E, Birnie K, Darzi A, Gedroyc WMW. Upright dynamic MR defaecating proctography in an open configuration MR system. Br J Radiol 2000; 73:152–155.

53. Barbaric ZL, Marumoto AK, Raz S. Magnetic resonance imaging of the perineum and pelvic floor. Top Magn Reson Imaging 2001; 12:83–92.

54. Lienemann A, Anthuber C, Baron A, Reiser M. Diagnosing enteroceles using dynamic magnetic resonance imaging. Dis Colon Rectum 2000; 43:205–213.
55. Law PA, Danin JC, Lamb GM, Regan L, Darzi A, Gedroyc WM. Dynamic imaging of the pelvic floor using an open–configuration magnetic resonance scanner. J Magn Reson Imaging 2001; 13:923–929.
56. Fielding JR, Versi E, Mulkern RV, Lerner MH, Griffiths DJ, Jolesz FA. MR imaging of the female pelvic floor in the supine and upright positions. JMRI 1996; 6:961–963.
57. Bertschinger KM, Hetzer FH, Roos JE, Treiber K, Marincek B, Hilfiker PR. Dynamic MR imaging of the pelvic floor performed with patient sitting in an open–magnet unit versus with patient supine in a closed-magnet unit. Radiology 2002; 223:501–508.
58. Hodroff MA, Stolpen AH, Denson MA, Bolinger L, Kreder KJ. Dynamic magnetic resonance imaging of the female pelvis: the relationship with the pelvic organ prolapse quantification staging system. J Urol 2002; 167: 1353–1355.
59. Singh K, Reid WM, Berger LA. Assessment and grading of pelvic organ prolapse by use of dynamic magnetic resonance imaging. Am J Obstet Gynecol 2001; 185:71–77.
60. Poon FW, Lauder JC, Finlay IG. Perineal herniation. Clin Radiology 1993; 47:49–51.
61. Felt–Bersma RJF, Cuesta MA. Rectal prolapse, rectal intussusception, rectocele, and solitary rectal ulcer syndrome. Gastroenterol Clin North Am 2001; 30:199–222.
62. Bartram C. Radiologic evaluation of anorectal disorders. Gastroenterol Clin North Am 2001; 30:55–76.
63. Yoshioka K, Matsui Y, Yamada O, Sakaguchi M, Takada H, Hioki K, Yamamoto M, Kitada M, Sawaragi I. Physiologic and anatomic assessment of patients with rectocele. Dis Colon Rectum 1991; 34:704–708.
64. Murthy VK, Orkin BA, Smith LE, Glassman LM. Excellent outcome using selective criteria for rectocele repair. Dis Colon Rectum 1996; 39:374–378.
65. Halligan S, Bartram CI. Is barium trapping in rectoceles significant? Dis Colon Rectum 1995; 38:764–768.
66. Aronson MP, Bates SM, Jacoby AF, Chelmow D, Sant GR. Periurethral and paravaginal anatomy: An endovaginal magnetic resonance imaging study. Am J Obstet Gynecol 1995; 173:1702–1710.
67. Klutke C, Golomb J, Barbaric Z, Raz S. The anatomy of stress incontinence: Magnetic resonance imaging of the female bladder neck and urethra. J Urol 1990; 143:563–566.
68. Mostwin JL, Yang A, Sanders R, Genadry R. Radiography, sonography, and magnetic resonance imaging for stress incontinence. Urol Clin North Am 1995; 22:539–549.
69. Carr LK, Herschorn S, Leonhardt C. Magnetic resonance imaging after intraurethral collagen injected for stress urinary incontinence. J Urol 1996; 155:1253–1255.

70. Tan IL, Stoker J, Zwamborn AW, Entius KAC, Calame JJ, Lameris JS. Female pelvic floor: Endovaginal MR imaging of normal anatomy. Radiology 1998; 206:777–783.

71. Strohbehn K, Quint LE, Prince MR, Wojno KJ, DeLancey JOL. Magnetic resonance imaging anatomy of the female urethra: a direct histologic comparison. Obstet Gynecol 1996; 88:750–756.

72. Quick HH, Serfaty JM, Pannu HK, Genadry R, Yeung CJ, Atalar E. Endourethral MRI. Magn Reson Med 2001; 45:138–146.

73. Kirschner-Hermanns R, Wein B, Niehaus S, Schaefer W, Jakse G. The contribution of magnetic resonance imaging of the pelvic floor to the understanding of urinary incontinence. Br J Urol 1993; 72:715–718.

74. Fielding JR, Dumanli H, Schreyer AG, Okuda S, Gering DT, Zou KH, Kikinis R, Jolesz FA. MR-based three-dimensional modeling of the normal pelvic floor in women: quantification of muscle mass. Am J Roentgenol 2000; 174:657–660.

75. Huddleston HT, Dunnihoo DR, Huddleston PM, Meyers PC. Magnetic resonance imaging of defects in DeLancey's vaginal support levels I, II, and III. Am J Obstet Gynecol 1995; 172:1778–1784.

76. Fielding JR, Hoyte L, Schierlitz L. Magnetic resonance imaging of pelvic floor relaxation. J Women's Imaging 2000; 2:82–87.

77. Lienemann A, Sprenger D, Anthuber C, Baron A, Reiser M. Functional cine magnetic resonance imaging in women after abdominal sacrocolpopexy. Obstet Gynecol 2001; 97:81–85.

78. Healy JC, Halligan S, Reznek RH, Watson S, Phillips RKS, Armstrong P. Patterns of prolapse in women with symptoms of pelvic floor weakness: assessment with MR imaging. Radiology 1997; 203:77–81.

79. Frohlich B, Hotzinger H, Fritsch H. Tomographical anatomy of the pelvis, pelvic floor, and related structures. Clin Anat 1997; 10:223–230.

80. Hoyte L, Schierlitz L, Zou K, Flesh G, Fielding JR. Two- and 3-dimensional MRI comparison of levator ani structure, volume, and integrity in women with stress incontinence and prolapse. Am J Obstet Gynecol 2001; 185:11–19.

81. Singh K, Reid WMN, Berger LA. Magnetic resonance imaging of normal levator ani anatomy and function. Obstet Gynecol 2002; 99:433–438.

82. Tunn R, Paris S, Fischer W, Hamm B, Kuchinke J. Static magnetic resonance imaging of the pelvic floor muscle morphology in women with stress urinary incontinence and pelvic prolapse. Neurourol Urodyn 1998; 17:579–589.

83. Hjartardottir S, Nilsson J, Petersen C, Lingman G. The female pelvic floor: a dome—not a basin. Acta Obstet Gynecol Scand 1997; 76:567–571.

84. Osaza H, Mori T, Togashi K. Study of uterine prolapse by magnetic resonance imaging: topographical changes involving the levator ani muscle and the vagina. Gynecol Obstet Invest 1992; 34:43–48.

85. Pannu HK, Genadry R, Gearhart S, Kaufman HS, Cundiff GW, Fishman EK. Focal levator ani eventrations: detection and characterization by magnetic resonance in patients with pelvic floor dysfunction. Int Urogynecol J Pelvic Floor Dysfunct 2003; 14(2):89–93.

86. Bo K, Lilleas F, Talseth T, Hedland H. Dynamic MRI of the pelvic floor muscles in an upright sitting position. Neurourol Urodyn 2001; 20:167–174.
87. Benson JT, Kelvin FM. Dynamic cystoproctography. In: Blaivas JG, Chancelor MB, eds. Atlas of Urodynamics. Baltimore: Williams & Wilkins1966:126–144.
88. Halligan S. Commentary: imaging of anorectal function. Br J Radiol 1996; 69:985–988.

Index